Vulnerable Populations in the United States

Vulnerable Populations in the United States

SECOND EDITION

LEIYU SHI
GREGORY D. STEVENS

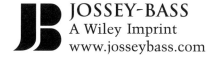

JOSSEY-BASS
A Wiley Imprint
www.josseybass.com

Published by Jossey-Bass
A Wiley Imprint
989 Market Street, San Francisco, CA 94103-1741—www.josseybass.com

Jossey-Bass books and products are available through most bookstores. To contact Jossey-Bass directly call our Customer Care Department within the U.S. at 800-956-7739, outside the U.S. at 317-572-3986, or fax 317-572-4002.

Jossey-Bass also publishes its books in a variety of electronic formats. Some content that appears in print may not be available in electronic books.

Library of Congress Cataloging-in-Publication Data

Vulnerable populations in the United States / Leiyu Shi, Gregory D. Stevens.—2nd ed.
  p.   cm.
  Includes bibliographical references and index.
  ISBN 978-0-470-59935-8; ISBN 978-0-470-87331-1 (ebk); ISBN 978-0-470-87332-8 (ebk); ISBN 978-0-470-87333-5 (ebk)
    1. Poor–Medical care–United States.   2. People with social disabilities–Medical care–United States.   3. Health services accessibility–United States.   I. Stevens, Gregory D., 1973- II. Title.
    [DNLM: 1. Health Services Accessibility–United States.   2. Vulnerable Populations–United States.   3. Quality of Health Care–United States. WA 300]
  RA418.5.P6S54 2011
  362.1086'9420973—dc22
                                                                              2010031898

Printed in the United States of America
SECOND EDITION
PB Printing 10 9 8 7 6 5 4 3 2 1

CONTENTS

Figures, Tables, Exhibits   xi

Preface   xvii

The Authors   xxiii

1   A General Framework to Study Vulnerable Populations   1
    Learning Objectives   1
    Why Study Vulnerable Populations?   3
    Models for Studying Vulnerability   8
    The Vulnerability Model: A New Conceptual Framework   18
    Summary   33
    Key Terms   33
    Review Questions   34
    Essay Questions   34

2   Community Determinants and Mechanisms
    of Vulnerability   35
    Learning Objectives   35
    Race and Ethnicity   36
    Socioeconomic Status   49
    Health Insurance   72
    Multiple Risk Factors   85
    Summary   90
    Key Terms   91

Review Questions   91
Essay Questions   92

3   **The Influence of Individual Risk Factors**   93
Learning Objectives   93
Racial and Ethnic Disparities   94
Socioeconomic Status Disparities   110
Health Insurance Disparities   124
Summary   135
Key Terms   135
Review Questions   135
Essay Question   136

4   **The Influence of Multiple Risk Factors**   137
Learning Objectives   137
Health Care Access   141
Quality of Health Care   152
Health Status   164
Summary   176
Key Terms   176
Review Questions   177
Essay Questions   177

5   **Current Strategies to Serve Vulnerable Populations**   179
Learning Objectives   179
Programs to Eliminate Racial and Ethnic Disparities   185
Programs to Eliminate Socioeconomic Disparities   198
Programs to Eliminate Disparities in Health Insurance   209
Summary   217
Key Terms   218
Review Questions   218
Essay Questions   218

6   **Resolving Disparities in the United States**   221

Learning Objectives   221

The Healthy People Initiative   222

Framework to Resolve Disparities   230

Resolving Disparities in Health and Health Care   234

Integrative Approaches to Resolving Disparities   256

Challenges and Barriers in Implementing the Strategies   267

Course of Action for Resolving Disparities   272

Summary   281

Key Terms   281

Review Questions   282

Essay Questions   282

References   283

Index   313

To our families

FIGURES, TABLES, EXHIBITS

Figures

Figure P.1   Organization of This Book   xix

Figure 1.1   Aday's Framework for Studying Vulnerable Populations   16

Figure 1.2   A General Framework to Study Vulnerable Populations   19

Figure 2.1   Projected Population Size in the U.S. by Race and Ethnicity, 2010 and 2050   40

Figure 2.2   Projected Distribution of the U.S. Population by Race and Ethnicity, 2010 and 2050   41

Figure 2.3   Conceptual Model Linking Race and Ethnicity with Health Care Experiences   42

Figure 2.4   Health Care Spending as a Percentage of Gross Domestic Product among Developed Countries, 2007   50

Figure 2.5   Household Monetary Income by Race and Ethnicity, 1967–2008   54

Figure 2.6   Number in Poverty and Poverty Rate, 1959–2008   56

Figure 2.7   Poverty Rates by Race and Ethnicity, 1968–2008   57

Figure 2.8   Gini Index of Income Inequality for the Thirty Most Developed Countries, 2007–2008   59

Figure 2.9   High School Completion Rates by Race and Ethnicity, Adults Twenty-Five Years and Over, 1968–2008   61

Figure 2.10   College Completion Rates by Race and Ethnicity, Adults Twenty-Five Years and Over, 1968–2008   61

Figure 2.11   Unemployment Rates by Race and Ethnicity, 1968–2009   63

Figure 2.12 Conceptual Model Linking Socioeconomic Status with Health   65

Figure 2.13 Uninsured Rates among Working Adults Ages 18–64 Years   76

Figure 2.14 Percentage of Individuals without Health Insurance Coverage, 2007   77

Figure 2.15 Uninsured Rates among the Nonelderly by State, 2007–2008   78

Figure 2.16 Conceptual Model Linking Health Insurance Coverage with Health Care Experiences   82

Figure 2.17 Simplified Interconnections between Risk Factors and the Cycling of Vulnerability   86

Figure 3.1 No Regular Source of Care among Adults Eighteen to Sixty-Four Years, by Race/Ethnicity, Poverty Status, and Insurance Coverage, 2006–2007   95

Figure 3.2 Receipt of Preventive Care by Race and Ethnicity, 2006–2008   99

Figure 3.3 Personal Interactions in the Health Care System by Race and Ethnicity, 2001–2004   102

Figure 3.4 Self-Reported Fair or Poor Health Status among Adults Eighteen to Sixty-Four Years, 2008   104

Figure 3.5 Infant Mortality Rates by Race and Ethnicity, 2005   105

Figure 3.6 Low Birth Weight Rates by Maternal Race/Ethnicity, 1980–2006   106

Figure 3.7 National Cause-Specific Mortality Rates by Race and Ethnicity, 2006   107

Figure 3.8 Health Risk Factors by Race and Ethnicity, 2005–2007   109

Figure 3.9 Type of Regular Source of Care among Adults by Educational Level, 2005   111

Figure 3.10 Receipt of Preventive Care by Education or Poverty Level, 2007–2008   113

Figure 3.11 Physician-Reported Perceptions of Patients According to Patient SES   115

Figure 3.12 Percentage Reporting High Satisfaction with the Overall Quality of Health Care in Five Nations by Income, 2001   116

Figure 3.13 Percentage Reporting That the Health System Is So Bad It
            Should Be Rebuilt, in Five Nations by Income, 2001   116

Figure 3.14 Reported Frequent Mental Distress by Income, Education,
            and Employment, 2007   118

Figure 3.15 Health Risk Behaviors by Educational Status,
            1999–2007   119

Figure 3.16 Clinically Indicated Preventive Services Not Received in the
            Past Year by Insurance Status, 2007   127

Figure 3.17 Health Care Experiences among Adults with Chronic
            Conditions by Insurance Status, 2008   129

Figure 3.18 Patient Satisfaction with Health Care by Health Insurance
            Plan Type, 1996–1997, 2003 and 2007   130

Figure 4.1   Overlap of Three Risk Factors among U.S. Adults and
            Children, 2007   138

Figure 4.2   No Regular Source of Care among Adults Eighteen to Sixty-
            Four Years by Race/Ethnicity and Insurance Coverage by
            Poverty Status, 2006–2007   142

Figure 4.3   Emergency Department Visit in the Past Year Among Adults
            Eighteen to Sixty-Four Years by Race/Ethnicity and Insurance
            Coverage, by Poverty Status, 2007   143

Figure 4.4   No Health Care Visits in the Past Year Among Children Under
            Eighteen Years of Age by Race/Ethnicity and Insurance
            Coverage, by Poverty Status, 2006–2007   145

Figure 4.5   Risk Profiles and Delayed Dental Care in the Past Year, Adults
            Eighteen and Over, 2007   151

Figure 4.6   Combinations of Risk Factors and Receipt of a Flu Shot in
            the Past Year, Adults Eighteen and Over, 2006   159

Figure 4.7   Ratings of Interpersonal Patient-Provider Relationships
            among Adults, by Race/Ethnicity, Income, and Health
            Status   161

Figure 4.8   Fair or Poor Health Status by Race and Ethnicity and Income,
            Adults Eighteen to Sixty-Four, 2006   164

Figure 4.9   Infant Mortality by Race/Ethnicity and Maternal Education,
            2005   168

Figure 4.10 Risk Factor Combinations and Proportion At Risk for
            Developmental Delay, Children Under Three, 2001   174

Figure 6.1   Goals of the Healthy People 2010 Initiative   224

Figure 6.2   Conceptual Framework for the Healthy People Initiative to Improve Health   225

Figure 6.3   An Action Model to Achieve Healthy People 2020 Overarching Goals   227

Figure 6.4   Conceptual Model of Points of Intervention for Vulnerable Populations   230

Figure 6.5   A Life Course View of Obesity and Health   264

Tables

Table 4.1   National Risk Factors and Access to Health Care, Adults Eighteen and Over, 2006   147

Table 4.2   National Risk Factor Prevalence by Race/Ethnicity, Adults Eighteen and Over, 2007   148

Table 4.3   Risk Factors Predicting Unmet Needs, Adults Eighteen and Over, 2007 (Odds Ratios and 95 Percent Confidence Intervals)   149

Table 4.4   Risk Profiles Predicting Unmet Needs, Adults Eighteen and Over, 2007 (Odds Ratios and 95 Percent Confidence Intervals)   150

Table 4.5   National Risk Factor Prevalence by Race/Ethnicity, Adults Eighteen and Over, 2006   154

Table 4.6   Risk Factors and Preventive Services in the Past Year, Adults Eighteen and Over, 2006 (Odds Ratios and 95 Percent Confidence Intervals)   155

Table 4.7   Risk Profiles and Preventive Services in the Past Year, Adults Eighteen and Over, 2006 (Odds Ratios and 95 Percent Confidence Intervals)   157

Table 4.8   Risk Factors and Health Literacy in California, Adults Eighteen and Over, 2007   162

Table 4.9   National Risk Factors and Self-Reported Health Status, Adults Eighteen and Over, 2006   165

Table 4.10   Risk Factors and Health Status, Children Eleven Years and Under, 2007   166

Table 4.11   Mortality Rates Among Black and White Populations in Selected Geographic Areas, 1989–1990 (per 100,000 Resident Population)   169

Table 4.12   Association of Risk Factors and Profiles with Health Status and Developmental Risk, Children Under Three Years, 2000 and 2007 (Odds Ratios and 95 Percent Confidence Intervals)   172

Table 6.1   Leading Health Indicators for the United States   229

Table 6.2   Differences between Traditional Research and Participatory Action Research   237

Exhibits

Exhibit 1.1   Measures of Predisposing, Enabling, and Need Attributes of Vulnerability at the Individual Level   22

Exhibit 1.2   Measures of Predisposing, Enabling, and Need Attributes of Vulnerability at the Ecological Level   24

Exhibit 1.3   Example Measures of Health Care Access   27

Exhibit 1.4   Example Measures of Health Care Quality   28

Exhibit 2.1   World Health Organization Rankings of International Health Systems   73

Exhibit 2.2   Remote Area Medical Event at the Los Angeles Forum, 2009   89

Exhibit 2.3   Variety of Mobile Clinics at the Los Angeles Forum, 2009   90

Exhibit 5.1   Contact Information for Current Major Programs to Serve Vulnerable Populations   181

PREFACE

We have written this book to call attention among policymakers, health care providers, social scientists, public health practitioners, students of these fields, and the general public to the persistent inequitable health and health care experiences of vulnerable populations in the United States. Achieving a high level of population health status is commensurate with the worldwide leadership position of the United States. Without attention to reducing these disparities within the nation, the United States will continue to spend more but have significantly poorer health across many indicators when compared with other industrialized nations. By providing this up-to-date account of disparities in access, quality, and health status of the nation's more vulnerable populations, this book heightens awareness of the challenges we face and measures progress that has been made toward reducing health and health care disparities.

The scientific and theoretical literature lacks a coherent, well-integrated, general framework to study vulnerable populations. Typically, vulnerable populations are studied as discrete population subgroups, but this method is problematic for developing and implementing truly effective health policy because these vulnerable subgroups are not mutually exclusive. This book contributes to the literature by introducing an integrated framework to study vulnerable populations. Operationalizing vulnerability as a combination or convergence of risk factors is preferred to studying risk factors separately because vulnerability, when defined as a convergence of risks, can best capture reality. This approach not only reflects the co-occurrence of risk factors but underscores our belief that it is futile to address disparities in one risk factor without addressing others.

Furthermore, the focus on vulnerable populations as a national health policy priority could be justified for political, social, economic, and moral reasons. Unfortunately, even with the health care reform law that was passed in 2010 to expand health insurance coverage to millions of additional Americans, today's health care delivery system is not designed to adequately address the health care needs of vulnerable populations. National policies and programs are at best patchworks of fragmented, uncoordinated, categorical, and inadequate initiatives. This book reviews existing programs, identifies their limitations, and proposes a course of action that aims to improve the health services system and addresses the multifaceted health needs of vulnerable populations.

As national, state, and local policies have gained momentum in addressing the needs of vulnerable populations, there has also been an increasing demand for knowledge about these populations. Not only is there interest in documenting the health and health care experiences of vulnerable populations, there is also growing interest in the mechanisms underlying these disparities. This book provides in-depth data on access to care, quality of care, and health status to meet this demand for data, and it tracks progress made toward reducing or eliminating disparities as identified in the Healthy People Initiative. It also updates and summarizes what is currently known and unknown regarding the pathways and mechanisms linking vulnerability with poor health and health care outcomes.

Finally, we intend for this book to provide a new perspective on a complex and important subject area. We hope that readers will gain a clear and sophisticated knowledge of the issues related to the health of vulnerable populations and draw inspiration for making significant improvements to the health care and social systems in the United States and other nations. For current practitioners, program administrators, and policymakers, we hope the book provides a practical guide to addressing the plight of vulnerable populations. For academics, social scientists, and health care researchers, we hope the book and the conceptual framework we propose will assist and guide their research on vulnerable populations and that the up-to-date literature review provides a comprehensive and substantive foundation on which to build future work. For students and the general public, we hope the book will enhance their awareness of the vulnerable populations amongst us and motivate their involvement in advocacy and programs to improve the situation of vulnerable populations.

ORGANIZATION OF THIS BOOK

The book is organized into six chapters (see Figure P.1). The first chapter discusses the definition and measures of a general conceptual framework used to study vulnerable populations. Chapter Two examines the determinants of vulnerability using a broad conceptual framework that includes both social and individual determinants and portrays the mechanisms whereby vulnerability affects access, quality, and health status. In Chapters Three and Four, we summarize the literature

FIGURE P.1   Organization of This Book

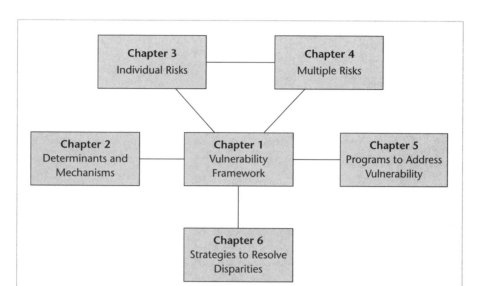

and provide empirical evidence of disparities in health care access, quality, and outcome for vulnerable populations, with particular emphasis on racial/ethnic disparities, socioeconomic status, and health insurance. We understand that current legislation to create a comprehensive national system of health insurance will significantly reduce the number of uninsured. Nevertheless, we still include lacking insurance as a measure of vulnerability because it will take years before the legislation takes full effect. And, even when that happens, millions of Americans will remain uninsured. Chapter Three focuses on influences of individual risk factors, and Chapter Four on influences of multiple risk factors. Chapter Five reviews programs currently in place for vulnerable populations; discusses the mechanisms of vulnerability addressed by these programs; and systematically critiques their potential to improve access to health care, the quality of care received, and the health of vulnerable populations. In Chapter Six, we review strategies and propose a course of action to address the needs of vulnerable populations and reduce or eliminate disparities. The course of action reflects the framework of determinants of vulnerability and takes into account the barriers and feasibility in its implementation.

Throughout the book, we present front-line experiences from health care practitioners who have had interesting and illustrative experiences in serving vulnerable populations. These experiences provide a practical sense of the theories and ideas we present. We also provide discussion questions and essay questions at the end of each chapter. There is a designated Web site for the book with ancillary materials for instructors. We hope that our integrated approach to writing about vulnerable populations will make this book particularly useful to students.

NEW IN THIS EDITION

This second edition retains the main features of the book, including the overall conceptual framework, chapter layout, and a heavy focus on empirical information. We have updated the text to incorporate the release of Healthy People 2020, the latest data and literature on health and health care disparities, and a detailed synthesis of the recent and increasingly expansive programs and initiatives to remedy these disparities. In addition to updating the many data tables, charts, and figures, the three major content changes to the text include the implications of Healthy People 2020 for vulnerable populations, discussion of health care reform legislation and considerations for vulnerable populations, and the addition of a new section to each chapter regarding clinical implications of each chapter topic. All chapters have been updated to reflect current evolutions in theory, our reflections on these changes, and all new data available. Where appropriate, we also have updated the front-line experiences with newly relevant contributions.

ACKNOWLEDGMENTS

We gratefully acknowledge the contributions of Phinney Ahn, Kena Burke, Lynda Burton, Paul Gregerson, Anthony Iton, Howard Kahn, Jane Marks, Lathran Woodard, Kynna Wright, and Vicki Young to the front-line experiences of this book. We also recognize the extensive assistance of the following research and administrative assistants for helping put this book together: Normalie Barton, Angeli Bueno, Heather Lander, Sheila Laqui, Paul Lee, Katharine Swartz, and Jinsheng Zhu. We acknowledge as well the valuable feedback that we received from faculty, instructors, and students who have used the book, the exceptionally thoughtful published professional reviews, and the contributions by the following peer reviewers to the first edition: Aram Dobalian, Charl du Plessis, Gail D. Hughes, and Bridget K. Gorman.

FEEDBACK AND SUGGESTIONS

We welcome comments and suggestions from our readers, including instructors and students in particular. We will carefully study suggestions with an eye to incorporating them into a future edition of the book. Communications can be directed to both of the authors:

Leiyu Shi
Department of Health Policy and Management
School of Public Health, Johns Hopkins University
624 North Broadway, Room 409
Baltimore, MD 21205–1996
lshi@jhsph.edu.

Gregory D. Stevens
Department of Family Medicine
Keck School of Medicine
University of Southern California
1000 S. Fremont Ave #80
Alhambra, CA 91803
gstevens@usc.edu.

THE AUTHORS

Leiyu Shi is professor of health policy and health services research from Johns Hopkins University Bloomberg School of Public Health Department of Health Policy and Management. He is co-director of Johns Hopkins Primary Care Policy Center. He received his doctoral education from University of California Berkeley, majoring in health policy and services research. He also has a master's degree in business administration focusing on finance. Dr. Shi's research focuses on primary care, health disparities, and vulnerable populations. He has conducted extensive studies about the association between primary care and health outcomes, particularly on the role of primary care in mediating the adverse impact of income inequality on health outcomes. Dr. Shi is also well known for his extensive research on the nation's vulnerable populations, in particular community health centers that serve vulnerable populations, including their sustainability, provider recruitment and retention experiences, financial performance, experience under managed care, and quality of care. Dr. Shi is the author of seven textbooks and more than 130 scientific journal articles.

Gregory D. Stevens is an assistant professor in the Department of Family Medicine at the Keck School of Medicine of the University of Southern California (USC). He is the associate director of research in the Center for Community Health Studies. He received a master's degree and a doctorate in health policy at the Johns Hopkins University Bloomberg School of Public Health. His research focuses on health care and social policy, with an emphasis on health equity for vulnerable populations. Dr. Stevens is best known for his work on child health and health care disparities, especially in the delivery of primary care and preventive services. At USC, he teaches courses on the U.S. health care system and comparative health policy in the master of public health program and works with family medicine residents to help them become familiar with community agencies in Los Angeles dedicated to improving the health of vulnerable populations.

Vulnerable Populations in the United States

CHAPTER ONE

A GENERAL FRAMEWORK TO STUDY VULNERABLE POPULATIONS

LEARNING OBJECTIVES

- To provide the rationale for studying vulnerable populations.
- To review frameworks used to study vulnerable populations.
- To introduce a new approach to study vulnerable populations.
- To describe how the new framework to study vulnerable populations might be used in research and practice.

VARIOUS terms have been used to describe America's vulnerable populations: the disadvantaged, *underprivileged*, medically underserved, poverty stricken, distressed populations, and the underclasses. Despite an extensive body of literature and the various national and state efforts at reducing disparity in health and health care between vulnerable populations and the general public, there is no explicit consensus as to what constitutes *vulnerability*. The eleventh edition of *Merriam-Webster's Dictionary* defines vulnerable as "capable of being physically wounded" or "open to attack or damage." In a broad medical sense, vulnerability denotes susceptibility to poor health. Based on the epidemiological notion of risk—the probability that a person will become ill over a given period of time—everyone is potentially vulnerable over an extended period of time. Yet researchers and policymakers obviously do not have everyone in mind when they refer to vulnerable populations.

The common practice by researchers and policymakers, when addressing vulnerable populations, is to focus on distinct subpopulations (Aday, 2001). Among many others, these include racial or ethnic minorities, the uninsured, children, the elderly, the poor, the chronically ill, the physically disabled or handicapped, the terminally ill, the mentally ill, persons with acquired immunodeficiency syndrome (AIDS), alcohol or substance abusers, homeless individuals, residents of rural areas, individuals who do not speak English or have other difficulties in communicating, and those who are poorly educated or illiterate. For example, in Healthy People 2000, a U.S. national prevention initiative strategy for improving the health of the American people, vulnerable populations were identified as those with low income, the disabled, and minority groups (U.S. Department of Health and Human Services, 1979). In Healthy People 2010, the U.S. federal government launched a targeted initiative to eliminate racial and ethnic disparities in health, specifically infant mortality, cancer screening and management, cardiovascular disease, diabetes, AIDS, and immunizations (U.S. Department of Health and Human Services, 2000). In Healthy People 2020, the definition of vulnerability is much more expansive, with the overarching national goals including increasing quality of life, promoting health for all, and eliminating *health disparities* across all groups, with a vision of a society where all people live long, healthy lives (Secretary's Advisory Committee on National Health Promotion and Disease Prevention Objectives for 2020, 2008).

A closer examination reveals that this approach is somewhat artificial. The distinctions between many of these vulnerable groups are often very thin, with vulnerable subpopulations sharing many common traits and experiencing a convergence or interaction of multiple vulnerable characteristics or risk factors. For example, racial/ethnic minorities are disproportionately distributed at the lower end of the socioeconomic ladder, are more likely to be uninsured, and have poorer health than white Americans (LaVeist, 2005). The subpopulations identified as vulnerable often lack the necessary physical capabilities, educational backgrounds, communication skills, or financial resources to safeguard their own health adequately. They have also been shown to bear increased burdens of illness, have poorer access to health care, and receive health care of poorer quality. These commonalities call for a renewed conceptualization of vulnerability.

This chapter introduces a *framework* to study vulnerable populations that reflects the convergence of vulnerable characteristics. The framework will serve as the organizing principle for the literature reviews, related analyses, discussions of health and social programs, and suggested solutions that are presented in this book.

WHY STUDY VULNERABLE POPULATIONS?

This book is about vulnerable populations, and we have chosen to highlight those with minority racial/ethnic backgrounds, low *socioeconomic status (SES)*, and no health insurance coverage. There are many reasons to focus national attention on the needs of vulnerable populations and reducing health and health care disparities experienced by these groups. We offer five reasons for enhancing the national focus on vulnerable populations:

1. Vulnerable populations have greater health needs;
2. The prevalence of vulnerable groups in the population is increasing;
3. Vulnerability is primarily a social issue that is created through social forces and therefore can only be resolved through social (as opposed to individual) means;
4. Vulnerability is intertwined with the nation's health and resources; and
5. There is a growing emphasis on equity in health.

Vulnerable Populations Have Greater Health Needs

Vulnerable populations are at substantially greater risk of poor physical, mental, and social or emotional health and have much higher rates of morbidity and mortality. Among many examples, they experience higher rates of asthma and diabetes, die at higher rates from cardiovascular disease and during infancy, and report more depression and social exclusion than other groups. Despite these greater health needs, they also typically face much greater barriers to accessing timely and needed care; and even when receiving care, they tend to have worse *health outcomes* than others. The magnitude and multifaceted nature of their health needs places a greater demand on medical care, public health, and related social and human services delivery sectors.

There Is an Increasing Prevalence of Vulnerability in the United States

The United States has become increasingly multiethnic. By the middle of the twenty-first century, the minority population is estimated to nearly equal the size of the non-Hispanic white population (U.S. Census Bureau Population Division, 2008). The national poverty rate has also increased since reaching a low in the early 1970s, and the number of individuals in poverty continues to increase steadily. The poverty rate in 2008 (13.2 percent) was the highest poverty rate since 1997, with 39.8 million people in poverty (U.S. Census Bureau, 2009a). The poverty rate remained the highest for blacks (24.8 percent), followed by Hispanics (23.2 percent), Asians (11.8 percent), and non-Hispanic whites (8.6 percent). The uninsured rate in 2008 was among the highest in the past decade.

Demographic shifts, immigration patterns, and socioeconomic trends in the United States and other nations will likely result in vulnerable groups becoming the majority population within this century. If nothing is done to improve their well-being, the health needs of these vulnerable populations will place an incredible strain on the capacity and resources of medical and social services to ensure a national population with a high level of health.

Vulnerability Is Influenced and Therefore Should Be Remedied by Social Forces

Vulnerability to poor health does not represent a specific personal deficiency but, rather, as described in Chapter Two, the interaction effects of many individual, community, and social or political factors, some of which the individuals involved have little or no control over. The creation of vulnerability in this way implies that society has a responsibility to assist these populations and actively promote the health of these individuals. Many programs are in place to address specific health disparities. The most effective approaches to mitigating the consequences of vulnerability and reducing levels of vulnerability in the first place must include broader health and social policies that address these social forces and environmental contexts.

Vulnerability Is Fundamentally Linked with National Resources

The well-being of vulnerable populations is closely intertwined with the overall health and resources of the nation. The United States continues to rank poorly compared with other developed nations on key national health indicators, including infant mortality, other mortality rates, and life expectancy. Poor health not only has an impact on individual families and lives but detracts from national productivity and economic prosperity. The poor health that vulnerable populations experience further subsumes national resources for social progress. For example, when negative health and social conditions (such as violence), which could have effectively been prevented, are left untreated or exacerbated by neglect, they end up costing society billions more dollars in treatment than in prevention. Fundamental improvement of the nation's health and resources cannot be accomplished without very specific efforts aimed at improving the health of vulnerable populations.

Vulnerability and Equity Cannot Coexist

Perhaps the most important reason for focusing on vulnerable populations is the guiding principle of *equity*. Equity is defined by *Merriam-Webster's* dictionary, eleventh edition, as "the quality of being fair." There are various ways in which fairness is conceptualized. In terms of medical care, policies that ensure equal access to health services, such as universal health insurance or health care programs such as the promotion of an AIDS surveillance system, may benefit the public equally. Fairness could also be defined in a relative way, such that the degree of access to health services is determined in direct proportion to the health needs of an individual or a population. By this definition, an equitable health care system is one in which the health need of an individual is the sole determinant of his or her access to and use of health care. By either definition, if equity is a guiding principle for the United States, then vulnerability cannot be allowed to persist.

Documents from the founding of the nation, in fact, identify equality as a governing principle. The U.S. Declaration of Independence states, "We hold these truths to be self-evident, that all men are created equal, that they are endowed by their Creator with certain unalienable Rights, that among these are Life, Liberty and the pursuit of Happiness." These principles of equity, while pursued and interpreted in ways that are sometimes inconceivable today (for example, slavery had been looked at as an exception, declaring those who were slaves would be counted in the census for purposes of representation as "three-fifths of a human"), have at critical points in history been markedly important for vulnerable groups.

The abolition of slavery in 1865 marked what was perhaps the first national legislation reflecting the guiding principles of equality, and it immediately changed the status of this vulnerable population. Perhaps the second landmark legislation for vulnerable groups was the winning of women's suffrage in 1920, giving women more, but still not fully equal opportunity for, political control in guiding the nation. While earlier public policy focused on equality in freedoms and political power, progressive policies in the 1960s enhanced race, gender, and SES equality in social and educational opportunities for U.S. citizens.

The Civil Rights Act of 1964, for example, made *discrimination* based on race, color, religion, and national origin illegal and has been updated several times to include other specific discriminatory factors, such as gender and sexual preference. The Johnson administration's War on Poverty during the 1960s further shifted public attention and social policies toward issues of social, educational, and *health inequalities*.

The past two decades have evolved to see a national and political interest in equality of results attained rather than just opportunity (Moss, 2000). In the social and medical realms, the Healthy People 2010 and 2020 initiatives explicitly identify health and health care equity as a public health objective and have called for a reduction in health disparities in the United States. The Institute of Medicine (IOM), in its landmark report, "The Future of Public Health," asserted that "the ultimate responsibility for assuring equitable access to health care for all, through a combination of public and private sector action, rests with the federal government" (Institute of Medicine Committee for the Study of the Future of Public Health, 1988, p. 13). Many federal and state government agencies also now have specific plans to remedy health disparities. Finally, the health care reform law of 2010 moves the United States further toward universal health insurance coverage for Americans that started with *Medicare* and *Medicaid* in the 1960s and the *State Children's Health Insurance Program* (now called the *Children's Health Insurance Program, CHIP*) in the 1990s.

Front-Line Experience: Managed Care Investing in Vulnerable Populations

Howard Kahn, the chief executive officer, and Phinney Ahn, special projects manager, at L.A. Care Health Plan, describe how one managed care organization, designed to serve vulnerable populations, has made substantial investments in reducing financial, geographic, and linguistic barriers to care. It has reached deep into the community to address a wide range of risk factors that contribute to poor access to care and poor health.

L.A. Care Health Plan is a community-accountable Medicaid *managed care organization* serving residents of Los Angeles County through a variety of programs including Medicaid and CHIP. With more than 800,000 enrolled members, L.A. Care is the nation's largest public, nonprofit health plan. Our mission to promote health by providing quality health care services to vulnerable populations and our commitment to support the safety net make us unique.

We understand that our members face many barriers to obtaining health care, including being low income, lacking health literacy, and having limited English proficiency. In our diverse community of Los Angeles County, approximately 70 percent of our members are non-white and about half prefer to speak a language other than English. The ability for patients to understand and communicate effectively with their health care providers is crucial to obtaining quality health services. We work with both patients and providers to help them connect in a common language by providing interpreter services and customer service training to providers and office staff.

It is also part of our mission to support the safety net. The safety net is a critical part of the health care system in L.A. County. Our support helps community clinics sustain operations, so that in addition to seeing our patients, they can care for the uninsured. We have worked with clinics to reduce wait times for appointments (through a scheduling system known as advanced access) and provided funding to extend their office hours to evenings and weekends. We have invested $80 million back into the community to promote dental care, health information technology, and accessibility for seniors and people with disabilities.

Recognizing that public health insurance programs are not enough to reach all the uninsured in L.A., we partnered with other public and private entities to lead the Children's Health Initiative of Greater Los Angeles, with the goal of covering as many uninsured children in lower-income families in the county as possible. Since 2004, the CHI has raised more than $140 million to fund health insurance for nearly 45,000 children through a program we call L.A. Care's Healthy Kids.

In an effort to promote *quality of care* and improved outcomes, L.A. Care offers a continuous calendar of provider education events that promote the use of evidence-based guidelines and improved provider practices. We were also one of the first Medicaid plans to offer a "pay for performance" program to align financial incentives with *preventive care*, chronic disease management, and use of health information technology. As a result of our efforts to raise the quality bar for health plans, we have been accredited by the National Committee for Quality Assurance.

Since we believe that positive change comes from within the community, we work with eleven regional community advisory committees that are composed of L.A. Care members, advocates, and providers who organize community events and advise us on local health care needs. The committees take a grassroots approach to developing realistic solutions to health issues while giving patients a sense of responsibility to their community and a voice to advocate for their health care. L.A. Care also reserves two spaces on our stakeholder board of governors for members to ensure that we stay accountable to the community. Having stakeholders serving on our board along with members creates a synergy that has resulted in creative ways to promote access to care. When funding for our Healthy Kids program was in jeopardy, our community advisory committee suggested to our board that members would be willing to pay a small premium to keep the program going. This small charge, which we had assumed would be too much for most families, had the potential to fill a large gap to keep thousands of children covered. We surveyed our members, who confirmed they would be willing to pay a small monthly premium, and implemented this option with broad support.

These multiple strategies work together to break down and overcome the multiple barriers our members face in navigating an increasingly complex system. We work directly with our community to develop innovative programs, to the extent that L.A. Care has become the go-to organization in L.A. for health care issues. By working together, we can promote access, quality, and most important, health.

MODELS FOR STUDYING VULNERABILITY

Over the years, studies of vulnerable populations have used different paradigms or models to examine why vulnerable groups experience poorer access to health care and poorer health status. Most of these models have focused on single explanations but increasingly have begun to acknowledge the multifaceted nature of vulnerability. Many have examined individual-level explanations for why vulnerability has negative influences on health. They highlight characteristics of individuals, their health-related behaviors, and their personal socioeconomic circumstances and health care access. Other models have suggested a broader community-level conceptualization of vulnerability, whereby individuals have poorer health due to community or social forces. Here, we summarize the major relevant models that have helped define and shape our understanding of vulnerable populations.

Individual Determinants Model

Perhaps the most foundational, and most common, model for understanding vulnerability is one that identifies specific population groups with certain individual characteristics as inherently more vulnerable than others. The model focuses on characteristics such as age, gender, race and ethnicity, education, income, and life changes (Rogers, 1997). The key to understanding the individual determinants model is that it very clearly delineates vulnerable populations from non-vulnerable populations based on a list of any number of personal characteristics and is not designed to reflect any aspects of community or society that might reflect vulnerability.

Rogers, for example, argued that both women and men could be considered vulnerable populations, depending on the purpose of the classification. Women could be considered vulnerable because they report poorer health status, while men could be considered vulnerable because of their higher mortality rates and overall shorter life expectancy. For women, vulnerability is derived from many factors including the stresses of childbearing, child rearing, and caregiving, reflected in a greater *incidence* of depression and injury from domestic conflict. Women also often have fewer financial resources at their disposal because they still unfairly earn less income on average than men do.

Rogers also considered three stages of life as inherently vulnerable: childhood, adolescence, and old age. Children are vulnerable because they depend on others for care, whereas adolescents engage in more risk-taking behaviors such as unprotected sexual intercourse and the use of drugs and alcohol. The elderly are at risk because of their decreased physical ability, and their risk can be compounded with the decline in financial resources and social support that may occur at this stage of life.

Minority race/ethnicity is considered a vulnerable characteristic in this model because certain groups have higher rates of poverty, morbidity (for example, both diabetes and hypertension are more common among African Americans than whites), and mortality. Educational attainment is considered a marker for vulnerability because those with higher education tend to have better health, which may be due to better access to medical care, a greater tendency to practice prevention, or other more subtle aspects of *social class*.

One of the most interesting components of the model is that major life changes, such as the loss of a job, the death of a loved one, the end of a close relationship, and other transitions (including a diagnosis of a major illness) impair individual health and functioning, making these transitions vulnerable periods.

Individual Social Resources Model

Another essential model of vulnerability has been proposed by Aday (Aday, 1994). It suggests that individual risks stem from lacking certain intrinsic social and personal resources that are essential to a person's well-being. According to this model, social status, *social capital* (or social support), and human capital (the productive potential of an individual) influence vulnerability. In this model, individual characteristics are not themselves the determinant of poor health but a reflection of larger issues related to their personal and social resources that contribute to vulnerability.

Social status is associated with biological characteristics such as age, gender, and race/ethnicity that can bring with them socially defined opportunities and rewards, such as prestige and power. African Americans, by this definition, are viewed as a vulnerable group because they experience more barriers to obtaining material resources (such as income) and nonmaterial resources (such as political power) that contribute to health and social advancement. Those with a combination of characteristics that are associated with poorer social status (for example, African Americans who are elderly) would be considered to have a higher level of vulnerability.

Social capital is defined as the quantity and quality of interpersonal ties a person has. These social ties reflect social resources that are instrumental in supporting psychological, physical, and social well-being. Aday (1994) provides an example of a single mother whose social capital (or social ties with friends) may be particularly helpful in offering child care so that she can direct energies toward personal advancements such as school or work. Examples of those with less social capital are those who live alone, single-parent families, the unmarried or those without life partners, those who do not belong to any organizations or groups, or those who have a limited network of family or friends. Having strong social ties in this model serves as a buffer against vulnerability.

Human capital refers to the skills and capabilities of an individual that enable the person to advance and make productive contributions within society. Without human capital, individuals may experience barriers to social advancement such as exclusion from the labor force, employment in low-wage or service sector jobs, or not being admitted to higher education. Higher social advancement is associated with better health (discussed in Chapter Two); without these opportunities, these populations may be considered vulnerable. This risk factor can certainly be modified through the provision of high-quality public education or vocational training.

Individual Health Behaviors Model

Many theories have been suggested for why the individual characteristics that both Rogers and Aday identified as vulnerable are associated with poor health. The next model explains this relationship through differences in personal health-promoting and *health risk behaviors*. It is argued that vulnerable populations engage in fewer health-promoting activities, such as regular physical activity, healthful eating, and wearing seat belts, and in more risky activities, such as smoking, excessive alcohol consumption, and substance abuse (Lantz and others, 1998; Power and Matthews, 1997; Power, Matthews, and Manor, 1998). These behaviors have direct influences on specific health conditions (for example, smoking and lung cancer, physical activity and obesity, and alcohol use and car accidents) and, thus, contribute to disparities in health.

Proponents of the health behavior model suggest that vulnerable populations engage in fewer health-promoting and more health risk behaviors due to psychosocial factors that create stress for individuals and lead to unhealthy behaviors. These factors include poorer social relationships and *social support*; reduced senses of life control and personal self-esteem; and racism, classism, or other stressors related to having less social power and resources (Lantz and others, 1998). These psychosocial stressors then create mental and physical barriers to the adoption of health-promoting behaviors (depressed individuals are less likely to exercise, for example) and lead individuals to adopt risky health behaviors as coping mechanisms, such as drinking alcohol and smoking tobacco to reduce stress. Chronic stress can also have direct physiological effects and reduce the likelihood that a person will be motivated to obtain medical care.

Several key publications support this health behavior model. The influence of health-promoting and health risk behaviors on health was first recognized among the major industrialized countries by the minister of health of Canada (Lalonde, 1974). Written by Marc Lalonde, the report suggested that lifestyle factors, or rather, "habits of indolence, the abuse of alcohol, tobacco and drugs, and eating patterns that put pleasing of the senses above the needs of the human body" (p. 5), are major contributors to poor health. In the United States, the first installment of the Healthy People reports in 1979 (U.S. Department of Health and Human Services, 1979) and two major IOM reports have summarized for U.S. audiences evidence of the association between certain behaviors and illness (Hamburg, Elliott, Parron, and Institute of Medicine, 1982; Institute of Medicine Committee on Health and Behavior: Research Practice and Policy, 2001). Nevertheless, the literature cautions that health behaviors explain only a modest portion of health disparities.

Individual Socioeconomic Status Model

Another explanation for why individual vulnerability characteristics are associated with poor health status is the influence of individual socioeconomic status (SES). In general, SES is defined by income, education, and occupation, but the same concept is often referred to as social class in other countries. In the United Kingdom, where social class is a common term, there is a standard measure of SES (the Registrar General's measure of occupation) using an individual's father's occupation to categorize one's social class (Hart, Smith, and Blane, 1998). Assessed in this way, social class is a less mutable individual characteristic, because no matter how much occupational promotion or financial wealth a person achieves, his or her social class remains largely determined by the previous generation. Despite differences in measurement, SES remains perhaps the most commonly encountered explanation for any linkage between vulnerable populations and poor health care access and health status.

There is extensive evidence of the relationship between poor health and individual SES. Studies have demonstrated a clear inverse relationship between levels of income, education, and mortality. The most prominent evidence comes from the Whitehall studies of British civil servants in London that demonstrated a nearly linear relationship between social class (defined by occupation) and mortality from most major causes of death (Adler and others, 2008; Marmot, 1993; Marmot, Shipley, Hemingway, Head, and Brunner, 2008; Marmot and others, 1991). Mortality was the lowest among high-level administrators and increased for each successively lower social class occupation, resulting in threefold differences in mortality for the highest and lowest social classes. Interestingly, behavioral risk factors for mortality, such as smoking prevalence, in these social class groups explained fewer than half of the differences in mortality, suggesting some clear limits to the ability of individual health behavior models in explaining the influences of vulnerability (Pincus, Esther, DeWalt, and Callahan, 1998).

In addition to the health behavior model, two major mechanisms have been proposed for the relationship between individual SES and poor health. First, low-SES individuals have fewer financial resources to maintain and promote personal health adequately. For example, low-income groups experience greater difficulty paying for basic health and social needs, including nutritious food, safe and adequate housing, reliable transportation, and child care services, which have been shown to promote health and child development. Second, low-SES groups also have less financial access to health care services. Although health insurance programs exist for poor individuals, there are still many financial barriers to accessing needed health services. The role of SES, in short, influences not only the ability to protect and promote health but also the ability to receive treatment when health problems occur.

Community Social Resources Model

The next set of models advances the concept of vulnerability beyond just individual risk factors and explores more of the community-level determinants of vulnerability. These models are particularly important because they emphasize that vulnerability is not simply a matter of individual bad luck or lack of personal will or resilience. Rather, they propose that community or social factors contribute to vulnerability and also highlight the responsibility that society has in addressing the consequences of vulnerability.

The first of these models, proposed by Flaskerud and Winslow (1998), suggests that community resources, defined broadly, strongly influence the health of a community and therefore contribute to the vulnerability of individuals living within the community. Although these social resources are similar to those proposed by Aday, the community social resources model is distinct in examining both community and individual-level social resources. Vulnerability in this model is therefore defined at the population level as social groups that experience differences in the availability of social resources and consequently have a higher risk for morbidity and premature mortality.

Flaskerud and Winslow use a very broad definition of resource availability, taking into account both socioeconomic and environmental circumstances. By socioeconomic resources, the authors refer to social status, social capital, and human capital factors, just measured at the community level. These include, for example, community unemployment and poverty rates, the availability of high-quality schools, and the presence of community organizations such as churches or social clubs that create opportunities for social connectedness. In particular, the community poverty rate has been one of the most consistent *predictors* of morbidity and mortality in the United States (Do and Finch, 2008; Erwin, 2008; Kaler and Rennert, 2008). Social status is also an important resource to consider in that the lack of political power associated with lower social status leaves them out of the decision-making process for community resource distributions.

The authors also discuss environmental circumstances that would create vulnerability for poor health, including poor access to health care and poor quality of care. Community violence and crime rates are considered environmental circumstances that would influence health, but the authors raise these issues only in regard to hindering access to health care and social services, since top-level health care professionals and social service providers are less inclined to work in these areas. Violence and crime in a community are also likely to have direct impacts on health, including through physical safety issues and even feelings of insecurity that may affect mental health. The authors finally highlight that poor health status of a population (the defining characteristic of vulnerability) may itself contribute to the poor resources in a population (for example, chronic illness may create difficulties with employment and social connectedness), creating a cycle of vulnerability. The authors suggest, however, that the influence of health on community resources seems to be relatively small.

Community Environmental Exposures Model

Other explanations for the influence of communities in creating vulnerability include the potential role of health-impairing environmental exposures. For example, it is hypothesized that lower-SES communities are exposed to more harmful environments, such as living in substandard housing with remnants of lead paint (contributing to lead poisoning in children), or living in inner-city or other crowded living areas that have much greater exposure to air pollution. Such living situations (for example, unventilated shelters) also promulgate the transmission of tuberculosis and increase the likelihood of exposure to violent crime. Workplace safety also varies by community, depending on the primary industry in the area. Rural areas, for example, offer jobs primarily in agriculture and meatpacking, which have high rates of manual labor injury.

One study provides a particularly cogent picture of the influences of environmental risk exposures on individual health over time. The study was designed to collect data longitudinally on a cohort of people from birth to thirty-three years of age (Power and Matthews, 1997). Accumulation of environmental risk factors during these years was measured by factors such as atmospheric pollution levels. Individual risk factors such as SES and smoking status were also taken into account, and both environmental and individual risk factors were clearly related to adult respiratory morbidity. The study demonstrated a strong occupational *gradient* for the prevalence of respiratory symptoms and several other measures, including health status, psychological distress, and job strain.

Community Medically Underserved Model

Community resources, as the community-focused models suggest, include the availability of medical care. The lack of available medical services in a community (referred to as medical underservice) has been commonly proposed as an explanatory factor for why certain populations have poorer health status. Although it is now generally recognized that medical care as a whole contributes only a small portion to the health of a population, the model suggests that the absence of health services directly impacts the population's health. For example, in this model, the poor health of rural populations is explained by the fact that there are fewer health care providers in these areas to help prevent health problems or treat health problems once they occur.

Wright, Andres, and Davidson (1996) have proposed a guideline for assessing medical underservice. Three components are used to define which populations might be medically underserved. The first is the limited physical availability of health care resources. For example, there are not enough health care workers, including doctors and nurses, to meet the demand for care. Second, there may be financial barriers to obtaining health services, such as patients who lack insurance or are underinsured, meaning that their insurance does not fully cover their costs. Third, there may be nonfinancial barriers such as the lack of transportation, language difficulties, or insufficient provider cultural sensitivity, which make it difficult for the community to access any health care providers that do practice in the area.

The current federal definition of a medically underserved area (MUA) is based on the measurement of the physician-to-population ratio, *infant mortality rates*, poverty rates, and proportion of the population that is elderly. The four criteria are used to decide which areas receive government assistance and Wright, Andres, and Davidson (1996) argue that these current definitions allow some populations who are medically underserved to be missed. Individuals may live in areas with high provider-to-patient ratios, but providers may not be willing to accept low-income patients or those covered by Medicaid, which reimburses physicians at rates much lower than private insurance. Women and children may be considered vulnerable but are not accounted for by the current criteria, and infant mortality rates are a relatively rare outcome that could be augmented by using rates of low birth-weight (which can cause substantial health problems for children and is much more common than infant mortality). Changes in these criteria have not yet occurred at the federal level, but they may provide a more realistic picture of medical underservice and may lead to greater action to address the health needs of vulnerable populations.

Individual and Community Interaction Model

Aday (1993) has developed perhaps the most comprehensive vulnerability model to date that combines many previous models and incorporates both individual- and community-level risk factors that determine vulnerability to poor physical, psychological, and social health (see Figure 1.1). Individual-level resources include social status, social capital, human capital, and health needs. Community-level resources include community cohesion (or ties between people), neighborhood characteristics (such as unemployment rates, availability of parks and recreation opportunities, and community violence), and community health needs. Based on these individual and community risk factors, Aday identifies nine specific subpopulations as those who are the most vulnerable: the physically vulnerable (high-risk mothers and infants, chronically ill and disabled, and persons living with HIV/AIDS), the psychologically vulnerable (mentally ill and disabled, alcohol or substance abusers, and those at risk for suicide or homicide), and the socially vulnerable (abusing families, the homeless, and immigrants and refugees). These specific groups, she argues, should be focal points for intervention.

FIGURE 1.1 Aday's Framework for Studying Vulnerable Populations

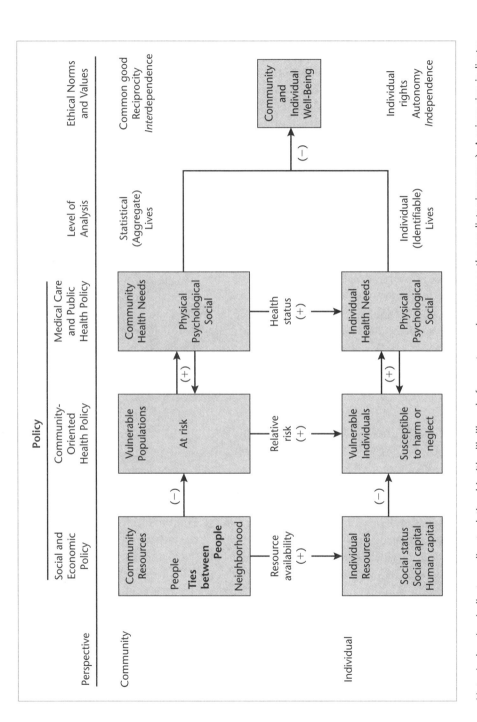

Note: A plus sign indicates a direct relationship (the likelihood of an outcome increases as the predictor increases). A minus sign indicates an inverse relationship (the likelihood of an outcome decreases as the predictor increases).

Source: Aday (2001, p. 3).

In considering interventions, Aday suggests that vulnerability is presumably influenced by ethical norms and values at both the individual level (for example, individual rights, independence, and autonomy) and the community level (for example, belief in the common good, a sense of reciprocity, and interdependence). Vulnerability is also influenced by both social and health policies (for example, welfare assistance, community regulations, public health programs, and health insurance coverage). Thus, interventions should take into account these factors when trying to prevent or modify the consequences of vulnerability.

Sinners and Victims Social Policy Model

Last, an even bigger-picture approach to understanding vulnerability considers the role of moral values in deciding whether or not a population is defined as vulnerable and ultimately how this affects social policy decisions. Based on the work of Morone (2003), this model describes how our view of a number of health issues today has been influenced by competing Puritanism and social gospel beliefs since the founding of the United States. As Morone (2005) describes, Puritanism was generally concerned with the negative effect that social and religious sinners had on the larger community. In comparison, social gospel followers were more concerned about the influence of societal trends, economics, and politics on members of the community. Mechanic and Tanner (2007) argue that this same moral division is at the heart of how society views the health problems of vulnerable populations, and even vulnerable populations themselves.

The issue of teen pregnancy is a good example to illustrate this model, with two polarized views. The first view is that teen pregnancy is an issue that results from the misbehavior (or sin) of the teenager. The teen had some understanding of the consequences of premarital sex, chose to have sex anyway, and did not to use protection (or did not use it correctly) during sex, and did not use emergency contraception afterward. From this point of the view, the teen was a sinner, potentially not only jeopardizing the well-being of the child and family but likely costing society (since single mothers constitute a large proportion of those living in poverty, receiving income assistance and food stamps, and qualifying for government health insurance). This was all preventable if the teen had simply chosen not to sin.

The other view is that teen pregnancy is the result of a very misguided society in which teens are victims of the social, economic, and political culture in which they live. From this point of view, teens have little choice but to engage in premarital sex, given their level of exposure to increasingly sexually oriented pop culture on television, in music, and in film. Further, society might be seen to offer few economic opportunities to women, leaving women with the belief that they are only to be valued for their sexuality and without any real motivation not to become pregnant. One might also view political culture as encouraging women to become pregnant, because some government assistance programs might appear to reward teens for having more children. This would be preventable if teens were simply not made victims by the social, economic, and political culture around them.

Which side is right? It is probably clear that neither side is perfectly correct, but it is certainly fair to debate whether one side better explains why teen pregnancy occurs. Mechanic and Tanner argue that whether society views a population (in this case, teens who become pregnant) more as sinners or as victims has major ramifications for whether society decides to help and particularly whether policymakers create social policy to intervene. If a particular legislator views teen pregnancy as an issue of sinners, the chance is slim that the legislator will spend tax dollars to prevent it (since teens should prevent this themselves). However, if a legislator views a teen mother as the victim of society, whether society has done harm to that teen, the legislator is much more likely to spend tax dollars to intervene.

There are many health issues like this for which disparities exist, such as obesity, cardiovascular disease, alcohol abuse, HIV and other sexually transmitted infections, medical marijuana, and the larger war on drugs. This model also likely explains why it is generally thought to be easier to convince legislators to spend tax money on children than on adults: society tends to view children as victims rather than sinners.

THE VULNERABILITY MODEL: A NEW CONCEPTUAL FRAMEWORK

Each of the models discussed in the previous paragraphs reflects an evolution in defining, researching, and developing approaches to reducing or eliminating the health effects of vulnerability. Some of the more progressive models have recognized the overlap between individual and community-level determinants of vulnerability, and others include the availability of medical care services as a predictor of vulnerability. The next evolutionary step, which we propose, requires a model that synthesizes previous work and recognizes the convergence of individual, social, community, and access-to-care risks that lead to vulnerability. We now turn to a discussion of a new model that we propose for both studying and assisting vulnerable populations (Figure 1.2).

In this book, vulnerability denotes susceptibility to poor health or illness. Poor health can be manifested physically, mentally, developmentally (as with language delays in children), socially (as with poor job performance), or

FIGURE 1.2   A General Framework to Study
Vulnerable Populations

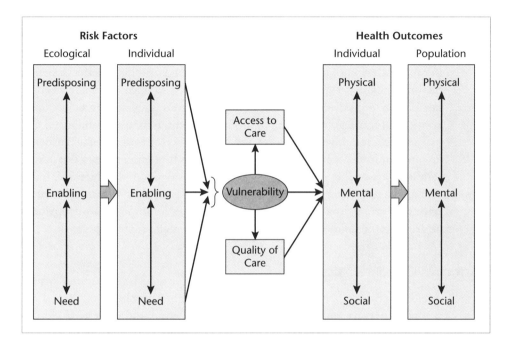

emotionally. Since poor health along one dimension can be compounded by poor health along others, health needs are considerably greater for those with multiple health problems than for those with single health problems.

Vulnerability to poor health is determined by a convergence of predisposing, enabling, and need characteristics at both the individual and ecological levels. In laying out the now well-known, access-to-care framework (Aday, 1993), Aday and Andersen (1981) have defined predisposing characteristics as those that describe the propensity of individuals to use services, which include demographic characteristics, such as age, sex, and family size; social structure variables, such as race/ethnicity, education, and occupation; and health beliefs, such as beliefs about health and the value of health care (Aday and Andersen, 1981). Enabling characteristics are the resources that individuals have available for the use of services, including those specific to individuals and families (examples are income and insurance coverage) and attributes of the community or region in which an individual lives (for example, the availability of health care services). Need factors are specific illnesses or health needs that are the principal driving forces for seeking health care.

These predisposing, enabling, and need characteristics converge and interact, and they work together to influence health care access, health care quality, and health status. Translated into the terms of our vulnerability model, health needs directly imply vulnerability, predisposing characteristics indicate the propensity for vulnerability, and enabling characteristics reflect the resources available to overcome the consequences of vulnerability. Therefore, individuals are most vulnerable if they have a combination of health needs, predisposing risk factors, and enabling risk factors. For example, individuals who have asthma (a need factor), are Latino (a predisposing factor), and uninsured (an enabling factor) would be considered more vulnerable than individuals who have asthma alone.

In our model, we emphasize the importance of vulnerability determinants at community or ecological levels. This implies that vulnerability does not represent any personal deficiency of the populations defined as vulnerable, but rather that they experience the interaction of many risks over which individuals may have little or no control. The model also implies an important role for society in addressing the health and health care needs of vulnerable populations.

Distinctive Characteristics

The vulnerability model has a number of distinctive characteristics. First, it is a comprehensive model, including both individual and ecological (contextual) attributes of risk. A person's vulnerability is determined not only by his or her individual characteristics but also by the environment in which he or she lives and the interactions among individual and environmental characteristics. Inclusion of ecological factors implies that attributes of vulnerability are beyond individuals' control, and their reduction requires societal efforts. Compared to models that focus on individual characteristics alone, a multilevel model (including both individual and ecological elements) not only more accurately reflects realities but also avoids a tendency to "blame the victim."

Second, this is a general model focusing on attributes of vulnerability for the total population rather than a specific model focusing on vulnerable traits of subpopulations. Although we recognize individual differences in exposure to risks, we also think there are common, crosscutting traits affecting many vulnerable populations. Due to current public funding options, a categorical approach to assisting vulnerable groups will likely continue. We believe such an approach is piecemeal, inefficient, duplicative, uncoordinated, and inadequate. It tackles symptoms rather than causes and is unlikely to substantively and fundamentally improve the situations of vulnerable populations. Our general model calls for a comprehensive and integrated approach that focuses on the most critical and common vulnerability traits in the community. Such a practice is more efficient and likely to bring more tangible improvement in the situations that vulnerable populations face.

Third, a major distinction of our model is the emphasis on the convergence of risk factors. The effects of experiencing multiple vulnerable traits may lead to cumulative vulnerability that is additive or even multiplicative. Individuals with multiple vulnerability traits may have especially poor health status. Examining vulnerability as a multidimensional construct can demonstrate gradient relationships between vulnerability and outcomes of interest and improve our understanding of how to intervene. The findings are likely to be more precise and can provide better guidance to policymakers. For example, if we see a gradient relationship between a set of vulnerability characteristics and, for instance, health care access and health outcomes, not only is our understanding of the patterns of vulnerability enhanced, but we learn what crosscutting characteristics (or combinations of characteristics) policymakers should target limited resources toward addressing to best help vulnerable populations and reduce disparities.

Components of the Model

Based on the overview presented above, we provide a graphical representation of our model of vulnerability (see Figure 1.2) and describe components of this model. Vulnerability, which is at the center of the figure, is most closely affected by individuals' predisposing, enabling, and need attributes (in the second left column) and is also influenced by these same risk factors at an ecological or community level. It is important to note that in our model, the predisposing, enabling, and need attributes are more than just risk factors for poor access; they also reflect risks for poor quality of health care and poor health status. These risk factors then combine, interact, and work together to create a level of vulnerability for each individual that is associated with negative health care access, quality of care, and health outcomes (see the columns on the right) at both individual and population levels.

Individual Risk Factors   Individual predisposing attributes in our model, reflecting risk factors for poor access to care, quality of care, and health status, include demographic factors, belief systems, and social structural variables that are associated with social position, access to financial and nonfinancial resources, and health behaviors that influence both health and health care access (Exhibit 1.1). Individual factors such as race/ethnicity, gender, sexual preference, or other factors may also be foci for discrimination. Individuals generally have little control over most predisposing attributes.

Exhibit 1.1   Measures of Predisposing, Enabling, and Need Attributes of Vulnerability at the Individual Level

Predisposing Factors

- Demographic characteristics associated with variations in health status, such as age or gender
- Inherited or cultivated belief systems associated with health behaviors, such as attitude, conviction, culture, or health belief
- Social structure variables associated with social position, status, and access to resources, such as race/ethnicity or gender

Enabling Factors

- Socioeconomic status factors (such as income, education, and occupation) associated with social position, status, access to resources, and variations in health status
- Individual assets (human capital) that enable one to be economically self-sufficient, such as inheritance, wealth, or skills
- Factors that enable the use of health care, such as health insurance, transportation, or language concordance with health care providers

Health Need

- Self-perceived or professionally evaluated health status, such as physical and mental health, diagnoses for diseases, and illness
- Quality-of-life indicators, such physical functioning, social limitations, cognitive limitations, and limitation in work, housework, or school
- Certain subpopulations defined by high health risks including physical health (chronically ill and disabled individuals, persons with AIDS), mental health (alcohol or substance abusers), and social well-being (abusing families, homeless people, and refugees)

Individual enabling attributes include SES, financial and nonfinancial social resources, and factors such as health insurance coverage associated with the use of health care services. Perhaps the most commonly cited enabling risk factors are low income or lack of health insurance coverage. Even with the passage of the health care reform, it is likely that certain subpopulations will remain uninsured. Although having a low income has some direct influences on health status (described in Chapter Two) that having health insurance does not, both risks create substantial barriers to obtaining needed health care.

Low educational level and language barriers are also commonly cited as important risk factors for poor health care access, quality, and health status. Education has a direct impact on health (for example, less-educated individuals are more likely to smoke), but both low education and difficulty speaking English produce substantial barriers to appropriate health care, including difficulty speaking with health care providers, communicating treatment preferences, reading health materials and prescription drug instructions, and following through on recommended treatments. Overall, enabling risk factors are generally more modifiable than predisposing factors; for example, educational opportunities can be expanded through programs such as *affirmative action* and Healthy Start.

Individual need attributes include self-perceived or professionally evaluated health status and quality-of-life indicators. Certain subpopulations are defined by their health; these include infants born with low birth weight, chronically ill or disabled individuals, persons with HIV/AIDS, those who are mentally ill and disabled, alcohol or substance abusers, and those who have been abused and have greater health care needs (Aday, 2001). For example, persons who are chronically ill or who have other functional disabilities, such as the frail elderly or children with disabilities, may have particular difficulty obtaining needed health services due to special challenges created by their physical illness or mental condition; examples are extensive reliance on caregivers for accessing health care or difficulty communicating health needs. Such individuals may be in need of highly specialized providers or even teams of providers, and access to these specialists is not always facilitated or well coordinated by insurance plans.

In our model, the bidirectional arrows linking predisposing, enabling, and need attributes at both the individual and ecological levels indicate that these risk factors influence one another. For example, racial/ethnic minorities (a predisposing attribute) are disproportionately represented in the low-SES groups (an enabling attribute). Having health insurance (an enabling attribute) is less available to low-income groups (an enabling attribute) and is essential for ensuring access to health care, particularly for subpopulations with chronic illnesses (a need attribute). Poorer health status (a need attribute) reduces the ability to maintain stable employment and earn income (an enabling attribute), and incomes are generally reduced for older individuals (a predisposing attribute) who are retired and may receive income only through the *Social Security* system.

Predisposing, enabling, and need attributes in our model each independently influence vulnerability status, as reflected by the three separate arrows. In addition, these three attributes converge and interact and jointly determine one's vulnerability status, as indicated by the larger bracket encompassing the three attributes. Indeed, the major difference between this framework and other models is the emphasis on the convergence of risks. Operationalizing vulnerability as a combination of disparate attributes is preferred to studying individual factors separately, because a population group that is considered vulnerable rarely experiences the risks in isolation. Those with one particular risk factor are more likely to have multiple risks.

Ecological Risk Factors   Since individuals live in communities, they are clearly influenced by the environment around them. Our model indicates that individual attributes of risk are influenced by ecological attributes of risk (the first left column in Figure 1.2) and that they combine to influence vulnerability. As with individual risks, there exist predisposing, enabling, and need risk factors at ecological levels (see Exhibit 1.2).

Exhibit 1.2   Measures of Predisposing, Enabling, and Need Attributes of Vulnerability at the Ecological Level

Predisposing Factors

- Residence or geographical location, for example, rural versus urban, and inner city versus suburban
- Neighborhood composition, for example, racial/ethnic integration or segregation
- Physical environment, for example, pollution, population density, and crime rates
- Political, legal, and economic system, for example, industrialization and market domination
- Cultural and social norms or beliefs, for example, religions, notions of justice, and level of tolerance for diverse cultures

Enabling Factors

- Socioeconomic status and social class, for example, neighborhood income level, high school or college education rates, and unemployment rate
- Resource inequalities, for example, the distribution of income or wealth within a population

- Workplace environment, for example, occupational safety, health promotion practice, workplace stress, and health insurance benefits
- Social capital and *social cohesion*, for example, characteristics of individuals' social network, such as family structure, friendship ties, neighborhood connections, religious organizations, and attributes of the community or region in which individuals live
- Health care delivery system, for example, availability and accessibility of medical care (both primary and specialty care), and public health or social services

Need Factors

- Population health behaviors, for example, smoking, exercise, diet, alcohol use, drug abuse, and seat belt use
- Population health status, for example, rates of mortality and morbidity for leading causes of death, life expectancy, infant mortality, and obesity
- Population mental health and social well-being, for example, rates of mental illness, homelessness, suicide, and quality of life
- Health disparities/inequalities, for example, racial/ethnic disparities in health, SES disparities in health

Ecological predisposing attributes include neighborhood demographic composition; the physical environment; political, legal, and economic systems; and cultural and social norms and beliefs. Geographical areas composed of larger populations of older individuals or inner-city areas with a larger number of teenage mothers create greater vulnerability because they require a higher intensity of medical care, financial, and social resources. For example, the low birth-weight rate is higher among teenage mothers, and low birth-weight babies require much more intensive care, monitoring, and social assistance than other infants, which draws resources from other medical or social services for the community. Similarly, areas that are characterized by dilapidated housing or substandard, public low-cost apartments have substantial health risks, such as lead poisoning from lead-based paint, and they may offer inadequate safety protections; there may be nonfunctioning smoke detectors and dark and unmonitored halls, for example. Social and political systems that tolerate high levels of health disparities (such as the United States) are also considered predisposing risks.

Ecological enabling attributes include socioeconomic position and social class in relation to others, workplace environments, social resources, and health care delivery system factors. For example, rural communities tend to have fewer economic opportunities besides agriculture and therefore tend to have higher rates of unemployment or employment in lower-wage sectors. Poor areas similarly tend to have fewer high-quality educational systems, since local taxes account for a substantial proportion of school system budgets, and revenues generated through taxes are lower in low-income areas. These community SES barriers also contribute to medical underservice, in part determining where health care providers will work (shortages are due in part to the lack of incentives for health care professionals to practice in rural and inner city areas) and limiting health insurance coverage opportunities, since large companies that offer coverage are less attracted to these areas.

Ecological need attributes include community health risk factors such as pollution levels, health-promoting community behaviors such as health fairs and recreational opportunities, and trends in health status and health disparities. For example, rural areas and inner-city urban areas experience much higher population rates of asthma due to the presence of dust and pollution in the air, which aggravates the lungs of potential asthmatics and increases the severity of conditions among those with asthma. Communities plagued with crime and violence create unsafe living conditions for community members, increase the risk of personal injury from violence (more so for teenagers), and may sabotage community feelings of solidarity and degrade mental health.

Like individual attributes, ecological attributes also influence one another. For example, compared with other industrialized nations, the United States (a predisposing attribute) tolerates a higher level of disparities in income, education, and access to health care (all enabling attributes), despite the fact that these SES and health care access disparities are causally linked to poor population health (a need attribute). Another example is that inadequate employment opportunities (an enabling attribute) may contribute to population health behaviors such as alcohol abuse (a need attribute) that are tolerated by a community based on cultural norms (a predisposing attribute) despite their contributing to neighborhood insecurity and levels of violence (a need attribute). Relationships such as these are demonstrated in the model with the bidirectional arrows; their independent and combined relationships with individual risk factors and, ultimately, vulnerability are also depicted.

The Consequences of Vulnerability   Vulnerability has direct influences on health care access, health care quality, and health status measured at the individual and population levels. The right side of our model in Figure 1.2 depicts aspects of health care access, quality, and health outcomes that vulnerability may impact. Whereas the ultimate effect of vulnerability is poorer health status, initial consequences may be observed in reduced access to health care and lower quality of care among those who are able to obtain access. Different types of access can be measured (see Exhibit 1.3), such as *potential access to care* (factors that facilitate obtaining care), *realized access to care* (actual receipt and use of health care services), and appropriate access to care (receipt of care in relation to recommended care or treatment guidelines) (Andersen and Aday, 1978). Quality of care may be measured in many ways (see Exhibit 1.4), including examining the appropriateness of care, efficiency and safety in care, particular experiences in the delivery of care, and satisfaction with care (Institute of Medicine Committee on Quality of Health Care in America, 2001).

Health status and health outcome measures represent a critical end point for assessing the influences of vulnerability. The World Health Organization (WHO)

Exhibit 1.3   Example Measures of Health Care Access

Potential Access to Care

- Insurance coverage, for example, whether insured and type of insurance
- Usual or *regular source of care*, such as whether an individual knows a provider or place where they can get needed health care
- Availability of health care facilities and providers, such as availability of needed provider types, hospitals, and affordable clinics

Realized Access to Care

- Preventive care, including visits for checkups, immunizations, and screenings
- Acute care, such as number of *primary care* visits
- Specialist care: receipt of needed care from specialists including mental health, obstetrics and gynecology, and other specialty-trained physicians
- Emergency care—number of emergency room visits
- Hospitalization—number of hospitalizations

Appropriate Access to Care

- Timeliness of care, for example, receipt of health care without delay when perceived as needed
- Obtaining all needed care and services such as screenings, lab tests, and prescription medications

Exhibit 1.4   Example Measures of Health Care Quality

Appropriate Care

- Receipt of preventive care in accord with professional or national guidelines, for example, receipt of childhood immunizations according to the recommendations of the American Academy of Pediatrics
- Receipt of acute care according to recommended treatment guidelines, for example, receipt of care for diabetes includes recommended screening and blood tests at regular intervals; counseling on nutrition, exercise, and self-management

Efficient and Safe Care

- The absence of duplicative tests and procedures, for example, not having to repeat immunizations because records of previous immunizations were lost
- Reduced hospital readmissions for preventable conditions such as due to the top two conditions for which hospitalization is considered preventable: heart failure and pneumonia

Experiences in Care

- Continuity of care, whether patient sees the same doctor or nurse each time for primary care and whether the doctor knows the patient well
- Coordination of care, whether someone at the primary care doctor's office helped the patient make a specialist appointment and whether the primary care doctor followed up with the patient on the specialist visit

Satisfaction with Care

- Reported satisfaction with the quality of health care delivered by the patient's doctor or nurse, for example, ratings of health care quality on a scale of 1 to 10
- Reported satisfaction with how well the doctor communicated with the patient, how well the doctor listened to the patient, and how well the doctor was able to explain things

has defined health as a "state of complete physical, mental, and social well-being and not merely the absence of disease or infirmity" (World Health Organization, 1948). This definition recognizes that health is influenced by a combination of biological, social, individual, community, and economic factors. In addition to its intrinsic value, health is a means for personal and collective advancement. It is not only an indicator of an individual's well-being, but a sign of success achieved by a society and its institutions of government in promoting well-being and human development.

Health status and outcomes can be measured along physical, mental, social, or emotional dimensions for individuals and can also be measured at the population level. Physical and mental health can be measured according to health symptoms, morbidity (the numbers and types of diseases people have), and mortality. Social and emotional health can be measured through social networks, *social participation*, and engagement with the larger community. Although mental, social, and emotional dimensions of health are less frequently measured, they are now recognized as important components of health status and outcomes. In addition, general measures of health are commonly used to more broadly reflect the sum total of physical, mental, social, and emotional health on perceptions of health, functioning and disability, and life achievements and satisfaction.

While positive health or health and life achievements are now believed to be part of broad conceptual definitions of health, the most commonly used indicators remain poor health or health deficits (Breslow, 2006). The major reason is that health status has been defined historically in terms of health problems, such as disease, disability, and death.

Measuring Vulnerability in Research

In research, vulnerability may be studied by using distinct population groups defined by one or more vulnerable attributes. Examples of vulnerable groups defined by one risk attribute are racial/ethnic minorities (predisposing characteristic), the uninsured (enabling characteristic), and the chronically ill (need characteristic). Examples of vulnerable groups defined by two risk attributes include uninsured racial/ethnic minorities (predisposing and enabling), children with chronic illness (predisposing and need), and low-income persons with AIDS (enabling and need). Examples of vulnerable groups defined by the convergence of predisposing, enabling, and need attributes of risk include children in low-income families with asthma or uninsured minorities who experience depression.

Sample sizes permitting, it is possible to include more than one risk attribute within predisposing, enabling, or need factors. For example, one can study minority children in low-income, uninsured families (two predisposing and one enabling attribute). Conceptualization of vulnerable populations should be guided by the study purpose and availability of sufficient sample sizes and accurate and reliable measures for both the vulnerable groups and the groups with which they are compared. Ultimately, however, the operationalization of vulnerability should always be based on the presumption that the interaction between multiple individual and ecological factors contributes to a higher level of vulnerability and a greater risk of poor health.

Focus on Vulnerability in Clinical Practice

Vulnerable populations require special considerations in the practice of clinical medicine. They often have limited access to medical care and live in areas with limited resources. Their communities are often characterized by poor schools, high crime rates, higher access to illegal drugs, and a lower-income environment, all of which can influence poor health (Mechanic and Tanner, 2007). While health care providers rarely receive any training about these social risk factors, and often feel that such issues are outside the realm of medicine, their strong influences on health are such that providers must find ways to become involved in these social issues if they truly want to improve their patients' health.

Similarly, clinical intervention programs to reduce health disparities are likely to be ineffective if their designers do not fully acknowledge the social and environmental factors that influence health and incorporate them into the design. In order to implement effective clinical intervention programs, they must be appropriate for the target vulnerable group and address the range of risk factors that lead to health disparity (Kilbourne, Switzer, Hyman, Crowley-Matoka, and Fine, 2006). If a clinic wanted to implement an effective clinical intervention to, say, reduce obesity rates, then in addition to simply screening for body-mass index and providing counseling on how to eat right and exercise, the following additional activities might be considered.

The clinic could develop special education sessions to improve "healthy literacy," such as how to read nutrition labels and provide tips and information about neighborhood resources (such as a local YMCA) to help families find ways to exercise during a busy day. The clinic might talk to the health plans with which they are contracted to find out what resources they offer to patients (for example, some health plans provide discounts to fitness centers or will even pay for Weight Watchers memberships for certain eligible adults), and then connect patients with those resources. Clinicians, who can have a particularly strong voice in public affairs, might also become involved with their local community center or talk with local city planners about improving local recreation leagues or local parks.

Of course, there are major barriers to serving vulnerable populations in the most effective ways. Health plans do not yet reimburse most of these activities, and primary care providers often find their offices extremely busy and generally understaffed. Nonetheless, such activities can make a career more personally rewarding, as health care providers often find it frustrating to have such sporadic contact with patients and find that their five-minute discussions with patients seem to have little or no effect. Things may change, however, as health plans, *foundations*, and governments are beginning to recognize the value of clinicians becoming involved in these activities.

Three Key Risk Factors

Although there are many predisposing, enabling, and need attributes of vulnerability, this book primarily focuses on three key risk factors—race/ethnicity, SES, and health insurance coverage—because they are three of the most powerful demographic predictors of poor health care access, quality of care, and health status, and therefore vulnerability. These three factors are closely intertwined but exert independent effects on health. They are also indirectly associated with, or contribute to, other vulnerability traits.

Race/ethnicity has long been a major basis of social stratification in the United States (LaVeist, 2005). While race and ethnicity are closely associated with SES and health insurance indicators, the effect of SES is not entirely equivalent across racial/ethnic groups. For example, even within categories of SES, racial/ethnic minorities often have higher rates of morbidity and mortality than whites. The failure of SES to completely account for racial variations in health status emphasizes the need to give attention to the unique factors linking race and ethnicity with health. Because race/ethnicity and SES in the United States are so closely intertwined, it is difficult to address SES or even health insurance disparities without examining racial/ethnic disparities.

The relationship between SES and health care access, quality of care, and health outcomes is quite well known. Variations in income and wealth, educational attainment, and occupational position as markers of socioeconomic inequality have long been associated with variations in health status and mortality (Adler and Ostrove, 1999; Mackenbach and others, 2008). Persons with high income, education, or occupational status live longer and have lower rates of diseases than those with lower SES. SES is also closely linked with health insurance status (due to health coverage provided primarily through employers and to income-based eligibility for *safety net insurance* programs like Medicaid), but both have independent effects on health.

Health insurance coverage has long been regarded as a marker for access to health care. The IOM concluded in 2009 that lacking health insurance contributes to excess mortality in the United States (Institute of Medicine Committee on Health Insurance Status and Its Consequences, 2009). The IOM's Committee on the Consequences of Uninsurance has concluded in multiple reports that providing health insurance to the uninsured would improve health and increase life expectancy (Institute of Medicine Committee on the Consequences of Uninsurance, 2002, 2003, 2004). The reports suggested that providing insurance would most greatly benefit the most vulnerable groups and thus would likely help to reduce health disparities. The health care reform law of 2010 will help to address this vulnerability. Since most of the features of the legislation begin in 2014, it will take many years before the full impact of the legislation is realized.

Given well-established disparities in race/ethnicity, SES, and health insurance in access to health care, quality of care, and health status, timely and accurate knowledge of these three aspects of diverse vulnerable population groups is of critical importance in developing interventions to reduce these disparities. Focusing on these disparities is also consistent with current long-term national health priorities. Healthy People 2010 focused national attention on racial/ethnic and SES disparities in health and health care and, in a bold step forward from Healthy People 2000, called for the elimination of disparities in health and health care access. Similarly, the overarching goals for Healthy People 2020 include increasing the quality of life, promoting health for all, and eliminating health disparities across all groups, with a vision of a society where people live long, healthy lives (Secretary's Advisory Committee on National Health Promotion and Disease Prevention Objectives for 2020, 2008).

There is ample health data available according to race and ethnicity, SES, and health insurance coverage, making it possible to demonstrate the disparities associated with these factors. National protocols have institutionalized the collection and reporting of health data according to these factors. For example, the U.S. Office of Management and Budget (1978) requires that federal agencies report health statistics for four race groups (American Indian/Alaskan Native, Asian and Pacific Islander, black, and white) and one ethnic category (Hispanic origin) (U.S. Office of Management and Budget, 1978). Regarding SES, in 1998, the U.S. Department of Health and Human Services (1998) issued its first annual report of U.S. health, which included a special chart book on SES and health, and later editions have continued to report health data using characteristics of SES (National Center for Health Statistics, 1998). Finally, almost all major national health surveys have included health insurance coverage data in addition to SES and race/ethnicity.

SUMMARY

Over the years, studies of vulnerable populations have used different paradigms or models in examining the characteristics that make populations vulnerable. These include individual demographic, behavioral, and socioeconomic characteristics; community characteristics; and the interaction of individual and community characteristics. Each of the models reflects an evolution in defining, researching, and developing approaches to reducing or eliminating the health effects of vulnerability. Some have recognized the overlap between individual and community-level determinants of vulnerability, and others include the availability of medical care services as a predictor of vulnerability.

In this book, we have defined vulnerability as a multidimensional construct reflecting the convergence of predisposing, enabling, and need attributes of risk at both individual and ecological levels. This broad definition of vulnerability presumes that vulnerable populations experience risks in clusters and that those susceptible to multiple risk factors, such as being of racial/ethnic minority background and living in poverty, are likely to be more vulnerable than those with a single risk, such as high-income minorities. Although there are many predisposing, enabling, and need attributes of vulnerability, this book primarily focuses on race and ethnicity, SES, and health insurance coverage because they are three of the most powerful predictors of poor health and health care access and, thus, vulnerability. These three factors are closely intertwined but exert independent effects on health. They are also indirectly associated with or contribute to other vulnerability traits.

In the next chapter, we delve into the mechanisms of vulnerability and the many pathways through which these influence health care access, quality, and health disparities.

KEY TERMS

Affirmative action
Discrimination
Equity
Foundations
Framework
Gradients
Health disparities
Health inequalities
Health outcomes
Health risk behaviors
Incidence
Infant mortality rate

Managed care organization
Medicaid
Medicare
Minority
Potential access to care
Predictor
Preventive care
Primary care
Quality of care
Realized access to care
Regular source of care
Safety net insurance

Social capital
Social class
Social cohesion
Social participation
Social Security
Social support
Socioeconomic status
State children's health insurance program (SCHIP)
Underprivileged
Vulnerability

REVIEW QUESTIONS

1. What is vulnerability? How can this concept be applied to the field of health care delivery?
2. Identify three possible risk factors that could be used to characterize vulnerable populations. Why might these risk factors be associated with vulnerability?
3. What are the five main reasons to focus our national attention on vulnerable populations? Briefly describe the rationale for each reason.

ESSAY QUESTIONS

1. Why should the concept of vulnerability focus not just on independent risk factors but also on profiles of multiple risks? How might this understanding change daily business in the pursuit of good health for everyone in the United States, including how politicians, health care administrators, local health programs, and health care providers operate or practice?
2. How is the concept of equity a guiding principle in focusing national efforts on vulnerable populations? What does equity mean in terms of health and health care access? How does the concept of health care as a right illustrate this concept of equity? Given that health and health care equity for vulnerable populations will likely require extensive political intervention and large costs, should this rationale of equity be prioritized over other factors, such as economics and politics? If so, why?

CHAPTER TWO

COMMUNITY DETERMINANTS AND MECHANISMS OF VULNERABILITY

LEARNING OBJECTIVES

- To become familiar with major demographic patterns in the United States that reflect vulnerable populations, including trends in racial/ethnic diversity, wealth and income distribution, education, occupation, and health insurance status.

- To understand the many ways in which race/ethnicity, socioeconomic status, and health insurance coverage make a person vulnerable to poor health care access, poor health care quality, and poor health or health outcomes.

I N the previous chapter, we outlined our general model of vulnerability, which highlights the interplay of multiple risk factors in creating barriers to receiving good health care and leading to poor health status. Before presenting the evidence of the impact of individual and multiple risk factors on health and health care access, sufficient knowledge is needed about why vulnerability factors exist and how risk factors can lead to inadequate health care access and poor health outcomes. Understanding the determinants and mechanisms of the main risk factors highlighted in this book (race/ethnicity, SES, and insurance coverage) will help guide the interpretation of the detailed data presented in Chapters Three and Four.

Such an understanding will also provide a basic foundation to assess the *effectiveness* of programs that aim to prevent the occurrence of these risk factors through primary prevention or to disrupt or negate the effects of vulnerability through secondary prevention. Developing more effective solutions will require understanding these determinants, so that interventions and policies can be developed to interrupt these mechanisms and pathways at critical junctures.

This chapter describes how vulnerability characteristics are produced and how they are allowed to persist in the United States. Vulnerability is a relative term that implies a particular susceptibility to adverse health and health care events beyond those normally experienced. How a population obtains the characteristics or risk factors that make it vulnerable must be viewed in relation to the community in which they occur, because many of these risks are based on interactions among members of the community and are affected by social policies. In this chapter, we examine each characteristic of vulnerability and discuss trends in occurrences, its determinants, and the potential mechanisms of its relationship with adverse health care experiences and health outcomes.

RACE AND ETHNICITY

Racial and ethnic differences are common societal divisions linked with disparity and conflict. Apartheid in South Africa, ethnic cleansing in Croatia, and tribal wars in Rwanda, for example, suggest a global preoccupation with racial and ethnic identity. In many countries, access to medical care breaks down across racial and ethnic lines (World Health Organization, 2001). Often, vulnerable populations in a country are minorities who are underserved in many ways, with health care delivery being only one issue.

Historical Development of the Importance of Race and Ethnicity

Although the preoccupation with race and ethnicity is not unique to the American culture, the United States has its own distinctive racial history that has contributed to tensions among diverse racial identities. Historically, race in the United States has played a significant role as a determinant of individual rights, opportunities, and social privilege. Laws and institutions catering to the interests of America's privileged class protected these rights and reinforced the significance of race. As a result, deficits in nearly every aspect of modern social life—education, employment, income, and health, for example—have accumulated for minorities throughout American history.

Starting in the 1950s, the national milieu began to improve for minorities as the civil rights movement ushered in proactive policies to reduce discrimination and level the playing field between whites and minorities. The Civil Rights Act of 1964 created equal employment opportunity, a law requiring federal contractors to provide minorities and women with a proportion of jobs equivalent to their representation in the labor force or population. In the 1970s, American universities sought to increase the diversity of their student bodies with affirmative action. The 1978 ruling by the Supreme Court in *University of California Regents v. Bakke* supported this effort by permitting race to be used as an admission criterion under certain circumstances. The intended result was to counter the earlier effects of discrimination in excluding minorities from higher education. Affirmative action policies have been successful in increasing minority representation in the nation's universities, and their continuing role in university admissions remains at the center of much debate even today.

The civil rights movement awarded value to minority status and provided minorities with the chance to compete against non-minorities for the same educational and professional opportunities; however, racial and ethnic identity continues to be associated with substantial vulnerabilities. In a report to the United Nations in 2000, the U.S. State Department noted a significant reduction in overt and institutionalized discrimination but acknowledged a strong "legacy of segregation, ignorance, stereotyping, discrimination and disparities in opportunity and achievement" for minorities (Lobe, 2000, p. 175). Racial and ethnic identity will likely continue to fragment the nation as long as race influences individual access to fundamental rights and privileges.

Defining Race/Ethnicity

Most policymakers, practitioners, and researchers are quick to use the term race/ethnicity in most discussions of disparities. But what does this term really mean? And why does it create such a division in society and politics?

At its simplest, race and ethnicity reflect skin color and, in some instances, cultural heritage or language. When measured as skin color, race/ethnicity is almost never the cause of disparities in health and health care (LaVeist and others, 2008;

LaVeist, Thorpe, and others, 2009; Link and McKinlay, 2009; Thorpe, Brandon, and LaVeist, 2008). Although there is evidence that the lightness or darkness of skin color may indeed be a risk factor for a few specific health issues, including incidence of skin cancer (Bradford, 2009; Dwyer, Blizzard, and others, 2002; Dwyer, Prota, and others, 2000; Fuller, 2000; Klag and others, 1991), there is little support for the direct correlation of skin color and health outcomes. For example, if we find that blacks are likely to receive fewer preventive services, can this be attributed to the color of skin? While the individual may experience discrimination based on skin color, skin color certainly does not cause the discrimination, nor does it transport a person to the doctor, or choose and pay for what preventive services are delivered. The differences in receiving preventive care are more likely to be explained by other factors, such as health insurance coverage, that are related to race/ethnicity.

It has been proposed that race/ethnicity frequently serves as a proxy measure for other factors that are more appropriate explanatory factors than skin color. Race/ethnicity can be a reflection of biological factors; socioeconomic status; cultural practices, beliefs, or acculturation; or political factors (King and Williams, 1995). Race/ethnicity may also serve as a proxy measure of experiencing discrimination. In the case of health outcomes, race/ethnicity may serve as a proxy for biological factors (blacks are more prone to sickle cell anemia, for example), cultural behaviors or practices regarding health, or access to material goods and services that support health. In the case of health care experiences, race/ethnicity may serve as a proxy for socioeconomic factors (enabling the purchase of services), language factors (creating barriers to accessing services), or discrimination based on skin color. This is not to say that race/ethnicity may not reflect other unmeasured or unknown factors, as is found in some research studies, but in any interpretation of the research literature, we seek to understand the mechanisms linking race/ethnicity with health and health care outcomes. LaVeist argues that where possible, measures of the actual mechanisms should be used instead of race/ethnicity so that more accurate interventions and health policies can be made. But in many cases, adequate measures such as cultural factors and measures of discrimination are only beginning to be developed, so we are left with race/ethnicity measures serving as relatively inaccurate proxies (LaVeist, 1994).

One final aspect of race/ethnicity to consider is how politics may influence the definition. While we have come to understand the complexity of race/ethnicity in modern research and now acknowledge combinations of racial/ethnic groups (such as white/Asian pairings) in national statistics as mixed-race groups, this highlights the political nature of how race/ethnicity is constructed. Starting in 2003, the U.S. Census attempted to capture some of this complexity in the self-reporting of race/ethnicity. Due to such changes in coding, there have been changes in the reported prevalence of racial/ethnic groups. Race/ethnicity is frequently used to determine affirmative action policies in universities, to decide funding allotments for health care workforce and other training programs, or to allocate money to underserved areas, and it is used in a range of national and local programs, so these coding changes are made with political scrutiny and not without political consequences.

Changes in simple terms such as "minority" will have to be redefined in the coming years to reflect these changes in racial/ethnic categories. For example, is a mixed-race individual who is both white and African American considered a minority? Is a Latino family living in Los Angeles County, which is predominantly Latino, considered a minority? Such changes in definitions could certainly influence the dynamics of health and social policies, how they are constructed, and to whom they are targeted. Although there isn't a clear answer to many of these questions, it is important to be aware of these challenges in discussions of vulnerable populations.

National Trends in Race/Ethnicity and Diversity

Minority racial and ethnic background has increasingly become an important consideration in the U.S. health care system. The creation of large national initiatives to reduce racial and ethnic disparities in health and health care has reaffirmed the nation's commitment to the elimination of one of its most entrenched problems. In the last decade, the former U.S. Surgeon General Dr. David Satcher worked to prioritize the elimination of racial and ethnic disparities at the top of the nation's health agenda (Satcher, 2000).

Even apart from the socioeconomic status factors that they are closely associated with, minority race and ethnicity have been shown to predict poorer health status, access to care, and quality of care. As discussed above, race/ethnicity is a relatively immutable personal trait that usually serves as a proxy for other factors such as language or culture that are correlated with health and health care experiences (LaVeist, 1994; Schulman, Rubenstein, Chesley, and Eisenberg, 1995). Understanding minority population trends is therefore essential.

Traditional use of the term minority is quickly becoming inapplicable in the United States. By 2006, a milestone had been reached where one in every ten U.S. counties had become "majority-minority," meaning the county had a population in which minorities combined to reflect more than 50 percent of the population (U.S. Census Bureau News, 2007). Much of this was due to the increase in immigration rates of Hispanic and Asian populations, and the trend is expected to continue (see Figure 2.1). The Hispanic population is projected to grow by more than 275 percent between 2010 and 2050, from 50 to 133 million

FIGURE 2.1   Projected Population Size in the U.S. by
Race and Ethnicity, 2010 and 2050

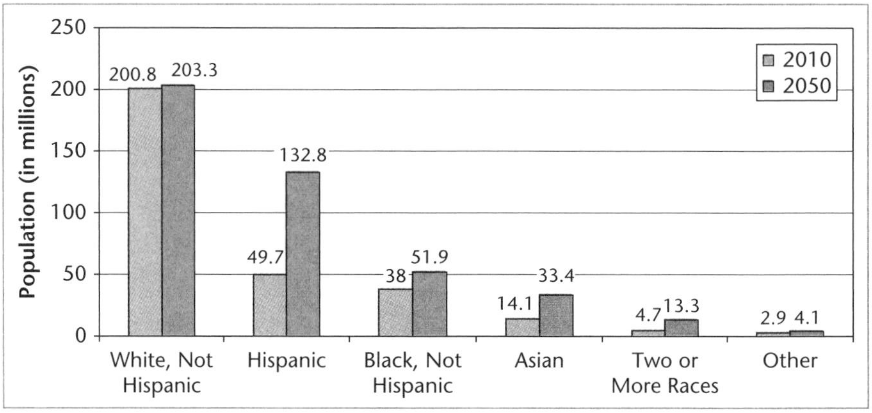

Source: U.S. Census Bureau Population Division (2008).

individuals in 2050. The Asian population is also expected to increase by about 220 percent over the same period, from 14 to 33 million individuals. At the same time, the number reporting two or more races is expected to nearly triple, from 5 to 13 million, reflecting greater intercultural mixing and *diversity*.

The projections of population growth by race/ethnicity translate into a major reshaping of the demographic picture of the United States, where by 2050 the country as a whole is majority-minority. While non-Hispanic whites account for 65 percent of the U.S. population in 2010, with a growth of only about 2 million individuals between 2010 and 2050, this is expected to decrease to 46 percent of the population in 2050 (see Figure 2.2). Contributing to whites accounting for a smaller proportion of the total population is the growth of the Hispanic population (projected to increase from 16 to 30 percent of the total population), the Asian population (increasing from 5 to 8 percent), and the number of whites who report themselves as being of two or more races.

Theoretical Pathways of Racial and Ethnic Vulnerability

We present a conceptual model in Figure 2.3 that builds on the original work of Stevens and Shi (2003), Aday and Andersen (1981), and King and Williams (1995) to describe several potential pathways linking race and ethnicity with health and health care (Aday and Andersen, 1981; King and Williams, 1995;

FIGURE 2.2   Projected Distribution of the U.S. Population by Race and Ethnicity, 2010 and 2050

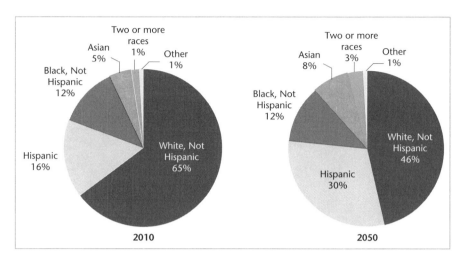

2010

2050

Source: U.S. Census Bureau Population Division (2008).

Stevens and Shi, 2003). The pathways begin with family characteristics that include socioeconomic status, cultural factors, discrimination, and health need. The model then traces the pathways through the health care delivery system and identifies provider and system factors that may contribute to disparities in care. Several pathways are likely to operate simultaneously, leading to adverse health and health care outcomes (Stevens and Shi, 2003).

Socioeconomic Status   One theory behind racial and ethnic differences in health care experiences is that they are attributable to differences in socioeconomic status such as income, education and occupation. African Americans, Hispanics, and certain other racial/ethnic groups are more likely than whites to have lower family income and lower education levels. They are also less likely to have insurance coverage, and when insured, they are more likely to be covered by public programs such as Medicaid and the Children's Health Insurance Program (CHIP) (Mills and Bhandari, 2003). These SES factors often combine to affect health care utilization, the presence and type of a regular source of care, and health status. Race/ethnicity is so closely intertwined with SES factors that it is often difficult to separate SES effects from the effects of other racial/ethnic pathways.

FIGURE 2.3 Conceptual Model Linking Race and Ethnicity with Health Care Experiences

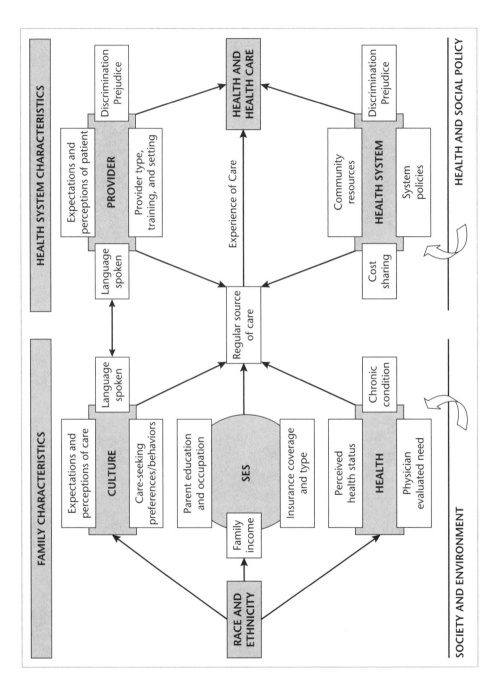

Source: Stevens and Shi (2003).

Cultural Factors   Perhaps offering the most potential for future research into racial disparities are family cultural factors, including language preference and ability, family preferences or beliefs leading to various health behaviors and health care-seeking practices, and differences in perceptions and expectations for health care. Language, in particular, is a well-known barrier to accessing health care (Aday, Fleming, and Andersen, 1984; Ferguson and Candib, 2002) and may also be an important barrier to developing a continuous patient-provider relationship. Language concordance between patient and provider, or accessibility of an interpreter, may be a more accurate explanatory variable (rather than patient language alone), but it is often absent from health care research.

Culturally based, care-seeking practices may also be associated with disparities in health and health care experiences. Controlling for SES, racial and ethnic minorities seek and obtain primary care more frequently from emergency departments. While appropriate sources of primary care such as community clinics and private physician offices tend to be lacking in areas where minorities live, a reliance on emergency departments may reflect a lack of knowledge about, or familiarity with, seeking regular preventive or primary care in more traditional settings. Moreover, cultural values and beliefs may influence the decision to seek health care and whether to adhere to medical advice (Flores, Abreau, Olivar, and Kastner, 1998; Flores and Vega, 1998). *Respeto* in Hispanic culture, for example, refers to the particularly high valuation of, and authority given to, physicians (American Medical Association, 1994). This may lead Hispanic patients to interact and collaborate with physicians differently than do other patients.

Racial and ethnic differences in family expectations or preferences for care are not yet well identified and cataloged, but they may uniquely affect individual ratings or experiences with care. There may be cultural differences in how families prefer to interact with health care providers, the types of questions they are comfortable asking and answering, and their expectations for treatments. For example, one study found that Asian and Latino parents are more likely than white parents to believe that antibiotics are necessary to treat the common cold (Mangione-Smith and others, 2004), even though antibiotics are ineffective. These beliefs not only affect whether physicians prescribe antibiotics (as physicians often feel compelled by parents to prescribe them) but can affect whether parents are satisfied with care if their children are not prescribed antibiotics. Without documentation and recognition of such cultural differences, it is difficult to know whether disparities in ratings of care reflect actual variations in the quality of care or whether they reflect differences in expectations.

Discrimination   Discrimination provides another potential pathway linking race and ethnicity to health and health care experiences. Defined as the differential action toward an individual or group based on race, discrimination is a manifestation of prejudice, the assumption of individual or group abilities, motives, and intentions according to race (Jones, 2000). Discrimination at the institutional level directly affects the health of minorities, who are treated differently once they enter the health care system. For example, in a study comparing bypass procedures given to a group with similar levels of severe illness and expected postoperative benefit, whites in the group received the surgery more often than black patients (Peterson, Shaw, and others, 1997). Another study found the same bias even after accounting for SES and health insurance (McBean and Gornick, 1994).

In some cases, differences in minority patient preferences for treatment have contributed to differences in health outcomes; however, a study by Hannan and others (1999) considered patient preferences and patient refusals for surgery as a cause for racial differences in the receipt of bypass surgeries and found that neither played a significant role in the differential treatment of minorities. In a synthesis of related studies, the Institute of Medicine reported that racial/ethnic minorities (most prominently African Americans) were less likely to receive necessary and appropriate medical tests, treatments, and procedures when compared to whites (Smedley, Stith, and Nelson, 2002). Further, this report found that health care systems, health care providers, and patients all contributed to the observed disparities.

Perceived discrimination and racism are also negatively associated with health. Recent research has shown a relationship between perceived discrimination and poor mental health, including conditions of psychological distress, major depression, and generalized anxiety (Brown, Williams, and Jackson, 2000; Jackson and others, 1996; Karlsen and Nazroo, 2002a, 2002b; Kessler, Mickelson, and Williams, 1999; Schulz and others, 2006; Williams, Neighbors, and Jackson, 2003). Studies have found that hypertension and poor self-rated health are associated with perceived discrimination (Dressler, 1990; Finch, Hummer, and Kolody, 2001; Guyll, Matthews, and Bromberger, 2001; Karlsen and Nazroo, 2002a, 2002b; Schulz and others, 2000). It is important to note that individual coping skills, however, can modify, for better or worse, negative effects of discrimination on mental and physical health (James, LaCroix, Kleinbaum, and Strogatz, 1984; Krieger, 1990; Krieger and Sidney, 1996; LaVeist, Sellers, and Neighbors, 2001).

Experiences of self-reported discrimination have also been linked to negative behavior patterns such as problem drinking and cigarette smoking, as well as low levels of compliance with medical recommendations (Cohen, Kessler, and Gordon, 1995; Landrine and Klonoff, 2000; Yen, Ragland, Greiner, and Fisher, 1999a, 1999b). Considering discrimination to be a form of stress, and perhaps a form of chronic stress, reveals one likely pathway that ultimately connects race/ethnicity with health. Current literature on stress suggests a process beginning with stress-induced anxiety or depression that either affects physical health directly or results in negative health behavior, which eventually worsens physical or emotional health.

Evidence suggesting that discrimination contributes to racial disparities in health and health care delivery continues to be challenged by limits in methodology and difficulty of standardizing a relatively subjective variable such as perceived discrimination. Some validated instruments have now been developed to better evaluate these experiences (Casagrande and others, 2007; Laveist, Isaac, and Williams, 2009; Sims and others, 2009), which will certainly help understand the impact of discrimination on minority health and how great a role it plays in racial disparities.

Health Needs   Health care needs drive the search for health care services. Health needs derive from both acute and chronic illnesses, as well as from public awareness of and recommendations for preventive care visits. Illness includes both clinically evaluated health problems and patient perceptions of health risks and needs. Racial and ethnic minorities generally have poorer health status than whites (National Center for Health Statistics, 2009). Thus, minorities have greater health needs that present both opportunities and challenges for the delivery of high-quality care. Even before entering the health care system, individuals are influenced and distinguished by family characteristics that will govern their health care experience and outcome.

Provider Factors   Individuals enter the health care system when they seek care from a provider or clinic of providers. Patients may identify the provider or clinic as a regular source of care, indicating they have prior experience with the source of care and will seek care in the future from this source. Alternatively, patients may obtain care from a variety of sources or in team care settings where there is no single regular provider of care. The presence or absence of and the type of regular source of care are determined by SES, cultural factors, and health needs (among other health system factors), which may influence both perceptions and actual delivery of care.

Once a person has entered the health care system, several provider factors may influence the delivery and experience of health care. Provider specialty, training, and setting of care may reveal differences in experience or preferences for delivering health care. Pediatricians may, for example, spend more time delivering preventive health services to minority children, whereas family practitioners may develop better knowledge of a minority family and then use that information when caring for the children. These differences by race/ethnicity in the types of providers who are seen are not well known but may contribute to some health care disparities.

In addition, providers have preferences and expectations for the delivery of care to their patients. Research suggests, in fact, that physician perceptions and beliefs about patients are affected by race, ethnicity, and socioeconomic status (van Ryn, 2002; van Ryn and Burke, 2000; van Ryn and Fu, 2003). These perceptions may affect physician treatment decisions, feelings of affiliation with patients, and beliefs about risk behaviors that influence the type and degree of care delivered. Perhaps for this reason, racial and ethnic concordance between provider and patient has been associated in some cases with better patient perceptions of partnership and satisfaction (Cooley, 2004; Cooper and Roter, 2002; Cooper and Powe, 2004; LaVeist and Carroll, 2002; Saha, Arbelaez, and Cooper, 2003; Saha, Komaromy, Koepsell, and Bindman, 1999). These measurably improved interactions may lead families to seek care from racially concordant providers (Gray and Stoddard, 1997). In a study among children, no disparities in primary care quality were found according to patient-provider racial/ethnic concordance, due perhaps to the attenuation in pediatric care of provider biases that may contribute to disparities (Stevens, Shi, and Cooper, 2003).

Health System Factors   Apart from provider characteristics, health care system factors such as community resources, health insurance deductibles and copayments, and other various health plan policies may influence the experiences of minorities in health care. The availability of health resources in the community may affect the ability of individuals to access care and may determine the setting in which care is delivered. Cost sharing has been shown to affect utilization of health services, and it may have a further impact on perceptions of the care received (Chernew and Newhouse, 2008). For example, patients in public health insurance programs that do not require copayments or deductibles may hypothetically feel less enfranchised to voice criticism of their health care simply because they are not directly paying for it.

Health care plan policies may be even more important in influencing the delivery of health care to families. For example, managed care policies that limit patient choice of providers may strengthen patient-provider relationships by linking patients with a specific provider. Alternately, restrictions in patient care may place an unnecessary burden on minority patients by reducing flexibility in finding race- or language-concordant providers. Either way, the effects of managed care are likely to be particularly pronounced for vulnerable populations and children (Miller and Luft, 1994, 1997).

Finally, health and social policies play an important role in mediating racial and ethnic minorities' experiences with health care. Health care policy shapes the nature and provision of safety net insurance coverage, regulates organizations such as managed care, and subsidizes the education and training of health care providers, particularly those of minority background. Many of the factors in this model are amenable to policy intervention, and thus policy may play an overarching role in reducing racial and ethnic disparities in health care.

Front-Line Experience: Wrapping Services Around the Homeless in Los Angeles

Dr. Paul Gregerson, the chief medical officer of the Weingart Foundation's Center for Community Health, explains how a new clinic on Los Angeles's infamous Skid Row has become part of a movement to transform a fragmented set of temporary-fix services into a coordinated, collective effort to alleviate the burdens of being homeless and even homelessness itself.

Los Angeles County's homeless population is the largest in the nation. It is estimated that there are more than 75,000 homeless people living on the streets, of which more than 5,000 are located in downtown Los Angeles's Skid Row. According to the Los Angeles Housing Authority, more than 74 percent are affected by depression, mental illness, substance abuse, physical disabilities, HIV/AIDS, or other chronic conditions. Many homeless individuals do not have health insurance or a primary care physician, or even recognize the need for these services.

A major barrier to treatment for homeless individuals is a lack of housing and supportive services in the area of housing. In many cases, the immediate goal of getting their most basic needs met, such as food and shelter, make health care a lower priority. Their days are usually filled by competing priorities such as waiting in meal lines, shelter lines, clothing lines, and traveling by foot back and forth from the welfare and unemployment offices, as well as to day jobs. Their struggle to obtain these basic necessities leaves homeless individuals little time for addressing their health care needs.

In Skid Row, these problems were compounded by a fragmented and duplicative system of care. Primary care, mental health, substance abuse, social service, and housing agencies were all operating independently, even though all were within walking distance of each other. There was no sharing of information, and this lack of coordination contributed to the continuous movement of Skid Row residents from one agency to another, leaving many to cycle between the streets, the shelters, the emergency room, and the jails.

This fragmentation prompted the Weingart Foundation and other philanthropic organizations to organize and fund an initiative (The Skid Row Homeless Healthcare Initiative) to address the ineffective healthcare delivery system. The initiative involved more than twenty-five agencies in and around Skid Row with the Center for Community Health the result of this collaboration. The Center provides comprehensive services under one roof, including medical, dental, mental health, substance abuse, optometry, HIV testing and counseling, and clinical pharmacy. Social services range from case management to housing placement, government benefits, and employment assistance. These built-in collaborations wrap services around the patient.

The Center's colocation of services at one site increases the chances that patients will receive and adhere to treatment plans needed to stabilize their situations. This care model has been achieved because of a structural integration of services across public and private organizations, supported by the physical proximity of care team members, regular case conferencing about patients and their needs, and the sharing of one chart for all participating providers. Integral are the enabling services, which entail consultation on entitlements and assistance in securing low-cost housing, employment, and training.

Each patient is assigned to a care team comprising a primary care physician, two medical assistants, a case manager, a psychiatrist, and a social worker. The team leader is the primary care physician. Exam rooms and social service offices are adjacent to each other. This facilitates a "warm hand-off" of patients from one care team member to another and allows the team to speak throughout the day about their patients. The single medical record shared by team members facilitates communication. This approach creates continuity and trust, as many homeless patients are mistrustful of the health care system or have a difficult time navigating it. In addition, the collaboration with the permanent supportive housing agencies helped achieve the ultimate objective of placing homeless patients into permanent housing.

Since there is still a greater need for services than is currently available, patients are prioritized according to need, and intensive case management is provided to those most vulnerable. The social worker conducts an initial assessment of the patient's needs for primary care, mental health, substance abuse, and/or social services, as well as information such as current housing, prior or current difficulties with law enforcement, life and vocational skills, and level of social support from family and friends. Patients are assessed every six months to monitor their level of functioning and perceived changes in their quality of life. When a patient is stabilized, he/she graduates to a less intensive level of case management, and another patient begins receiving the higher intensity care.

Mildred (name has been changed) is one success story of this integrated approach. When she presented to the center for medical care, Mildred had completed a five-year prison sentence for possession of heroin a few weeks earlier, but was homeless at the time and living with breast cancer. While in prison, she was placed on pain management for a gunshot wound she had sustained prior to her incarceration. At Mildred's initial visit, her primary care provider referred her to the social worker. During his evaluation, she reported the following: (1) she was staying at a local shelter, but on a limited stay; (2) she had no income and was not receiving public assistance; (3) she had recently lost her California ID; (4) she was about to be terminated from a pain management program unless she obtained Medicaid; (5) she had not contacted her new parole agent due to a case transfer; and (6) she had not talked with her sister (her only family contact) for months. Based on the assessment, an action plan was created with specific goals and deadlines.

The social worker talked with the shelter to extend her stay while he assisted Mildred with her application to a recuperative care program, where she currently resides. The program provides transitional housing and medical care for patients not sick enough to be in the hospital but not well enough to stay in a shelter. He also referred Mildred to the Department of Public Social Services for temporary cash relief and food stamps, and to the local Social Security Insurance (SSI) office. Her Medicaid and SSI applications were completed by her care team. He contacted her parole agent and hosted a visit between her and her agent in his office. The center provided her with a voucher to lower the cost of obtaining her new state ID. With Mildred's permission, her sister was contacted, and she agreed to house Mildred once she completes parole. The team continues to provide primary care and coordinates with specialty care for her breast cancer. Her entire care team monitors her for symptoms of depression secondary to her medical problems and economic situation and continues to provide social support for her as she completes her parole.

Without the integrated services provided by the multidisciplinary care team, Mildred could have fallen down any number of alternative paths. She may have received medication for her breast cancer at a local medical center but may have missed follow-up appointments or not adhered to her medication regimen. Her medical, mental health, and substance abuse problems may have been exacerbated if she had lost access to her shelter and not received public aid. Her insurance applications may have never been completed, and she may have violated her parole by not contacting her officer. In addition, Mildred may have never contacted her sister and would have never had the option to stay with her once her parole was complete.

SOCIOECONOMIC STATUS

An unfortunate truism in the United States, and in nearly every other developed and developing country, is that individuals with the greatest financial resources have the best health. They also have the greatest ability to access health services and obtain the highest quality care. The apparent explanation is that income translates into purchasing power for health care services. In fact, based on national spending in the United States, one would think that purchasing medical care is the only determinant of a population's health, since the U.S. spends the most on health care per person and as a percentage of gross domestic product (GDP) in the world (see Figure 2.4).

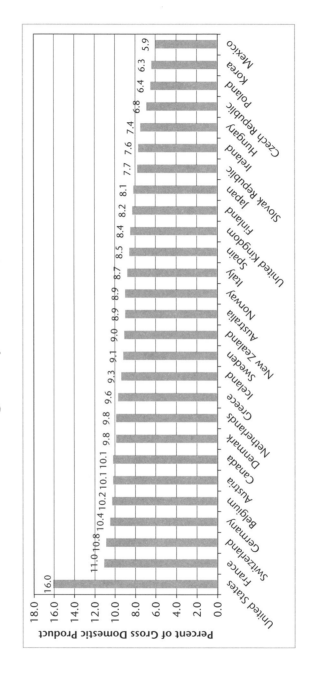

FIGURE 2.4 Health Care Spending as a Percentage of Gross Domestic Product among Developed Countries, 2007

Source: Organisation for Economic Co-operation and Development (2009).

However, research has revealed much more substantial and complex effects of income on health than just purchasing power. On closer review, income appears to be just part of a larger concept of social position, generally referred to as socioeconomic status (SES) that most commonly incorporates measures of income, education, and occupation, to provide a broader picture of a person's status in a community or society.

Historical Development of the Importance of Socioeconomic Status

Before examining the relationship between SES and health, it is important to take a step back and consider what determines an individual's socioeconomic status. Because SES has a significant impact on health, it is essential to understand what factors influence it and how modifying these factors could improve population health well before public health efforts or medical care are required. Environment and place of residence, in particular, influence all three measures of an individual's SES: income, education, and occupation. Changes made at the environmental level may ultimately improve community health by improving the SES of the population.

First, in the United States, residence dictates which public school students can attend. Because public school funding depends on the local tax base, a community's financial resources partially determine the quality of a neighborhood's public school. In areas of concentrated poverty, where financial resources are limited, public schools have lower average test scores, more restricted curricula, fewer qualified teachers, less access to more experienced academic advisers, less interaction with potential colleges and employers, higher levels of teen pregnancy, and higher dropout rates than public schools in middle-class areas.

Minorities are the most common residents in areas of high poverty concentration and disproportionately suffer the consequences of low-quality educational opportunities compared with whites (Orfield and Eaton, 1996; Willms, 1999). Differences in educational opportunities contribute to racial/ethnic disparities in educational attainment, competency levels among graduates, and preparation for enrollment in college or employment, all factors that shape an individual's ability to seek higher education, stable employment, and steady income (Acevedo-Garcia, Lochner, Osypuk, and Subramanian, 2003; Williams and Collins, 2001).

Second, residence further dictates employment opportunities by determining access to convenient and well-paying, entry-level job opportunities. Since the 1950s, low-skilled, higher-paying jobs have been migrating out of poor, urban communities to suburban areas (Kasarda, 1989; Wilson, 1996). Minorities living in urban areas are the most affected by this migration, what has been termed "spatial mismatch." Among minorities, African Americans are the most disadvantaged by their geographical distance. In fact, sociologists argue that spatial mismatch is a significant factor contributing to the consistently low employment rates of African Americans, lower SES, and poorer health status (Raphael and Stoll, 2002; Schulz, Williams, Israel, and Lempert, 2002).

Discrimination based on negative racial stereotypes may also be a factor in low employment rates and fewer opportunities for minorities. Corporations seeking to expand, relocate, or build new facilities have used geographical racial composition in deciding where to place these facilities. The location of African American communities, in particular, has been a significant negative factor in some of these decisions (Cole and Deskins Jr., 1988; Kirschenman and Neckerman, 1991; Neckerman and Kirschenman, 1991; Wilson, 1987, 1996). Thus, it follows that white residential areas have more convenient and well-paying job opportunities than African American residential areas (Raphael and Stoll, 2002).

The effect that residential segregation has on employment opportunities further demonstrates the role that discrimination plays in creating poor labor markets for African Americans. Cities such as Detroit, New York, and Chicago, which have high levels of residential segregation, have greater spatial mismatches between African Americans and job locations. Conversely, African Americans living in cities with less residential segregation such as Portland, Oregon, and Charlotte, North Carolina, have better access to jobs. This relationship persists even as cities change over time. Cities that became less segregated from 1990 to 2000 showed a concurrent improvement in spatial mismatch between African American residents and job opportunities (Raphael and Stoll, 2002). Corporate and geographical discrimination contributing to segregation leaves inner-city communities isolated and further impoverished by high unemployment.

Communities with high unemployment are entangled in a cycle of poverty, as fewer employment and job-networking opportunities limit an economic escape and fewer consistently employed adults are able to act as role models for young adults in the next generation (Wilson, 1987). Furthermore, living in areas of concentrated poverty over an extended period of time can weaken a strong work ethic, devalue academic achievement, and reduce the social stigmas of incarceration, low educational attainment, and economic failure (Shihadeh and Flynn, 1996). Moreover, such devaluations and lower achievement may discourage future companies from moving into economically deprived areas, extending the cycle.

Factors leading to limited educational and employment opportunities in poor communities are made worse by political neglect. Social services have the potential to buffer disadvantaged communities from the stress and circumstances of poverty. Politicians, however, are more likely to cut funding for services in poor areas because these communities are less politically organized and less empowered to successfully protest the funding cuts compared with more economically and socially advantaged communities (Wallace, 1990, 1991; Wilson, 1987). Even for conscientious politicians, providing essential social services in areas of concentrated poverty is challenging. As individuals who are able to afford better neighborhoods move from urban to suburban areas, the urban tax base contracts, making it difficult to continue to fund social services (Bullard, 1994; Wilson, 1987).

In short, environmental factors, including racial and ethnic segregation and political neglect, influence the education, employment, and income of individuals residing in a community. Not only do these factors determine where individuals will rank along the SES gradient, they also govern mobility up and down the social classes.

National Trends in Income and Poverty and Their Distribution

The importance of SES to health has been recognized in Europe since the early 1900s when mortality statistics were first reported according to occupation. The United States has been slower to adopt this practice. In 1976, the U.S. Department of Health and Human Services released its inaugural report of the nation's health, revealing substantial differences in mortality, morbidity, and access to care according to SES. Numerous studies since the 1976 report have concluded that lower-SES populations have a higher incidence of chronic disease, disability, and mental health problems. How prevalent is low SES in the United States, and what populations are the least well off?

Household income has changed substantially in the past forty years. In 1968, the median adjusted household income in the United States was equivalent to about $40,500 in 2008 dollars. By 2008, the annual household income had reached $50,300, just lower than the highest median income recorded in the nation's history in 2007. Per capita income grew similarly during this period, increasing from about $12,300 in 1970 to $26,900 in 2008. Changes in annual income, however, have not been consistent across all demographic groups (DeNavas-Walt, Proctor, and Lee, 2009).

Some of the most striking differences in income are across racial/ethnic groups. Since 1970, Asians and whites have consistently had higher annual household incomes than blacks and Hispanics. In 2008, the median household income of Asians and whites reached $65,637 and $55,530, respectively, compared with Hispanic and African American households with incomes of $37,913 and $34,218 respectively. These incomes may seem high, but they are in fact slightly lower (in fact, 3.6 percent lower) than in 2007, as the United States had just begun to enter its first recession since 2001. Moreover, in comparison to the respective income peaks prior to the 2001 recession, 2008 household income was actually 4.3 percent lower for all races combined (from $52,587 in 1999), 2.7 percent lower for non-Hispanic whites (from $57,059 in 1999), 5.8 percent lower for Asians (from $69,713 in 2000), 7.8 percent lower for African Americans (from $37,093 in 2000), and 8.6 percent lower for Hispanics (from $41,470 in 2000). This suggests a troubling, longer-term downward trend in real household income, particularly for African Americans and Hispanics (see Figure 2.5).

These racial differences in household income look somewhat different when one considers per capita income, as household sizes may differ. Although Asians had the highest median household income in 2008, income for each household member was lower for Asians ($30,300) compared with whites ($31,300). Asian and Pacific Islander households are typically composed of more members than white households (3.1 versus 2.5 members), partly explaining the higher household income for Asians. Similarly, Hispanics and African Americans had much lower per capita income ($15,700 and $18,400, respectively).

Another important way to examine household income is through the concept of poverty. The U.S. poverty threshold was first developed in 1963 by the Social Security Administration as a measure of whether families were earning enough money to afford the cost of living in society. The measure was created rather crudely from the U.S. Department of Agriculture's estimate of what it cost a

FIGURE 2.5   Household Monetary Income by Race and Ethnicity, 1967–2008

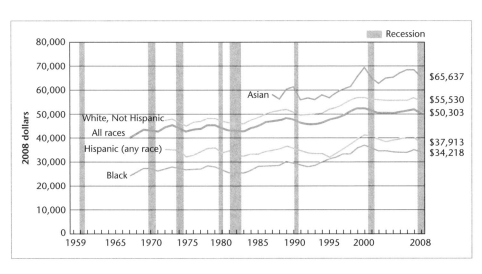

Source: DeNavas-Walt and others (2009).

family to buy enough food to feed its members in the most economical way (called the "economy food plan" at the time). This cost was then simply multiplied by three, based on an estimate at the time that buying food required about one-third of a family's income in a given month. That amount was annualized and adjusted upward or downward based on the number of family members. Families annually earning less than that amount of money were, thus, considered to be living in poverty. The threshold has been adjusted upward to account for inflation in the cost of living using the Consumer Price Index. Even today, the poverty threshold is still based on that original calculation in 1963 and remains a simple reflection of annual inflation adjustments in the cost of living since that time.

The poverty threshold still varies by family size to account for the amount of money needed to support different-sized families. For example, the poverty threshold in 2008 for a three-person family was $17,600 and a four-person family was $21,200 (U.S. Department of Health and Human Services, 2008). In 2009, the poverty threshold was adjusted upward to $18,310 for three family members and $22,050 for four (U.S. Department of Health and Human Services, 2009). The poverty thresholds are important because they are used by government agencies as eligibility criteria for particular assistance programs. There are many programs that use the poverty thresholds, including *Head Start*, the Food Stamp Program (formally known as the Supplemental Nutrition Assistance Program), the National School Lunch Program, the Low-Income Home Energy Assistance Program, Medicaid and the Children's Health Insurance Program (CHIP).

One important point to understand is that each program (and often each state) sets its own eligibility, typically based on a percentage of the federal poverty threshold, more commonly known as the federal poverty level (FPL). For instance, to be eligible for CHIP in one state, the state government may decide that families have to earn less than 150 percent of the FPL, meaning less than 1.5 times the federal poverty threshold, while eligibility may be set at 250 percent in another state (2.5 times the FPL). To illustrate this, a family of three in the first state would need to earn less than 1.5 times the $18,310 federal poverty threshold in 2009, a cut-off of $27,465.

Even more interesting (or frustrating, depending on your point of view) is that each agency and program may use different income and family size calculations. For some programs, income may be limited to after-tax dollars, while others may require gross, pre-tax income. For other programs, there may be distinctions in how family size is calculated by accounting for differences between the number of children and number of adults in the family. It is important to remember that these differences across programs do not affect the poverty thresholds themselves or how the government reports the number of families living in poverty, but just the eligibility for a range of assistance programs.

FIGURE 2.6   Number in Poverty and Poverty Rate, 1959–2008

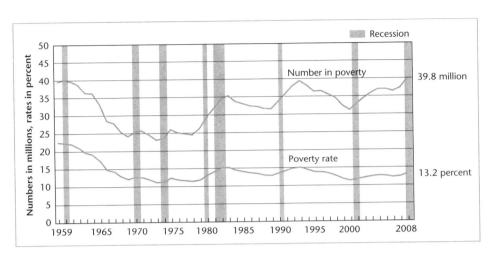

Source: DeNavas-Walt and others (2009).

Trends in poverty generally mirror the changes in income (Figure 2.6). In 2008, 13.2 percent of the population was living in poverty, up from 11.3 percent in 2000, which was then statistically similar to the lowest recorded rate of poverty in history (11.1 percent), set in 1979. Even the seemingly small change in the poverty rate from 2000 to 2008 reflects an increase of more than 5 million people living in poverty, from 34.6 to 39.8 million. Substantial variation in the rates of poverty between 1960 and 2002 shows that it is closely tied to the changes in the national economy and strongly impacted by the presence of a recession (DeNavas-Walt and others, 2009).

As with income, some of the most striking differences in poverty rates are across racial and ethnic groups. African Americans and Hispanics have traditionally experienced the highest rates of poverty. In 2008, 24.8 percent of African Americans and 23.2 percent of Hispanics were living in poverty, the highest rates since 2000, and much higher than the 11.8 percent rate for Asians and 8.6 percent rate for non-Hispanic whites (see Figure 2.7). However, the disparity in poverty rates between African Americans and whites has decreased over the past forty or so years. In 1968, for example, nearly 35 percent of African Americans were poor compared with 10 percent of whites, a difference of 25 percentage points. This gap has narrowed significantly since that time, with the size of the disparity in poverty rates between African Americans and whites just 16.1 percent in 2008.

FIGURE 2.7   Poverty Rates by Race and Ethnicity, 1968–2008

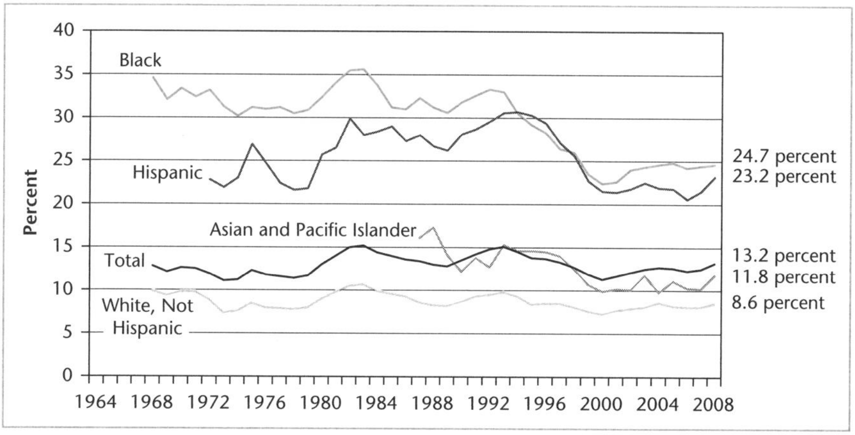

Note: Hispanics could be of any race. For all years, census data on African American and Asian or Pacific Islander races were not available by Hispanic ethnicity. Prior to 1993, census data did not separate Hispanic whites from non-Hispanic whites.
Source: U.S. Census Bureau (2009a).

The difference between Hispanics and whites has also decreased slightly from 16.5 percent in 1973 (the first year poverty status was measured for Hispanics) to 14.6 percent in 2008 (U.S. Census Bureau, 2009a).

Finally, there are several interesting, smaller trends in both income and poverty according to region and household type. Single-parent households headed by women have generally had lower incomes and higher rates of poverty than other household types. There had been a trend of increasing household income for these families—by 2000 their poverty rate (although still very large) had decreased to 24.7 percent, its lowest level in history. But by 2008, this rate had climbed to 28.7 percent, compared to just 5.5 percent of married-couple households. Nativity is also a major predictor of poverty status. Among the 87.8 percent of the population that was born in the United States, 12.6 percent lived in poverty in 2008. Among the 12.2 percent of the population that was foreign born, those who were naturalized citizens had a lower poverty rate of 10.2 percent, but among those who were not citizens, the rate was 23.3 percent (DeNavas-Walt and others, 2009).

Children are an important consideration because they are more likely than adults to live in families in poverty, due mainly to lower-income families having more children on average than higher-income families. The number of children living in poverty has been rising. In 2008, 19.0 percent of children lived in poverty compared with 16.7 percent in 2000. This varied considerably by race/ethnicity. Just 10.6 percent of non-Hispanic white children lived in poverty compared to 14.5 percent of Asians, 25.0 percent of Native Hawaiian or Pacific Islanders, 30.6 percent of Hispanics, 34.7 percent of African Americans, and 37.0 percent of American Indians or Alaska Natives. To put this in perspective, this means that in 2008, one of every four Hispanic and Native Hawaiian or Pacific Islander children and more than one in every three African American or American Indian and Alaska Native children lived in poverty (U.S. Census Bureau, 2009a).

Trends in Income Inequality   As we will discuss shortly, both absolute income and the distribution of income in a population are important considerations in determining the health of a population. The U.S. Census Bureau has traditionally used two measures of income distribution to describe the income inequality in the population. The first measure is the *Gini index*, which uses a single statistic (ranging from 0 to 100) to summarize the degree of income dispersion across a population. A score of 0 indicates perfect equality, where everyone receives an equal share of income, and a score of 100 indicates complete inequality, where all of the income is received by a single person.

The second measure of income distribution uses shares of income to describe the level of income inequality in a population. This approach ranks households according to income and divides them into groups of equal population size, such as quartiles or quintiles. The aggregate income of the group is then described as a proportion of the total income, such that each quartile or quintile holds a certain percentage of all the income. The more income that a single group holds, the greater is the level of income inequality.

According to both of these measures, income inequality in the United States has increased significantly in the past forty years. In 1968, the top quintile of U.S. households held 42.6 percent of all the U.S. income. By 2008, the amount of total income held by the top quintile increased to 50.0 percent. According to the Gini index, the degree of income inequality increased between 1968 and 2008 from 38.6 to 46.6 (DeNavas-Walt and others, 2009).

Although there is some difficulty in comparing income inequality rates across countries with varying frequencies of data reporting, the United States appears to have much greater income inequality than other developed countries. Among the thirty countries ranked highest in the degree of human development in the 2009 Human Development Report, the United States had a Gini coefficient of 46.6 (rounded to 47), followed by Singapore and Hong Kong, both with a rounded coefficient of 43. Sweden, Japan, and Denmark had the three lowest levels of

FIGURE 2.8 Gini Index of Income Inequality for the Thirty Most Developed Countries, 2007–2008

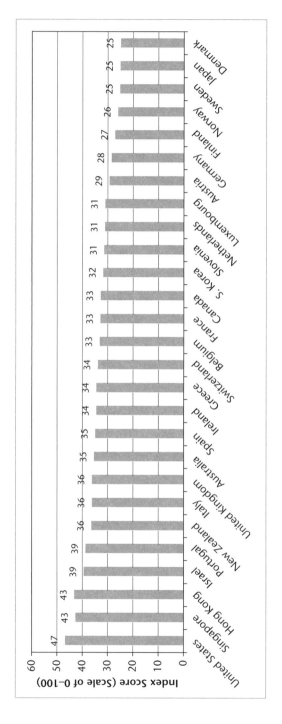

Note: An index score closer to 100 indicates a more unequal distribution of wealth.

Source: United Nations Development Programme (2009).

inequality, each with a coefficient of just 25 (see Figure 2.8) (United Nations Development Programme, 2009).

Global distribution of wealth is even more dramatically disproportionate. According to the same United Nations report, the richest 5 percent of the world's population has income 114 times higher than that of the poorest 5 percent (United Nations Development Programme, 2009). The United States earns much of this global wealth. The income for the wealthiest 25 million Americans is equivalent to the aggregate income of the 2 billion poorest people in the world, suggesting significant income inequality among the world's nations. Since the mid-1980s, income inequality measured across countries has risen 20 percent, to just under 54. This global income inequality was relatively constant between 1960 and the early 1980s, with an average Gini coefficient of 46. After the 1980s, the greater level of inequality in the world has been attributed to recessions among Latin American countries and weaker economies in Eastern Europe and the former Soviet Union in the 1990s.

Trends in Education   Income and education are strongly correlated, such that more highly educated individuals generally earn higher wages. Trends in education, however, vary somewhat from trends in income. The most commonly reported measure of education is whether a person has completed high school, and statistics on this measure have changed dramatically over the years. In 1940, only 24.5 percent of the population age twenty-five and over had completed high school (see Figure 2.9). By 1968, high school completion had more than doubled to 52.6 percent and by 2008 the rate had increased to 86.6 percent for all races. Similarly, college participation and completion have accelerated dramatically in the past sixty years (see Figure 2.10). In 1940, only 4.6 percent of the population age twenty-five and over had completed college. By 1968, college completion had more than doubled to 10.5 percent. Like high school completion, even greater increases occurred in college completion in the forty years after 1968, nearly tripling by 2008 to 29.4 percent for all races.

Like income, educational attainment is unequally distributed across demographic groups. In particular, there have been dramatic differences in education across racial/ethnic groups. In 2008, 91.5 percent of whites and 88.7 percent of Asian Americans completed high school, but only 83.0 percent of blacks and 62.3 percent of Hispanics had done so. Even greater disparities existed in college education in 2008, with completion rates ranging from 52.6 percent for Asians and 32.6 percent for whites, to 19.6 percent for African Americans and 13.3 percent for Hispanics.

Similar disparities in educational attainment also exist according to gender. In 2000, men age twenty-five and over completed college at a rate 3.4 percent

FIGURE 2.9   High School Completion Rates by Race and Ethnicity, Adults Twenty-Five Years and Over, 1968–2008

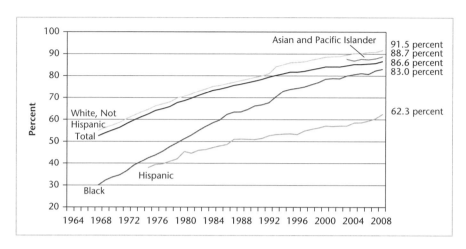

Note: Hispanic individuals could be of any race. For all years, census data on African American and Asian or Pacific Islander races were not available by Hispanic ethnicity. Prior to 1993, census data also did not separate Hispanic whites from non-Hispanic whites.

Source: U.S. Census Bureau (2009b).

FIGURE 2.10   College Completion Rates by Race and Ethnicity, Adults Twenty-Five Years and Over, 1968–2008

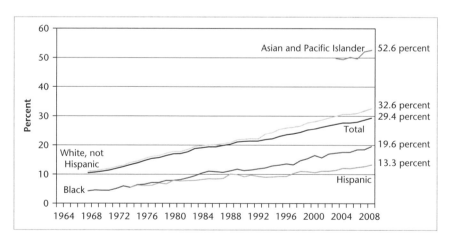

Note: Hispanic individuals could be of any race. For all years, census data on African American and Asian or Pacific Islander races were not available by Hispanic ethnicity. Prior to 1993, census data also did not separate Hispanic whites from non-Hispanic whites.

Source: U.S. Census Bureau (2009b).

higher than the rate for women (28.5 percent versus 25.1 percent), but this disparity is closing with each passing year. In 2008, 30.1 percent of men had completed college compared to 28.8 of women, a difference of only 1.3 percent. Moreover, women have been outpacing men in high school graduation rates. In 2000, 84.4 percent of women had graduated from high school compared with 83.8 percent of men (a difference of 0.6 percent), which was the first statistically significant gender difference in high school completion rates since the 1980s, when men graduated from high schools at higher rates than women. In 2008, 87.2 percent of women had graduated from high school compared with 85.9 percent of men, a difference of 1.4 percent. Interestingly, the gap between female and male graduation rates increases as income decreases, suggesting that men's chances of completing high school are much lower in areas that are economically deprived (Horn, 2006).

To compare how well the United States ranks globally in education is difficult because of diverse educational systems and variations in education data collected in different countries. Using adult functional literacy rates as a proxy for education, it is interesting to note that 10 to 20 percent of people in most OECD (Organisation for Economic Co-Operation and Development) countries are functionally illiterate. Among the thirty most highly developed countries, Sweden and Norway have the lowest functional illiteracy rates (7.5 and 7.9 percent, respectively). Germany, Canada, and New Zealand were in the middle range of illiteracy rates with 14.4, 14.6, and 18.4 percent considered functionally illiterate. The United States (20.0 percent), United Kingdom (21.8 percent), and Ireland (22.6 percent) had the highest functional illiteracy rates (United Nations Development Programme, 2009).

Trends in Occupation   Occupation is closely tied to income and education. In general, higher education is associated with the ability to obtain higher-level occupations with higher salaries and greater benefits. Understanding the trends in employment and occupation is particularly important because occupation plays a major role in determining aspects of personal lifestyles and because it is a primary source of health insurance coverage for most Americans.

The unemployment rate in the United States has fluctuated significantly over the years, most typically in response to variations in the national economy. In 2009, about 9.5 percent of the workforce reported being unemployed. This reflects an increase of about 5.5 percent compared with 2000, when the unemployment rate was just 4.0 percent, the lowest rate of unemployment in the past forty years. The rate of unemployment in 2009 was nearly equivalent to the highest rate of unemployment reached in the past forty years, a high of 9.7 percent in 1982 (Bureau of

Labor Statistics, 2009a). Relative to nine other industrialized countries reporting unemployment rates that are comparable in methodology, the United States had a higher average unemployment rate than all but one. In late 2009, 9.5 percent of the U.S. population was unemployed, and only France had a higher unemployment rate, of 9.7 percent. Netherlands, Australia, and Japan had the three lowest rates of unemployment (3.3, 5.5, and 5.8 percent, respectively) (Bureau of Labor Statistics, 2009c).

As with income and education, there are differences in unemployment rates across racial/ethnic groups. African Americans and Hispanics have had higher rates of unemployment than whites, and these disparities have remained consistent over the past forty years (see Figure 2.11). In 2009, the rate of unemployment was 15.3 percent for African Americans, 12.4 percent for Hispanics, 8.7 percent for whites, and 7.5 percent for Asian and Pacific Islanders. These rates are much higher than their lowest points for Hispanics and Asians in 2006 and for African Americans and whites in 1999. Though substantial differences remained in 2009, these disparities were smaller than those experienced in the late 1970s through the

FIGURE 2.11   Unemployment Rates by Race and Ethnicity, 1968–2009

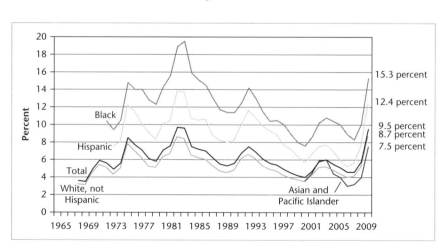

Note: Hispanic individuals could be of any race. For all years, census data on African American and Asian or Pacific Islander races were not available by Hispanic ethnicity. Prior to 1993, census data also did not separate Hispanic whites from non-Hispanic whites.

Source: Bureau of Labor Statistics (2009b).

mid-1980s, when differences in unemployment were as much as 10 percentage points between African Americans and whites.

There are also some differences in employment rates across genders. Among labor force participants, men have had slightly higher unemployment rates than women. In 2008, for example, the unemployment rate in the civilian labor force age sixteen and over for males was 6.1 percent compared with 5.4 percent for females. Perhaps more interesting are the gender differences in labor force participation. In the 1970s, the participation rate for males was 79.7 percent but only 43.3 percent for females. By 2008, this has changed considerably to 73.0 percent for males and 59.5 for females, a narrowing in its largest gap of 36.3 percentage points in the 1970s to just 13.5 percent in 2008 (Bureau of Labor Statistics, 2009d).

Unemployment rates are lowest in managerial or professional occupations (1.7 percent) compared with service occupations (5.3 percent) and blue-collar positions (6.3 percent). Technical and administrative support positions, along with production, craft, and repair positions, all have rates of unemployment of 3.6 percent. Not only do individuals in service and blue-collar occupations experience greater rates of unemployment, but the incomes for these individuals (often based on the minimum wage) are shrinking. Adjusting for inflation, the minimum wage has decreased steadily over the past thirty years, dropping from $7.10 per hour in 1970, $6.48 in 1980 and $5.15 in 2000, to just $4.41 in 2007. Finally, these jobs are also less likely to offer basic, good-quality employee benefits. Health insurance coverage, for example, is available in 79 percent of professional and managerial positions, but only in 74 percent of full-time service and blue-collar positions. While this difference may seem small, the type of health insurance coverage offered in service and blue-collar positions tends to be much less comprehensive, and employees tend to have to pay a greater share of the cost.

Theoretical Pathways of Socioeconomic Status

Levels of income, education, and occupation together characterize an individual's relative position along the socioeconomic gradient. But by what means does this position or status affect health outcomes and health care experiences? We present a model (Figure 2.12) that synthesizes the work of Evans, Barer, and Marmor (1994); Seeman and Crimmins (2001); Starfield and Shi (1999), and researchers from the MacArthur Network on SES and Health (Adler and Ostrove, 1999) to describe potential pathways linking socioeconomic status with disparities in health and health care. In its simplest form, SES is related to health and health care in two ways, *material deprivation* and lack of social participation (Marmot, 2002).

FIGURE 2.12 Conceptual Model Linking Socioeconomic Status with Health

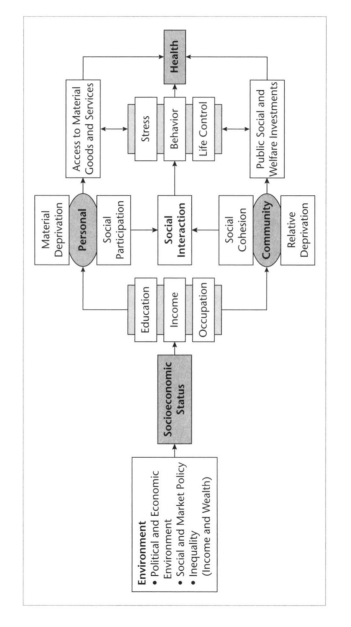

Material deprivation encompasses access to material goods that are required for good health, including clean water and good sanitation, adequate nutrition and housing, reliable transportation, and a safe and comfortable environment. Social participation includes having time for leisure activity and group participation, having friends or family around for entertainment and support, receiving chances for professional achievement, and ultimately having sufficient opportunities and control over one's life to lead a fulfilling and satisfying life. Without access to material goods and supportive social participation, health may falter, and greater barriers may be experienced in obtaining needed health care services. In the following section, we take a closer look at the pathways linking material deprivation and social participation to population health.

Material Deprivation   Material deprivation is the lack of material resources that enable the protection or promotion of health. These resources also enable a person to obtain adequate health care when faced with ill health. Steady income is fundamental to obtaining clean water and adequate housing, proper nutrition, electricity and heat, and a safe environment. These factors are most clearly associated with health in developing countries, but they also play an important role in areas of developed countries, such as many rural and inner-city areas of the United States, that experience poverty and deprivation resembling that of developing countries.

In addition to affording basic life necessities, absolute personal income allows the purchase of health insurance coverage and specific health care services. Education and occupation also play an important role in obtaining health insurance coverage and health care. Most people in the United States receive their health insurance coverage through their employer, though there has been a decline in the percentage of employers offering this benefit, particularly in lower-paying, nonprofessional positions. The U.S. government provides safety net health insurance coverage to many low-income individuals. Many individuals, however, do not qualify for safety net coverage because they are employed and earn just a bit too much income but not enough to purchase health insurance.

A unique consideration with regard to SES and health is the likely presence of an income threshold above which simple material deprivation may no longer play a primary role in determining health. Above this proposed threshold, people are universally able to afford basic material necessities, and any higher income is less likely to affect or improve health through the purchase of material goods. Interestingly, however, there still exists a stark SES gradient in health above this income threshold, suggesting the presence of SES effects other than material deprivation.

Social Participation   There is substantial debate regarding the correlation of SES and health above the proposed income threshold. Social participation provides a possible explanation for the SES gradient above the income threshold, with greater income being associated with greater social participation. At the individual level, there is substantial evidence of the effects of social participation on health across all levels of income. Social participation includes having time for leisure activity and group participation, support of family and friends, chances for professional achievement, and sufficient opportunities and control to lead a fulfilling and satisfying life.

Specifically, there are three main mechanisms through which social participation may be correlated with health: the effects of stress and coping, health-related behaviors, and life control. Other mechanisms have been proposed, including reciprocal influences of health on SES, such that being in poor health limits the ability to earn income and participate in society. There is some evidence of this direction of causality, but this is likely limited to only the most disabling, long-term conditions (Adler and Ostrove, 1999).

Social participation links SES to health by providing a protective effect against the deleterious health effects of chronic stress associated with lower incomes. It has been demonstrated that stressful life events or high levels of stress that persist over time result in physical and psychological strains, enhancing vulnerability to infectious diseases, heart disease, cancer, HIV, and depression (Baum, Garofalo, and Yali, 1999; Kaplan and Manuck, 1999). There is also substantial evidence to suggest that these strains can be reduced or even reversed when effective coping mechanisms are present (Taylor, Katz, and Moos, 1995; Taylor, Repetti, and Seeman, 1997; Taylor and Seeman, 1999). Coping mechanisms can be individual coping behaviors or skills, or they can be buffers such as social support from family and friends. Therefore, the lack of social participation that may be associated with lower income may also weaken the ability of low-SES individuals to cope with stress, placing their health at even greater risk.

The second mechanism by which social participation links SES with health is the presence of socioeconomic differences in deleterious health-related behaviors. Extensive research has documented an SES gradient in health risk behaviors, such that individuals of lower SES are more likely to smoke, drink excessively, and participate in less physical activity than individuals of higher SES (Colhoun and others, 1997; Marmot, 1998; Seeman and Crimmins, 2001; Winkleby, Cubbin, Ahn, and Kraemer, 1999). Why these differences exist is not entirely clear, but one likely hypothesis is that risk behavior is a negative coping response to the chronic stress that is more common in lower-SES groups (Gallo and Matthews, 1999, 2003). If this hypothesis is true, there may be a particularly important role for social participation in protecting against the adoption of health risk behaviors.

In fact, social support is associated with lower rates of smoking and drinking, better nutrition, and higher rates of health prevention behaviors and of seeking preventive care (Franks, Campbell, and Shields, 1992; Geckova and others, 2003; Ross and Mirowsky, 2002; Yarcheski, Mahon, and Yarcheski, 2001; Yarcheski, Mahon, and Yarcheski, 2003).

The third mechanism linking SES with health is the presence of socioeconomic differences in feelings of personal control over life circumstances. Research has shown that populations with low SES are more likely to lack a sense of control over their life, particularly with regard to the daily work environment. Studies have shown that SES differences exist in employment security, opportunities for occupational advancement, control over work, and the variety and pace of work (Marmot and Theorell, 1988; Marmot and others, 1991; Steenland and others, 2000; Steptoe and Appels, 1989; Taylor and Seeman, 1999).

There is a large body of empirical research showing that these aspects of control in the work environment are related to cardiovascular disease and other measures of health (Karasek, 1990; Lundberg, 1999; Marmot and others 1997; Seeman and Lewis, 1995; Syme, 1989). In addition, there is evidence that a lack of social support at work, when coupled with high demands and low control, substantially increases health risks (Johnson and Hall, 1995). It is plausible that these feelings of control affect health through additional stress or health-related behavior mechanisms, making it difficult to delineate the separate effects of each.

Community and Relative Deprivation   So far, we have considered the pathways between individual SES and health that operate through either the ability to purchase goods and services (material deprivation) or through the interrelated elements of social participation (such as stress, health behaviors, and control). Interestingly, a large body of literature now suggests that individual determinants of health have their community-level counterparts and that these may play an even larger role in determining the health of a population.

The first mechanism by which community-level socioeconomic inequalities may be associated with health is through community-based material deprivation (sometimes termed relative deprivation). With community-based deprivation, the socioeconomic characteristics of the community play an important role in determining health above and beyond the effects of personal income. A growing number of studies have demonstrated this relationship between disadvantaged communities and poorer health outcomes, even after controlling for individual-level demographic and socioeconomic factors (Bird and others, 2009; Diez Roux, 2003; Diez Roux and others, 2001; Diez-Roux, Nieto, Muntaner, and others, 1997; Do, 2009; Lang and others, 2009; LeClere, Rogers, and Peters, 1998; Lee and Cubbin, 2002).

Exploring the potential pathways between community deprivation and health, studies have shown that both adults and youth living in disadvantaged communities have poorer dietary habits, less physical activity, higher rates of smoking, and greater exposure to environmental risks compared with those living in more advantaged communities (Chichlowska and others, 2008; Diez-Roux, Nieto, Caulfield, and others, 1999; Diez-Roux and others, 1997; Evans and Kantrowitz, 2002; Shishehbor, Gordon-Larsen, Kiefe, and Litaker, 2008; Yen and Kaplan, 1998). Although these intermediary factors provide an explanation for the relationship between community disadvantage and health, they fail to offer an explanation for why these higher risk factors occur in disadvantaged communities.

No one would dispute that absolute poverty is bad for health. But a major change in thinking about the health effects of socioeconomic status is revealed in evidence showing that mortality rates in a population are strongly related to the degree of inequality (typically income) in a population (Backlund and others, 2007; De Vogli, Mistry, Gnesotto, and Cornia, 2005; Wilkinson, 1996; Wilkinson and Pickett, 2008). Such findings have been reported in the United States, the United Kingdom, Canada, and a dozen or more European and Latin American developed and developing countries. Repeated corroboration that inequitable distribution of resources in a population is associated with poorer health has prompted research into the mechanisms underlying this relationship.

Social Cohesion   One frequently proposed explanation of the relationship between inequality and health is the intermediary role of social cohesion (Kawachi and Kennedy, 1997, 1999; Kawachi, Kennedy, and Glass, 1999; Kawachi, Kennedy, Lochner, and Prothrow-Stith, 1997). Social cohesion is the community-level equivalent of social participation and is used to characterize social relationships on a larger scale. Social cohesion (also often referred to as social capital) reflects concrete elements of the social fabric—such as the forming of associations, church groups, and political organizations—and also less tangible aspects of social interaction—such as interpersonal trust and community norms—that shape individual identities, norms, beliefs, and practices (Lindstrom, 2009; Mansyur, Amick, Harrist, and Franzini, 2008; Schultz, Corman, Noonan, and Reichman, 2009; Snelgrove, Pikhart, and Stafford, 2009; Subramanian, Lochner, and Kawachi, 2003).

There is abundant literature suggesting that as social status differences in society and community deprivation increase, the quality of social relations deteriorates. Circumstantial evidence was derived from analyses of a number of countries (including Japan and the Kerala state in India) that were found to be unusually egalitarian, socially cohesive, and healthy (Wilkinson, 1996). Additional studies have confirmed this pattern, showing that areas with greater inequality and deprivation are less socially cohesive: they have lower trust, less participation in community and civic groups, greater hostility, and more violent crime (Abel, 2008; Hanks, 2008; Hseih and Pugh, 1993; Huisman and Oldehinkel, 2009; Oksanen and others, 2008; Perry, Williams, Wallerstein, and Waitzkin, 2008; Stafford, De Silva, Stansfeld, and Marmot, 2008). Moreover, income inequality has been related to mortality from homicides and alcohol-related causes, both of which are health outcomes that have strong social roots, which suggests that social mechanisms are involved (Wilkinson, 1997).

The evidence linking social cohesion to health outcomes is still somewhat sparse, reflecting the relatively recent application of this concept to the field of population health. It is now well established that socially isolated individuals are at an increased risk of mortality, reduced survival after major illness, and poor mental health (Barger, Donoho, and Wayment, 2009; Berkman, 1995; House, Landis, and Umberson, 1988; House, Robbins, and Metzner, 1982; Sato and others, 2008). Two studies, however, have strongly linked social cohesion at the community level to health outcomes (Kawachi, 1999; Kawachi and others, 1997), and it is plausible that social cohesion affects health through the same mechanisms through which social participation operates at the individual level, such as anxiety and stress, health-related behaviors, and life control (Wilkinson, 1997).

There have been several key criticisms of the community deprivation and income inequality determinants of health theories. One of these recognizes the close association between wide income disparities in SES and lower public investments in social welfare, education, and health care (Kaplan and others, 1996; Ross and others, 2000). It is argued that disparities in health and health care are more attributable to the public health and welfare safety nets in place to assist those of lower SES than to any psychosocial mechanisms of inequality. While not refuting the effects of income inequality, additional critiques have pointed to the importance of including race, the political context, and class relations in analyses of social inequalities in health (Muntaner and Lynch, 1999; Navarro and Shi, 2001; Williams, 1999).

Health Care System   Although the literature indicates some skepticism as to the overall contribution of medical care to the improvement of population health worldwide (McKeown, 1976), there is evidence that access to certain types of medical care may be more beneficial than others in reducing a country's overall burden of disease (Starfield, 1994, 1998). In particular, primary care, defined as "that level of a health service system that provides entry into the system . . . provides person-focused care over time, provides care for all but very uncommon or unusual conditions, and coordinates or integrates care provided elsewhere or by others" (Starfield, 1998, p. 19), has been shown to have an important impact on health outcomes for some of the most common medical problems. Several studies have demonstrated that the higher proportion of practicing primary care physicians in a given geographic area (as opposed to practicing physician specialists), the better a wide range of health outcomes, such as infant and other mortality rates, particularly among the disadvantaged (Shi, 1992, 1994, 1995).

Moreover, studies have found that greater access to primary health care can mediate some of the effect of the SES differentials (Macinko and Starfield, 2001; Macinko, Starfield, and Shi, 2003; Shi, Macinko, and others, 2003; Shi, Macinko, and others, 2004; Shi, Starfield, Kennedy, and Kawachi, 1999). Shi, Macinko, and others (2003), in an ecological study in the United States, found that income inequality and primary care (measured by primary care physicians per 10,000 population) exerted a strong and statistically significant influence on state mortality rates and life expectancy. The study also suggested that high levels of primary care might overcome some of the adverse health impacts of income inequality on population health.

In a multilevel model including individual, community, and state-level variables, researchers presented stronger evidence for the ability of primary care to partially attenuate the adverse health effects of income inequalities (Shi and Starfield, 2000). Adjusting for many community demographic variables, higher income inequality was associated with poorer self-rated health, whereas higher community primary care was associated with better self-rated health. Primary care seemed to significantly attenuate the effects of income inequality on self-reported health status. Adding individual-level SES variables somewhat reduced the magnitude of the association between income inequality, primary care, and self-reported health. The study found that an increase of one primary care physician per 10,000 individuals was associated with a 2 percent increase in the odds of reporting excellent or good health.

Although the authors do not propose any specific mechanisms, there may be several possible explanations for the observed relationship between income inequality, primary care, and health. One mechanism is that access to a regular source of primary care may improve prevention and early detection of diseases such as hypertension (Shea and others, 1992). Another may be that the preventive aspects of primary care interrupt some of the negative health effects of inequalities that are likely to develop from long-term stressors into chronic ailments. Because primary care implies ongoing care, it is expected that in the best of circumstances, individuals living in areas with high levels of primary care may develop an important social tie with their primary care provider that assists with catching problems early. And last, such primary care may function as a sensitive measure of social transfer that allows individuals to compensate for their relative income deprivation with the receipt of an essential social service.

HEALTH INSURANCE

The United States is the only developed nation that does not yet guarantee all of its citizens access to health care through a system of *universal health coverage*. In 2000, the World Health Organization released a report ranking countries on the quality of their health systems (see Exhibit 2.1). The report placed the United States in the thirty-seventh spot for health system performance and seventy-second for health outcome performance (out of 191). This was primarily because of its failure to ensure access to care for the uninsured and because of the relatively low life expectancy and high infant mortality, despite the fact that the United States spends more than all other nations on health care (World Health Organization, 2000). Although there was controversy surrounding the methodology of the report (Almeida and others, 2001; Braveman, Starfield, and Geiger, 2001; Navarro, 2000), few contest the placement of the United States far below most other developed countries.

Historical Development of the Importance of Health Insurance Coverage

Policymakers have not ignored the irony of spending more than any other industrialized nation on health care without providing universal coverage. There have been numerous attempts by various presidents to establish universal coverage. Administrations under Presidents Truman, Kennedy, Nixon, and Clinton have all tried and failed (Bodenheimer, 2003). In 2010, President Obama and the Democrat-controlled Congress barely succeeded in another effort at ensuring universal coverage through a mix of private and public health insurance expansions. However, until the major elements of the Patient Protection and Affordable Care Act, signed into law in March 2010, are implemented in 2014, tens of millions of Americans will remain uninsured.

There are at least two major reasons that universal coverage has been so difficult to establish in the United States. First, a majority of the American public and the politicians who represent them have not decided that health care is a fundamental right. The belief in a personal "right" to health care that is the foundation for universal access to health care in other countries is not well established in the United States (Brown and Sparer, 2003). Second, inherent in American culture is the belief that government-run programs tend to be invasive and inefficient (Tooker, 2003).

Another major barrier to establishing universal coverage has been determining the best way to extend health care to the uninsured. Even during the health care reform debates that occurred in 2009 and 2010, politicians were

Exhibit 2.1 World Health Organization Rankings of International Health Systems

Performance on Health Level (DALE)					Overall Performance				
Rank	Uncertainty Interval	Member State	Index	Uncertainty Interval	Rank	Uncertainty Interval	Member State	Index	Uncertainty Interval
1	1–5	Oman	0.992	0.975–1.000	1	1–5	France	0.994	0.982–1.000
2	1–4	Malta	0.989	0.968–1.000	2	1–5	Italy	0.991	0.978–1.000
3	2–7	Italy	0.976	0.957–0.994	3	1–6	San-Marino	0.988	0.973–1.000
4	2–7	France	0.974	0.953–0.994	4	2–7	Andorra	0.982	0.966–0.997
5	2–7	San-Marino	0.971	0.949–0.998	5	3–7	Malta	0.978	0.965–0.993
6	3–8	Spain	0.968	0.948–0.989	6	2–11	Singapore	0.973	0.947–0.998
7	4–9	Andorra	0.964	0.942–0.980	7	4–8	Spain	0.972	0.959–0.985
8	3–12	Jamaica	0.956	0.928–0.986	8	4–14	Oman	0.961	0.938–0.985
9	7–11	Japan	0.945	0.926–0.963	9	7–12	Austria	0.959	0.946–0.972
10	8–15	Saudi Arabia	0.936	0.915–0.959	10	8–11	Japan	0.957	0.948–0.965
11	9–13	Greece	0.936	0.920–0.951	11	8–12	Norway	0.955	0.947–0.964
12	9–16	Monaco	0.930	0.908–0.948	12	10–15	Portugal	0.945	0.931–0.958
13	10–15	Portugal	0.929	0.911–0.945	13	10–16	Monaco	0.943	0.929–0.957
14	10–15	Singapore	0.929	0.909–0.942	14	13–19	Greece	0.933	0.921–0.945
15	13–17	Austria	0.914	0.896–0.931	15	12–20	Iceland	0.932	0.917–0.948
16	13–23	United Arab Emirates	0.907	0.883–0.932	16	14–21	Luxembourg	0.928	0.914–0.942
17	14–22	Morocco	0.906	0.886–0.925	17	14–21	Netherlands	0.928	0.914–0.942
18	16–23	Norway	0.897	0.878–0.914	18	16–21	United Kingdom	0.925	0.913–0.937
19	17–24	Netherlands	0.893	0.875–0.911	19	14–22	Ireland	0.924	0.909–0.939
20	15–31	Solomon Islands	0.892	0.863–0.920	20	17–24	Switzerland	0.916	0.903–0.930

(Continued)

Exhibit 2.1 (Continued)

| | Performance on Health Level (DALE) | | | | | Overall Performance | | | |
Rank	Uncertainty Interval	Member State	Index	Uncertainty Interval	Rank	Uncertainty Interval	Member State	Index	Uncertainty Interval
21	18–26	Sweden	0.890	0.870–0.907	21	18–24	Belgium	0.915	0.903–0.926
22	19–28	Cyprus	0.885	0.865–0.898	22	14–29	Colombia	0.910	0.881–0.939
23	19–30	Chile	0.884	0.864–0.903	23	20–26	Sweden	0.908	0.893–0.921
24	21–28	United Kingdom	0.883	0.866–0.900	24	16–30	Cyprus	0.906	0.879–0.932
25	18–32	Costa Rica	0.882	0.859–0.898	25	22–27	Germany	0.902	0.890–0.914
26	21–31	Switzerland	0.879	0.860–0.891	26	22–32	Saudi Arabia	0.894	0.872–0.916
27	21–31	Iceland	0.879	0.861–0.897	27	23–33	United Arab Emirates	0.886	0.861–0.911
28	23–30	Belgium	0.878	0.860–0.894	28	26–32	Israel	0.884	0.870–0.897
29	23–33	Venezuela, Bolivarian Republic of	0.873	0.853–0.891	29	18–39	Morocco	0.882	0.834–0.925
30	23–37	Bahrain	0.867	0.843–0.890	30	27–32	Canada	0.881	0.868–0.894

Source: World Health Organization (2000).

mired down by a complex array of potential solutions, including the expansion of public programs, such as the extension of Medicaid and CHIP; an individual mandate to purchase health insurance (similar to state laws that all drivers must have car insurance); increasing funding for *community health centers*; or creating new health insurance exchanges where individuals can shop for coverage (and even potentially purchase coverage through a proposed public health plan).

National Trends in Public and Private Health Insurance Coverage

Before the 1960s, the U.S. government was mostly uninterested in assisting its citizens with the ability to access health care. In 1965, however, a monumental change occurred. As part of President Lyndon Johnson's Great Society, the federal government enacted two major health insurance programs that would help the poor (Medicaid) and the elderly (Medicare) obtain care. These *entitlement programs* have expanded over the years into major federal and state efforts, so much so that they have consistently occupied the top spots in the federal budget. In 1997, the federal government took another incremental step toward universal coverage by enacting a program to provide health insurance coverage for children who are from low-income families but were not categorically poor. After discussing demographic trends in insurance coverage, we review these programs separately. The promotion of community health centers for the uninsured and medically underserved will be discussed in Chapter Five.

In 2008, an estimated 15.4 percent of the population (46.3 million people) did not have health insurance coverage. This was up from a low in the past decade of 14.6 percent of the population in 2001, an increase of nearly 8 million uninsured people (DeNavas-Walt and others, 2009). The percentage of the population with no coverage is correlated very strongly with changes in employment rates—since the majority of the population receives insurance through their employer—and to expansions of public coverage programs. An important note is that over the past decade, employers have been less likely to offer insurance coverage because of major increases in health care costs. This has translated into subtle but consistent changes in the proportion of the population covered by private insurance. In 1998, 62.0 percent of the U.S. population was covered by employment-based insurance (Campbell, 1999), but by 2008 this had declined to 58.5 percent (a decrease of 3.5 percentage points). The pace of decline has also accelerated. From 2007 to 2008, the decline was a sizeable 0.8 percentage points (reflecting nearly one-quarter of the total decline over the past decade), translating into a decrease of 1.1 million covered by their employer (DeNavas-Walt and others, 2009).

Because of this trend, the problem of the uninsured has evolved into an issue primarily among the working poor. The working poor are generally employed in lower-paying jobs that typically do not offer health insurance coverage or do not provide sufficient income to enable individuals to purchase insurance on the private market. These individuals also tend to have earnings too high to qualify for government insurance programs like Medicaid. So while the United States has insured the poorest individuals, there are still many families living on meager wages for which health coverage remains out of reach. Figure 2.13 shows the dramatic picture of uninsured rates among those who are employed and demonstrates very clearly that working individuals at lower levels of pay are much more likely to be uninsured. One exception is that individuals at the very lowest level of pay (making less than $10,000 per year) were more likely to be insured than other lower-income individuals, due entirely to their eligibility for Medicaid.

Because health insurance coverage is closely tied to education, occupation, and income, there are substantial demographic disparities in insurance coverage (Figure 2.14). For example, Hispanics were the most likely racial/ethnic group to be uninsured (33.2 percent) in 2008. African Americans and Asians had similar rates of being uninsured (19.0 percent and 18.2 percent, respectively), which were much higher than the rate for whites (10.0 percent). Coverage rates also vary

FIGURE 2.13   Uninsured Rates among Working Adults
Ages 18–64 Years

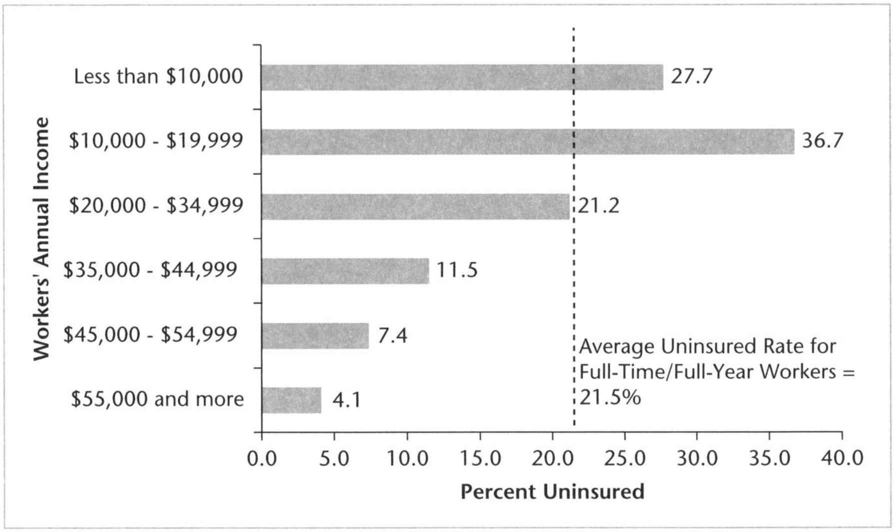

Source: New analysis of the National Health Interview Survey (2008).

FIGURE 2.14   Percentage of Individuals without
Health Insurance Coverage, 2007

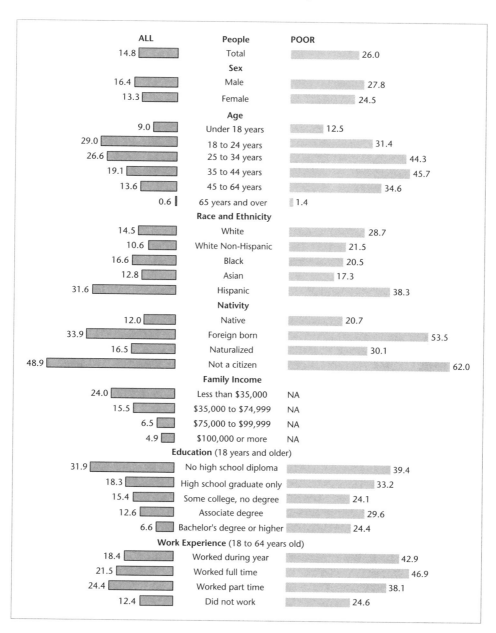

Source: New analysis of the National Health Interview Survey (2008).

FIGURE 2.15   Uninsured Rates among the Nonelderly
by State, 2007–2008

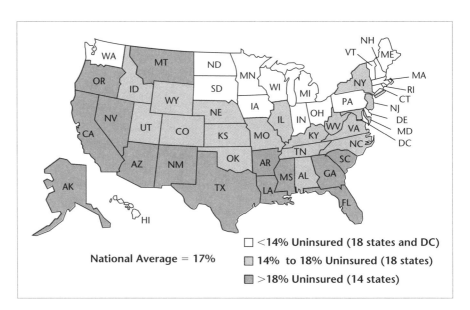

National Average = 17%

□ <14% Uninsured (18 states and DC)
▨ 14% to 18% Uninsured (18 states)
▦ >18% Uninsured (14 states)

Source: Kaiser Commission on Medicaid and the Uninsured (2009b).

significantly across states, reflecting differences in local economies and income levels, employment opportunities, immigration patterns, and differences in the generosity of eligibility for Medicaid and CHIP (see Figure 2.15). Most prominently, southern states tend to have higher uninsured rates than middle states, and middle states have higher rates of uninsured than northern states.

Despite the presence of Medicaid and CHIP safety net insurance programs, 26.0 percent of poor individuals (10.1 million) were still uninsured in 2008. Among the total population, foreign-born individuals and individuals who were not citizens (including legal and illegal immigrants) were at particularly high risk of being uninsured (33.9 percent and 48.9 percent, respectively). In the general population, young adults ages eighteen to twenty-four years old were more likely than other age groups to be uninsured (29.0 percent), but among the poor, older age was generally associated with being uninsured. For the general population, this trend is attributable to the transitional period between when insurance coverage through a parent generally ends and when young adults find employment that offers coverage. For the poor, this trend is explained by the more generous eligibility criteria for public programs for children and young adults.

Medicaid   Medicaid is a major combined federal and state initiative to provide health insurance for the poor. Authority over the Medicaid program is somewhat complex, with the federal government paying 50 to 80 percent of the costs of the program, depending on the state and its per capita income. Following broad national guidelines, the states are allowed to establish the eligibility for the program, the range of covered services, and the rate of payment to providers for those services. Medicaid was initially tied to state welfare programs (to simplify administration of the program), but this was undone in the 1990s so that being classified as poor no longer automatically makes a person eligible for Medicaid. In fact, most people become eligible for the program by meeting a specific criterion: advanced age, blindness, disability, or membership in a single-parent family with dependent children. Within this rubric, states may set very different eligibility criteria (Kaiser Commission on Medicaid and the Uninsured, 2009c). Because Medicaid is cofunded by state governments, eligibility for the program is heavily dependent on the state's economic situation, as well as the amount of federal funding provided to help expand Medicaid enrollment.

In 2007, approximately 13.9 percent of Americans received health insurance coverage through the Medicaid program, up from 9.7 percent in 1998 (National Center for Health Statistics, 2009). Among poor individuals under age sixty-five years in 2007, nearly 47.6 percent was covered by Medicaid. There are differences in Medicaid enrollment according to race and ethnicity. African Americans (27.3 percent) and Hispanics (23.1 percent) were more likely than whites (11.4 percent) and Asians (8.7 percent) to be covered by Medicaid. More than one in every four children in the United States are covered by Medicaid (29.8 percent).

Medicare   By the time Medicare was enacted in 1965, the legislative contributors envisioned the combined programs of Medicaid and Medicare as only a preliminary step toward achieving the inevitable goal of universal health insurance coverage. Although this goal has never materialized, Medicare alone has become the nation's single largest payer for medical care services, covering about 46 million beneficiaries (Kaiser Commission on Medicaid and the Uninsured, 2010). Most of these recipients are over sixty-five years of age, but the architects of the program included eligibility for two smaller categorical groups: those who are permanently disabled and those with end-stage renal disease.

Medicare is financed through a form of social insurance that requires employers and employees to contribute to a fund that finances the coverage for those who are currently enrolled in the program. Medicare offers two major benefit categories: Part A, which covers hospital and limited long-term care costs, and Part B, which covers physician services and most other health care services outside a hospital setting. Those who are eligible for Medicare are automatically enrolled in Part A and are offered the opportunity to purchase Part B through monthly premiums. Medicare allows elderly individuals to voluntarily enroll in private managed care plans (known as Medicare Part C or Medicare Advantage), and the U.S. Congress in 2004 passed a prescription drug bill to allow seniors to optionally enroll in private prescription drug coverage under Medicare, known as Medicare Part D.

Because Medicare is nearly universally available after age sixty-five, there are few differences in coverage rates across racial or socioeconomic groups. There are, however, challenges to maintaining the solvency of the program. Since its creation, spending in this program has increased by a factor of twenty, reaching $504 billion in 2010 (Kaiser Commission on Medicaid and the Uninsured, 2010). Predicted continuing growth of the elderly population, longer life expectancy, and increasing rates of chronic illness are expected to place considerable strain on the Medicare program. In 1997, Congress opened the program more substantially to managed care plans in order to contain costs, but due to low reimbursement rates and substantial administrative burden, initial participation was weak. This changed when the federal government increased payment rates to these private plans to encourage participation, and as a result Medicare Advantage plans now receive payment rates that are 114 percent of the cost of similar benefits in traditional Medicare (Kaiser Commission on Medicaid and the Uninsured, 2010). This payment rate will convert back to the standard Medicare rates as the health care reforms of 2010 are implemented.

Children's Health Insurance Program   Despite the large safety net role of Medicaid, children were continuing to account for a large proportion of the uninsured in the early 1990s. Recognizing this and building on the work of several states, such as Massachusetts, that had successfully and inexpensively expanded coverage to children (McDonough, Hager, and Rosman, 1997), the federal government passed the State Children's Health Insurance Program (now known as CHIP) as part of the Balanced Budget Act of 1997. CHIP provided about $40 billion for states to expand coverage to children in low-income families for a ten-year period. In 2007, the program came up for reauthorization. After former President Bush and Congress could not agree on CHIP reauthorization details, the program was extended through 2009.

Upon taking office, President Obama and Congress immediately reauthorized CHIP through 2013 and expanded funding by nearly $33 billion during this period by increasing tobacco taxes. Prior to reauthorization, the program allowed states to cover children in families up to 2.5 times the FPL with full federal matching funds. States could expand their eligibility higher, but with reduced federal funding. With the reauthorization, states are now allowed to cover children up to three times the FPL with full federal matching funds. Within broad federal guidelines, CHIP allowed states the choice of expanding coverage through the Medicaid program, through a new child health insurance program developed by the state, or a combination of both (Rosenbaum and others, 1998). By 2009, coverage was available for children in families whose income was 200 percent of the FPL or higher in forty-three states (up from thirty-nine states in 2002), and between 100 and 200 percent of the FPL in seven states (Kaiser Commission on Medicaid and the Uninsured, 2009a).

In 2000, CHIP was providing comprehensive insurance coverage to 3.3 million uninsured children. By 2008, about 7.4 million children were enrolled in CHIP programs across the country. Twelve states had also obtained federal permission to use some CHIP funds to insure parents of eligible children, in order to spur child enrollment and improve the retention of children in the program. These states enrolled more than 334,000 adults through the CHIP program by 2008 (Centers for Medicare & Medicaid Services, 2009).

Theoretical Pathways of Health Insurance Coverage

We present a model (Figure 2.16) that synthesizes a large body of literature on the role of health insurance coverage in supporting health and determining experiences in the health care system. With some exceptions for individuals living in close proximity to free health care clinics or community health centers, the uninsured are particularly vulnerable to financial barriers to care. Once a person is insured, there are three mechanisms by which insurance may be related to health and health care experiences: (1) health plan policies may affect care-seeking and cost-sharing behaviors of beneficiaries, (2) providers' incentives and reimbursement strategies may influence provider behavior, and (3) patient perceptions of health insurance programs may create feelings of stigma and affect the use of services and reports of quality.

Health Plan Policies   Insurance companies have developed a variety of plans that implement various care-seeking and cost-sharing policies that are intended to improve care and reduce costs simultaneously. Plans range from fee-for-service (FFS) coverage (which pay providers for each service rendered) to a variety of prepaid health plans (which generally pay providers a specified monthly amount to care for all of a given patient's health care needs). The most common prepaid plans are *health maintenance organizations (HMOs)*, point of service (POS) plans, and preferred provider organizations (PPOs). These prepaid plans, referred to categorically as managed care, reflect an insurance company that has contracts with (or even owns and operates) a network of providers and oversees the care they

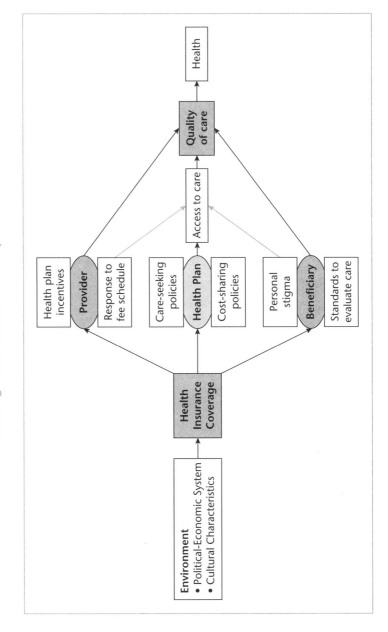

FIGURE 2.16 Conceptual Model Linking Health Insurance Coverage with Health Care Experiences

deliver. Managed care organizations (MCOs) have been on the rise since the late 1970s and currently cover about 90 percent of the nonelderly population, including many of those enrolled in Medicaid.

Many MCOs and some FFS plans have adopted a range of care-seeking policies that may affect access to and quality of health care. The most common policies include *gatekeeping*, where a beneficiary is required to seek primary care and obtain referrals for specialty care only from a preselected provider. Another common policy is to require that beneficiaries seek care only within a network of health plan providers. Although such policies are generally intended to improve the quality and efficiency of health care by improving coordination between providers and eliminating duplication of effort, some concern has been raised about unnecessarily limiting or restricting access to particular primary care and specialty care services.

Despite a vast literature on the effects of managed care, the evidence is mixed on how health plan policies affect access to care and quality. Compared with FFS plans, MCO plans with gatekeeping and network restrictions generally have more physician office visits per beneficiary, less use of expensive procedures and tests, and greater provision of preventive services, but also poorer *patient-provider relationships* and lower patient satisfaction (Miller and Luft, 1994; Miller and Luft, 2002; Starfield, 1973, 1993, 1997; Stevens and Shi, 2002a; Szilagyi, 1998a, 1998b; Szilagyi, Rodewald, and Roghmann, 1993). Although studies have shown that these care-seeking policies reduce the use of specialty care by restricting direct access to these providers, the debate is far from over (Dusheiko, Gravelle, Yu, and Campbell, 2007; Ferris and others, 2002; Forrest and others, 1999; Halm, Causino, and Blumenthal, 1997; Hodgkin and others, 2007; Merrick and others, 2008). Moreover, because most states have used managed care to serve an extensive proportion of their Medicaid populations, there remains some concern about whether MCOs make care sufficiently accessible to these vulnerable populations (Draper, Hurley, and Short, 2004; Landon and others, 2007).

Health plans generally require that beneficiaries share some portion of the costs of care, through premiums, deductibles, or copayments, or a combination of these. Although contributions are usually fairly small, they serve the purpose of making consumers sensitive to the costs of care and have been shown to reduce use of services significantly. Though this may reduce some costs for health insurance plans, *cost sharing* has been shown to reduce use of needed services in addition to unnecessary care (Anderson, Brook, and Williams, 1991; Chernew and Newhouse, 2008; Leibowitz and others, 1985; Valdez and others, 1985). In response, Medicaid has a regulation that does not allow any patient cost sharing; state CHIP programs have very low cost sharing; and many private health plans have eliminated service costs for the receipt of preventive care.

Health Plan Influences on Providers   Not only do most modern health plans place some restrictions on care seeking and usually require some cost sharing by beneficiaries, many managed care plans and their variants place similar restrictions on providers. Though not exactly restrictions, there are a handful of incentives and reimbursement mechanisms that may influence the behaviors of providers in both positive and negative ways. Some MCOs have offered providers financial bonuses for limiting the number of referrals or for seeing more patients to reduce costs or increase revenue. Other plans offer education or systems of peer review that are intended to improve the quality of care. Studies have indeed found that incentives to increase productivity or limit referrals may compromise patient care (Grumbach and others, 1998; Mechanic and Schlesinger, 1996; Williams, Zaslavsky, and Cleary, 1999). This approach is criticized because most physicians contract with many different health plans and are not able to remember the incentives attached to each patient. But this finding has been debunked by research showing that the presence of any health plan incentive increases the perception of pressure to alter services for patients.

The most common incentive that MCOs use to influence the behavior of primary care physicians is reimbursement through *capitation*, which is paying a physician a specified monthly amount to provide all the necessary care for a particular patient. From the perspective of the health plan, shifting the financial risk of care to providers helps predict and stabilize the MCO's expenditures. For the provider, this helps stabilize income (albeit capitation rates are generally low, often in the range of $10 to $30 per member per month) but also places the provider in an awkward position of needing to provide all necessary primary care for a patient versus losing personal income. The more care the provider refers, the less income he or she takes home. From the perspective of the patient, knowledge of this provider role may reduce patient trust in the physician and inhibit development of the patient-provider relationship.

Reimbursement is also a factor for physicians not providing services to Medicaid beneficiaries. Physician surveys show that the primary reason for a physician not to accept Medicaid is the low reimbursement rates. When Medicaid payment rates lag too far behind private insurance or Medicare payments, physicians stop accepting new Medicaid patients. It is interesting to note that physicians in areas of high market saturation (those with a higher proportion of Medicaid patients in the population) are more willing to accept Medicaid patients (Tooker, 2003).

Health Plan Influences on Beneficiaries   Although Medicaid and CHIP provide health insurance coverage to many low-income families, some advocacy groups have recognized the possible presence of stigma created by the long-standing correlation between Medicaid and welfare programs. Not much research has been conducted on this issue, but it is plausible to recognize that beneficiaries of such programs for low-income families may have some reservations about seeking care for fear of judgment about their socioeconomic position.

In the same regard, it has been proposed that beneficiaries of public programs may be less likely to voice concerns about their experiences in medical care. Researchers have argued that because these beneficiaries are paying relatively little for their coverage, they may not feel they have a right to evaluate the care they receive negatively. Again, this has not been well researched but does suggest some caution when interpreting ratings of health care quality or satisfaction among beneficiaries in public programs.

MULTIPLE RISK FACTORS

Vulnerability characteristics or risk factors, while having independent influences on both health status and health care access and quality, tend to be very closely associated. Although most of this chapter has been devoted to describing these individual risk factors and how they affect a range of health care access, quality, and health status outcomes, it is not trivial to discuss how the risk factors we have studied tie together, overlap, and often recycle themselves across decades in families and populations.

One very simplified model demonstrates the linkage between minority race/ethnicity, low SES, and health insurance coverage (see Figure 2.17). This model incorporates some additional risk factors as stepping-stones or bridges between the three main risks, highlighting an important point: that there is a range of other risk factors for poor health care access, quality, and health status that could be appropriately addressed in this book. Although this book attempts to be as comprehensive as possible with regard to the range of risk factors, addressing more than a handful of risks in the context of this review is not feasible to allow sufficient detail and focus.

This model of interconnections can be interpreted as follows: Because of a long history of social segregation and exclusion from educational resources, African Americans and Hispanics remain less likely than other racial/ethnic groups to obtain higher education. Without higher education, employment opportunities for these individuals are frequently limited to low-wage or service sector jobs. These jobs rarely pay sufficiently well to support a family and also frequently do not provide health insurance coverage. Although insurance is available

FIGURE 2.17   Simplified Interconnections between Risk Factors and the Cycling of Vulnerability

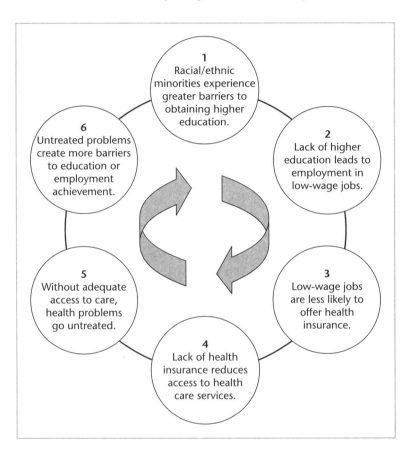

for private purchase, individuals working in low-wage jobs are less able to spend their already sparse dollars on insurance to protect against incurring future possible health care costs.

This interconnection of risk factors can be carried through even further, such that lacking health insurance coverage creates major barriers to obtaining high-quality medical care and reduces the chances that needed preventive and acute health care services will be obtained. For adults, this likely means more sick days from work, and for children this means more sick days from school, and ultimately for both a greater likelihood that both major and minor health problems will go undetected or untreated. For adults, this means that common problems such as hypertension, depression, and diabetes go untreated, and for children this means that some learning problems may go undiagnosed, and a host of other social barriers to achieving at school may remain unaddressed.

These interactions and pathways between risk factors create the potential for a vicious cycle where vulnerable adults and children have much greater difficulty obtaining higher education, obtaining jobs that can provide sufficient income to support a family and offer health insurance, and obtaining needed health care services. While this one model is oversimplified and it assumes a continuous and uninterrupted flow from each of the risk factors to another, it describes a general process by which risks may co-occur, interact, and recycle across generations.

Many other risk factors could easily be used to constitute vulnerability. A list of a range of predisposing, enabling, and need-based risk factors might include genetics (which influence the biological likelihood of developing health conditions), marital status and social support (which have been shown to predict adult mortality), and primary language and cultural beliefs about medical care (which affect how health care needs are reported and may create barriers to obtaining and using health services). Additional risk factors include depression, which not only creates a need for health services among adults but influences child development and also reduces the chances that a person will effectively seek health care for self or family.

Many health system factors may also constitute vulnerability. Geographical inaccessibility (a rural or inner-city setting) of health services may limit the availability of medical providers from whom to seek care, health insurance type (managed care versus fee for service) may influence how and what services are obtained, and both cost sharing and provider type could potentially influence the technical quality of care. Community factors such as community SES and community social cohesion may influence health status through factors such as stress and the availability of basic health and social resources, such as recreational parks and community safety.

Granted, this list is just the beginning of enumerating potential vulnerability factors. This book details many of the most commonly cited risk factors in the process of discussing the mechanisms and pathways of race/ethnicity, SES, and health insurance. Some of these additional risk factors are also discussed in Chapter Four, where we present data from other studies on the influences of multiple risk factors.

Focus on Vulnerability in Clinical Practice

Every day in Los Angeles, many community clinics provide free services to hundreds of poor, underserved families. But in August 2009, when Remote Area Medical (RAM), a well-known Tennessee-based nonprofit organization known for providing medical missions in developing countries and rural parts of America, decided to try their hand at offering free medical services in a large, urban setting, people came from all over Los Angeles and swarmed the organization for help.

RAM set up their services at the Los Angeles Forum, a large arena that used to be home of the L.A. Lakers basketball team. The setting was striking, with large, mobile clinics parked on the floor of the arena, and long rows of tables set up as stations for medical care, dental care, and vision services (see Exhibit 2.2 and 2.3). Rows of chairs were set up as waiting rooms inside the arena, and bleachers were provided outside the arena to accommodate the originally expected hundreds of patients each day. Instead of hundreds, the organization received more than 1,500 patients each day, many more than RAM could accommodate.

Patients lined up for hours, usually starting the night before, hoping to be one of a lucky few to receive a number to be served that day. Those who didn't get a number could wait another day for services, and many did. The media quickly latched onto the event because the sheer number of individuals showing up for care was more than most of the general public in Los Angeles had fathomed. The event revealed a vast need for health care that had previously gone unnoticed by the general public.

With extra emergency calls for volunteers, RAM was able to attract 3,800 volunteers, including doctors, dentists, nurses, opticians, and lay people. Over eight days, RAM was able to provide more than 14,000 services to about 7,000 patients. Still, RAM was not sufficiently staffed to help everyone who needed help, as only 10 percent of all doctors who signed up to participate actually showed up.

Perhaps the most striking thing about this effort was its ability to reach needy families where they lived. In many ways, this effort reflects the concepts presented in this chapter because it recognized the many pathways by which health disparities are created. First and foremost, it provided services free of charge, which removed many of the financial barriers to obtaining medical care. But it turns out that as many as one-quarter of the individuals who sought care from RAM actually had health insurance, predominantly Medicaid. Making the services available in the South L.A. community opened up new doors for accessing care, even among the insured, since many insured individuals often need to wait days, weeks, or even months for care from local doctors and at community clinics.

Third, the services were all provided at a single site, so that individuals could move from medical care directly over to dental care and later even get glasses made on the spot. Over the eight days, there were 9,000 medical services provided, 3,800 dental visits (with 5,500 cavities filled and 2,300 teeth extracted), and 2,000 pairs of glasses made (Remote Area Medical Volunteer Corps, 2009). Fourth, care was made available in many different languages and formal arrangements were made with language translation services through local nonprofit medical plans. This was essential, as about one-quarter of all patients spoke a language other than English (mostly Spanish).

Finally, a range of health and social services–related booths were set up around the arena for individuals to visit while waiting for services. These included the county health department, the local nonprofit Medicaid health plan, family resource centers, and many different nonprofit agencies handing out social service information and health education materials.

Of course, the main problem with all volunteer agencies (including RAM) is that there is little opportunity for continuity. This was a sporadic intervention at best, and while it helped many people, it is unlikely to alleviate (even to a slight extent) any disparities in health or health care. While RAM returned to Los Angeles in 2010 and may do so annually, there is no easy way to help families establish any continuity with local services, as such services are already overwhelmed.

Exhibit 2.2   Remote Area Medical Event at the Los Angeles Forum, 2009

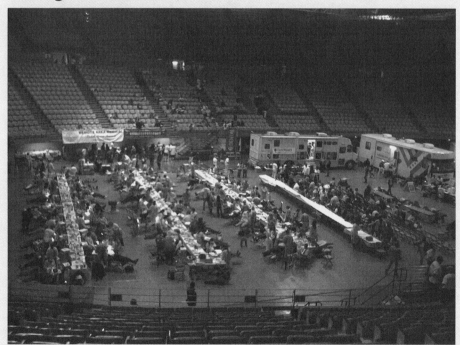

Source: Photo by G. Stevens (2009).

Exhibit 2.3   Variety of Mobile Clinics at the Los Angeles Forum, 2009

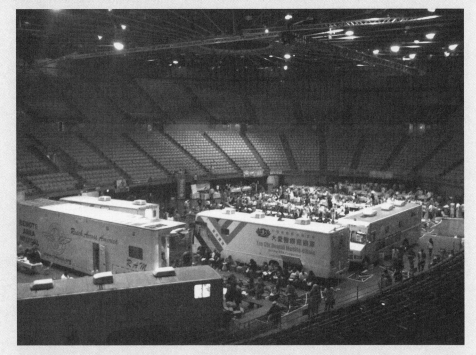

Source: Photo by G. Stevens (2009).

SUMMARY

This chapter described how vulnerability characteristics (race/ethnicity, SES, and health insurance coverage) are produced and how they are allowed to persist in the United States. It then discussed the mechanisms or pathways by which these vulnerability characteristics are associated with negative health and health care experiences. The models we presented summarize the relationships between the vulnerability characteristics and either health or health care experiences, but the mechanisms tend to be similar for both outcomes.

In the pathways of racial and ethnic vulnerability, we present a summary conceptual model that describes several potential pathways linking race and ethnicity with health and health care. The pathways begin with family characteristics that include SES, cultural factors, discrimination, and health need. The model then traces the pathways through the health care delivery system and identifies provider and system factors that may contribute to disparities in care. Several pathways are likely to operate simultaneously, leading to adverse health and health care outcomes.

In the pathways of SES, levels of income, education, and occupation together characterize an individual's relative position along the socioeconomic gradient. SES is related to health and health care in two ways: material deprivation and lack of social participation. In the pathways of health insurance coverage, we present a model of the role of health insurance coverage in supporting health and determining experiences in the health care system. Uninsured individuals are particularly vulnerable to financial barriers in accessing health care.

By understanding these mechanisms and pathways, we can begin to show why disparities persist and how they influence health and health care within the United States. In the next chapter, we present current evidence of the individual contributions of risk factors to health care access, quality of care, and health status. Interpreting these findings with a broader grasp of how these disparities are created will improve the ability to design more effective ways to enhance equity in health and health care.

KEY TERMS

Capitation

Community health centers

Cost sharing

Diversity

Effectiveness

Entitlement program

Fee for service

Gatekeeping

Gini index

Head Start

Health maintenance organization (HMO)

Material deprivation

Patient-provider relationship

Proxy measure

Universal health coverage

REVIEW QUESTIONS

1. Define race and ethnicity. Identify three factors for which race/ethnicity is often used as a *proxy measure*. Why is skin color rarely the main reason that race/ethnicity is associated with health status or health care access and quality?

2. What is socioeconomic status, and how is it usually measured? Briefly describe two possible individual-level pathways through which SES is related to health care access (that is, getting health care when needed).

3. Define Medicaid and CHIP. What are the main criteria that determine eligibility for these programs, and how large a proportion of the population is covered by these programs? Does this proportion vary by race/ethnicity?

ESSAY QUESTIONS

1. Describe how vulnerability is created through social (as opposed to personal) forces. Identify these social forces for risk factors such as race/ethnicity, SES, and health insurance coverage. What are the strengths and weaknesses of focusing national efforts on both social determinants and individual determinants of vulnerability? Make sure to discuss how a focus on these social determinants of vulnerability creates a societal obligation to address the consequences of vulnerability on health.

2. Vulnerability can be composed of many different risk factors. Identify three risk factors besides race/ethnicity, SES, and health insurance coverage for poor health care access. Examine some of the peer-reviewed research literature on these risk factors, and present a short synopsis of why and how these factors are related to access to care. Be sure to describe how strongly these factors are related to health care access in comparison to race/ethnicity, SES, and health insurance.

CHAPTER THREE

THE INFLUENCE OF INDIVIDUAL RISK FACTORS

LEARNING OBJECTIVES

- Become fluent with the most important research demonstrating health and health care disparities by race/ethnicity, SES, and health insurance coverage.

- Understand how prevalent health care disparities are in the United States and recognize how broadly affected individuals' lives are by these disparities.

- Recognize that differences in health care and health outcomes are moving targets, and where some improvements may be seen in certain areas, other areas may become worse.

IN this chapter, we present findings regarding disparities according to the three main vulnerability characteristics addressed in this book: race/ethnicity, socioeconomic status (SES), and health insurance coverage. For each characteristic, we present evidence of disparities in access to health care, quality of care, and health. Doing so reflects an overarching concern for equity. Vulnerable populations are groups for which the current system is not equitable. In the past decade, there has been a growing interest in the concept of equity in health and health care (Caplan, Light, and Daniels, 1999; Glazier, Agha, Moineddin, and Sibley, 2009; Glick, 1999; Siegel and Nolan, 2009; Starfield, 2002, 2005; Taylor, 2009). Much of the literature reviewed presents findings on health, health care access, and utilization for vulnerable groups relative to nonvulnerable groups or the population as a whole. These comparisons not only help in understanding whether there is an equitable distribution of health across populations but whether vulnerable groups have access to health services commensurate with their level of need.

The evidence for this review comes from a variety of sources. First, a systematic review of MEDLINE was conducted to identify empirical studies addressing disparities in access to health care, quality of care, and health across racial/ethnic, SES, and insurance groups. We have chosen to present data from nationally representative studies when they are available because they are the most useful starting points for policymakers and can be supplemented with state or regional data. Preliminary or innovative research on disparities is usually available only from smaller, non-representative samples. Second, we incorporated our own analyses of national surveys sponsored by the federal government (for example, the National Health Interview Survey and the Medical Expenditure Panel Survey) and private foundations (such as the Community Tracking Survey). Third, many of the sources of evidence in this chapter are derived from annual reports by the National Center for Health Statistics that synthesize many of these national data sources. We do not attempt to present an exhaustive review of the literature. Rather, the goal of this chapter is to present the most recent and seminal research that best illustrates the pervasive influence of vulnerability.

RACIAL AND ETHNIC DISPARITIES

Because of the recent national attention given to eliminating racial/ethnic disparities in health and health care, there has been an explosion of research documenting these disparities. The available evidence strongly suggests that racial/ethnic minorities have poorer access to health care, receive poorer quality of care, and experience greater deficits in health status and health outcomes.

Health Care Access

One of the most consistent findings across decades of research is that minorities have poorer access to health services compared with their white counterparts, even after controlling for SES, insurance coverage, and health status. A commonly used measure of access to care is whether a person has a regular source of care (RSC). In most research studies, an RSC is defined as a single provider or place where patients obtain, or can obtain, the majority of their health care. Having an RSC is associated with greater coordination of care, a greater likelihood of receiving preventive care, better treatment for chronic and acute health conditions, and fewer delays in care (Carpenter and others, 2009; Corbie-Smith, Flagg, Doyle, and O'Brien, 2002; DeVoe, Fryer, Phillips, and Green, 2003; DeVoe, Saultz, Krois, and Tillotson, 2009; Hoilette, Clark, Gebremariam, and Davis, 2009; Rodriguez, Bustamante, and Ang, 2009; Xu, 2002).

Figure 3.1 shows the likelihood of having an RSC by race and ethnicity. According to 2006–2007 national data, about 18.5 percent of the total adult population does not have a regular source of health care, reflecting an increase from 16.4 percent in 2001–2002. Minorities are less likely than whites to report having an RSC. More than one-third of Hispanic adults (34.8 percent) reported not having an RSC, followed by 24.4 percent of American Indians and Alaska Natives (up from 15.9 percent in 2001–2002), 18.9 percent of African Americans, and 17.3 percent of Asians. These rates of lacking an RSC are higher than for whites (15.2 percent).

FIGURE 3.1   No Regular Source of Care among Adults Eighteen to Sixty-Four Years, by Race/Ethnicity, Poverty Status, and Insurance Coverage, 2006–2007

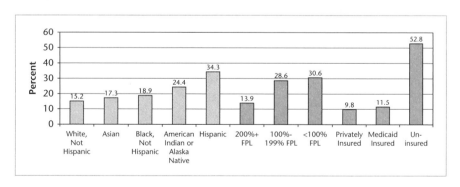

Source: National Center for Health Statistics (2009).

Similar results have been found specifically among children. A study by Weinick and Krauss (2000) examined racial/ethnic differences in having an RSC for children. The study controlled for different sets of variables and found that Hispanic, African American, and Asian children were significantly less likely than white children to have an RSC (OR = 0.35, 0.54, and 0.85; all p < .01). Even after controlling for insurance coverage, family income, maternal education, and employment status (all factors strongly associated with adult access to care), the disparities in having an RSC remained nearly the same for African American children (OR = 0.57, p < .01) and decreased slightly, but remained significant, among Hispanic children (OR = 0.52, p < .001). Finally, after controlling for the potential influences of language on access to care, the disparities in having an RSC decreased further for Hispanic children (OR = 0.71) such that they became nonsignificant, and increased slightly for African American children (OR = 0.55, p < .01). This suggests that many, but certainly not all, of the racial/ethnic disparities in having an RSC for children are attributable to factors such as health insurance coverage, family income, and language (Weinick and Krauss, 2000).

One recent study compared differences in health care access among Latinos living in the United States based on their nativity and immigration status. Using data from a nationally representative survey of 4,016 Latino adults conducted in 2007 the study found that U.S.-born Latinos and foreign-born citizen Latinos were equally likely to report having an RSC (79 percent), but foreign-born permanent resident Latinos and undocumented Latinos were less likely to report having an RSC (69 percent and 58 percent, respectively) (Rodriguez, Bustamante, and Ang, 2009). Other studies have shown similar results for access to medical and dental care (Marshall, Urrutia-Rojas, Mas, and Coggin, 2005; Mohanty and others, 2005; Nandi and others, 2008) and specifically for children (Guendelman and Schwalbe, 1986; Stevens, West-Wright, and Tsai, 2008).

There are many reasons that individuals do not have a regular source of health care. In an important analysis of the 2000 Medical Expenditure Panel Survey (MEPS), the authors found that among adults who did not have a usual source of care, two-thirds (66.2 percent) reported that they were seldom or rarely sick and so did not need a regular source of care; 10.2 percent reported not being able to afford health care; and 6.3 percent reported having recently moved and not yet found a new source of care (Viera, Pathman, and Garrett, 2006). Providing more insight, Weinick and Drilea (1998) analyzed the 1996 MEPS and found that Hispanics were more likely to report being unable to afford health care as the reason for not having an RSC (16.4 percent versus 7.1 percent for African Americans and 7.4 percent for whites) (Weinick and Drilea, 1998). This provides further evidence of the importance of ensuring adequate health insurance coverage and keeping cost sharing low to improve access to care.

Even among individuals who have an RSC, racial/ethnic minorities still report much less flexibility in their choices of where to seek medical care. Factors including language difficulty, poor geographical proximity to health care providers, and the absence of providers and clinics offering *culturally appropriate* services may be the reasons for the lesser flexibility in where minority individuals can obtain care. Data from the 2001 Commonwealth Fund Health Care Quality Survey show that 18 percent of all adults report "very little" or "no choice" of where to seek medical care. Hispanic and Asian respondents are the most likely to report having very little or no choice (28 percent and 24 percent, respectively), compared to 22 percent of African Americans and only 15 percent of whites (Collins and others, 2002). Lesser flexibility in where to seek medical care may lead to greater dissatisfaction and lead individuals to delay or forgo obtaining some needed medical services.

Although a person may have a regular source of care, organizational or health system barriers may prevent the timely and appropriate use of primary health care services. Forrest and Starfield (1998), in a key study reviewing barriers to access and their effects on seeking primary care, found that Hispanic and African American adults faced significantly more barriers to timely access compared with whites. Five barriers to primary care access were measured: no after-hour care, a wait time of five or more days for an appointment, a wait time of thirty or more minutes in the office, travel time of thirty or more minutes to the health care site, and no insurance for part or all of the year. The study showed that racial/ethnic minorities faced more barriers than whites. Whites faced an average of 0.96 access barriers per person, while Hispanic and African American respondents faced an average of 1.22 and 1.14 ($p < .001$) barriers, respectively (Forrest and Starfield, 1998).

Poor access to care is also frequently documented through delayed or forgone health care. These *unmet health care needs* can be measured directly by asking patients if they had delayed or did not seek care for any health problems that they believed required medical attention. Alternately, waiting times for appointments can be compared across demographic groups. The importance of short waiting times for appointments is shown in a study among adults using the Veterans Administration health system that found 20 percent higher rates of mortality associated with physician appointment wait times longer than thirty-one days (Prentice and Pizer, 2007).

In a 2009 national study comparing unmet health care needs among children 0–17 years according to race and ethnicity, Latinos and Asian/Pacific Islanders had 1.4 and 3.0 times the odds of reporting difficulty getting specialty care compared with whites (Flores and Tomany-Korman, 2008). Native American and multiracial children were more likely than whites to "not receive all needed medical care" in the past year (OR= 3.0 and OR= 2.83, respectively); and African American, Native American, and multiracial children all were less likely than whites to have received all needed dental care among all children who had a dental visit in the past year (OR = 2.1, OR = 2.2, and OR = 2.4, respectively). Earlier studies have not found the same pattern of disparities for children once health insurance coverage is accounted for (Newacheck and others, 2000; Newacheck, Hughes, and Stoddard, 1996; Stoddard, St. Peter, and Newacheck, 1994).

Health Care Quality

Recognizing that assessments of disparities in access to care are likely to reveal only the tip of the iceberg of racial disparities in health care, there has been a movement to monitor racial/ethnic disparities in the quality of care that patients receive (Smedley, Stith, and Nelson, 2002). There are many approaches to assessing quality of care. Quality can be measured by the receipt of care in accordance with national recommendations or care guidelines. It may also be measured by looking at more *qualitative experiences* such as patient-provider interactions and patient satisfaction with care. Some outcomes of care may also reflect quality, such as hospitalizations for certain conditions that should have been adequately managed in primary care.

One seminal study examined adults who received recommended care for a set of thirty medical conditions and preventive care (Asch and others, 2006). Medical records were reviewed for 6,712 adults who had participated in the Community Tracking Study health survey in twelve metropolitan communities. Overall, the adults received on average just 54.9 percent of all recommended care, raising major concerns about both access to needed care and the quality of care being delivered. Higher income was associated with slightly better care (56.6 percent versus 53.1 percent, $p < 0.001$), and there were only slight differences in quality across racial/ethnic groups, with differences that favored African American adults (57.6 percent) and Hispanic adults (57.5 percent) compared with whites (54.1 percent, $p < 0.001$ for both comparisons). When the measures of quality were divided into categories of screening, diagnosis, treatment, and follow-up, Hispanic adults were more likely than whites to have received recommended screening (55.9 percent versus 51.6 percent, $p = 0.02$) and African American adults were much more likely than whites to have received recommended treatment (64.0 percent versus 56.3 percent, $p < 0.001$). Though the absence of disparities for African Americans and Hispanics is positive, it runs somewhat counter to other research presented in this book. It is nonetheless troubling that all groups received the correct care only about half of the time.

FIGURE 3.2   Receipt of Preventive Care by
Race and Ethnicity, 2006–2008

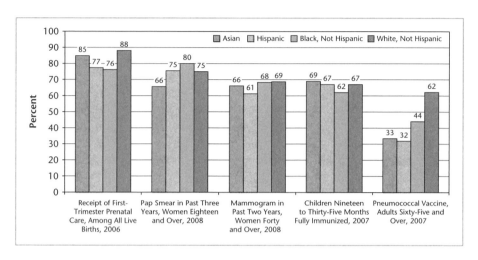

Source: National Center for Health Statistics (2009).

Figure 3.2 shows recent estimates of racial/ethnic disparities in the receipt of preventive services. In general, racial and ethnic minorities are less likely than whites to receive preventive services, including early childhood immunizations, receipt of prenatal care in the first trimester, mammography for women forty years of age and over, and smoking cessation counseling for current smokers. Hispanics and Asians were least likely to receive these preventive services, with the exception that Asian children were more likely to be fully immunized than whites and Asian women were similar to whites in the likelihood of obtaining prenatal care. African American women were more likely than white women, and Hispanic women were equally as likely as white women, to receive a Papanicolaou smear (Pap smear) in the past three years. It is interesting to note that despite universal financial access to immunizations, less than 70 percent of all children ages nineteen months to thirty-five months were up-to-date with their immunization schedule.

Numerous additional studies have evaluated racial and ethnic disparities in receipt of preventive services such as immunizations, *well-child care*, health screenings, type 2 diabetes checkups, and others. Ronsaville and Hakim (2000) used a nationally representative sample of all births that occurred in 1988 along with 1991 longitudinal follow-up data to determine factors associated with incomplete compliance with well-child guidelines. The study found that 58 percent of white, but only 35 percent of African American and 37 percent of Hispanic infants, obtained or received all recommended well-child care. After adjustment for SES, demographic factors, the number of children in the family, parent smoking, and main site of care, the strongest risks for incomplete compliance were being African American (OR 1.7; confidence interval [CI]: 1.5–1.9), Hispanic (OR 1.7; CI: 1.4–2.1) and having low family income measured as a percentage of the federal poverty level (FPL): 100–200 percent of FPL (OR 1.3; CI: 1.1–1.6) and less than 100 percent of FPL (OR 1.6; CI: 1.3–2.0).

A study of adolescents in California to examine the health counseling topics received during their routine medical care found a different pattern (Adams, Husting, Zahnd, and Ozer, 2009). Among adolescents ages twelve to seventeen years old who had at least basic access to medical care (they had attended a physical exam within the past six months), the study found that physicians were more likely to discuss sexually transmitted diseases, violence, nutrition, and the use of seatbelts and bike helmets with Hispanics (ORs ranging from 1.34 for nutrition to 2.61 for violence). Similarly, African American youths were more likely than whites to receive counseling on nutrition, but less likely than whites to receive counseling on violence (OR = 0.45, CI: 0.21–0.95). Lower income and uninsured youths were more likely to receive counseling on most topics, but there were no differences by race/ethnicity, income, or insurance in counseling on tobacco, alcohol use, drug use, or physical activity.

In order to better understand racial/ethnic differences in preventive care, Fiscella, Franks, Doescher, and Saver (2002) evaluated the receipt of preventive services by race/ethnicity and language for adults covered by either private insurance or Medicaid. The study found that the receipt of preventive care for English-speaking Hispanic patients was not much different from that of white patients. Spanish-speaking Hispanic patients were 23 percent less likely than whites to have had a physician visit, 50 percent less likely to have a mental health visit, and 70 percent less likely to have received an influenza vaccination. Adjustment for predisposing, enabling, and need factors revealed that Spanish-speaking Hispanic patients had significantly lower use than whites across all four measures. African Americans were 27 percent less likely to have received an influenza vaccination and were 54 percent less likely than white patients to have had a visit with a mental health professional. The ethnic disparities observed in some preventive care services may be explained by differences in English-language fluency, but other racial and ethnic disparities in care still persist despite adjustment for language and other common enabling, predisposing, and need factors (Fiscella, Franks, Doescher, and Saver, 2002).

Major disparities have also been found in screening for cancer. Gaps in breast cancer screening rates between African Americans and whites have been demonstrated, even among those with insurance (Gornick and others, 1996;

Rahman, Dignan, and Shelton, 2003). Among women in Massachusetts diagnosed with early stage breast cancer, African American women were 25 percent less likely than white women to receive care according to the recommended guidelines, such as the receipt of mastectomy or breast conserving surgery plus radiation (Berz and others, 2009). After adjusting for insurance coverage, SES, and hospitals (in case differences exist in the quality of hospitals performing the surgeries), these disparities in care did not persist. But even after controlling for all other factors, African American women had nearly 1.6 times the odds of death from early stage breast cancer than white women. Similar findings of poorer-quality breast cancer treatment for African American women have been reported elsewhere, and higher mortality rates have been widely confirmed (Du, Fang, and Meyer, 2008; Grann and others, 2006; Short and others, 2009; Smith-Bindman and others, 2006).

There are now many studies documenting racial and ethnic disparities in the treatment of heart disease, a leading contributor to mortality for minorities. One major study analyzed more than 2.5 million patients to summarize trends in the rate of adherence to practice guidelines from the American Heart Association and American College of Cardiology in the treatment of acute myocardial infarction (Peterson, Shah, and others, 2008). The study found that from 1990 to 2006, overall rates of adherence to the practice guidelines improved, increasing by more than 30 percentage points for the use of beta blockers and more than 50 percent for anticoagulant therapies. In most cases, however, adhered-to recommendations still fell short for one in every five patients. The study further revealed that disparities between African American and white adults in the rates of receipt of recommended treatments remained at least 10 percentage points throughout the sixteen-year study period, rarely decreasing, and in some cases slightly increasing (such as for percutaneous coronary intervention and coronary artery bypass grafting).

Another study used hospital discharge data from ten states to evaluate racial/ethnic differences in preventable hospitalization rates as an indicator of poor access to and quality of primary care (Gaskin and Hoffman, 2000). Preventable hospitalizations are hospitalizations for conditions such as asthma or diabetes that can usually be easily managed through high-quality primary care and that rarely require hospitalization if managed appropriately. After adjustment for individual demographics, SES, and county-level health care factors such as availability of health centers and hospital beds, the authors concluded that in 44 percent of the study's possible comparisons across states and insurance types for African Americans, Hispanics, and white patients, Hispanic children and African American adults were significantly more likely than whites to experience a preventable hospitalization.

Newer explorations in quality of care have been examining the variations in racial/ethnic group perceptions of personal interactions in the health care system.

Most of the studies include a measure of patient-provider communication, aspects of the interpersonal relationship, or trust in the provider. Some of these studies have shown that personal interactions in the health care system are influenced by factors such as provider race/ethnicity and gender concordance between patients and providers, but little evidence yet exists to show that the differences contribute to differences in health outcomes (Cooper and Roter, 2002; Cooper-Patrick and others, 1999; Meghani and others, 2009; Saha, Arbelaez, and Cooper, 2003; Stevens, Shi, and Cooper, 2003).

Figure 3.3 presents two unique findings regarding racial/ethnic differences in personal interactions in the health care system. National data from various sources reveal that Asian, Hispanic, and African American adults are more likely than whites to report a lack of trust in their physician, feel looked down upon or treated with disrespect, and believe they were treated unfairly due to both race and language. Nearly half of Asian adults (46 percent) report lacking trust in their physician (compared to 28 percent of whites), and feel looked down upon or treated with disrespect (20 percent versus 9 percent of whites). Hispanics (5 percent) and African Americans (11 percent) were also more likely than whites (2 percent) to say that in seeking health care their experience was worse than for

FIGURE 3.3   Personal Interactions in the Health Care System by Race and Ethnicity, 2001–2004

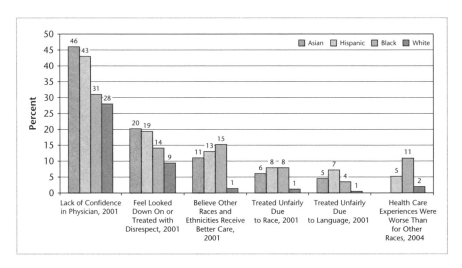

Source: Data on confidence in physicians is from Collins and others (2002). All other data from 2001 are from Blanchard and Lurie (2004). Data from 2004 are from Hausmann, Jeong, Bost, and Ibrahim (2008).

other races. These experiences of perceived discrimination have been shown to negatively impact health (Ahmed, Mohammed, and Williams, 2007; Williams and Mohammed, 2009; Williams, Neighbors, and Jackson, 2008).

A study examining the 1996, 2001, and 2002 Medical Expenditure Panel Survey evaluated race/ethnicity disparities in both objective and subjective health care experiences (Shi and Macinko, 2008). After adjustment for health insurance coverage, health status, and many other demographics variables, the study found that Asian and Hispanic adults were less likely to report positive experiences than whites. In 2001, for example, Asian adults had 2.11 times the odds (CI: 1.43–2.53), and Hispanic adults had 1.30 times the odds (CI: 1.06–1.60) of whites of saying they were not satisfied with the quality of care. In 2002, Asian adults had 1.45 times the odds (CI: 1.02–2.08) and Hispanic adults had 1.32 times the odds (CI: 1.08–1.62) of whites of saying their regular provider does not listen to them. African American adults were similar to whites in their reported health care experiences. Moreover, it appears that differences between whites and both Asian and Hispanic adults had narrowed slightly between 1996 and 2001/2002. Similar patterns of racial/ethnic disparities in experiences have been reported elsewhere (Armstrong and others, 2008; Rodriguez and others, 2008; Schnittker and Bhatt, 2008; Shi, 1999; Stevens, Pickering, Seid, and Tsai, 2009; Stevens, Seid, Pickering, and Tsai, 2009; Stevens and Shi, 2002b).

Health Status

Health status and health risk behaviors both contribute to driving the use of medical care. Health status is also an important tool for assessing the effects of health care services, since protecting and improving health is the main purpose of health services. Many studies document that racial/ethnic minorities experience much higher incidence rates of morbidity and mortality compared with whites. Disparities in health exist between white and nonwhite Americans in terms of perceived health status as well as traditional indicators of health, such as infant mortality rates and general population mortality rates. Racial/ethnic disparities in health status are so significant that the federal government has named the elimination of racial/ethnic disparities as a primary goal for the *Healthy People initiative* (Secretary's Advisory Committee on National Health Promotion and Disease Prevention Objectives for 2020, 2008; U.S. Department of Health and Human Services, 2000).

Some of the earliest efforts in revealing racial/ethnic disparities in the United States were through the use of national statistics on health status and health risk factors. The disparities were so prominent in early studies that now nearly all vital statistics and reports of health conditions are routinely reported according to race and ethnicity, although not all racial/ethnic subgroup populations are consistently represented in each statistic. In this section, we present key evidence illustrating racial/ethnic disparities in perceived health status, health risks, and mortality.

Figure 3.4 presents self-assessed health status by race and ethnicity. The most common way of assessing patient perceptions of health status is to use a Likert-type response scale with response options ranging from "poor" to "excellent." This method is frequently used because it has been very closely linked to future health outcomes and health care utilization among adults (McGee, Liao, Cao, and Cooper, 1999). The figure, using data from the 2008 National Health Interview Survey shows large racial/ethnic differences in individual age-adjusted assessments of health status. For example, American Indians and Alaska Natives were the most likely to say their health status was "fair" or "poor" (16.8 percent), followed by African Americans (14.4 percent), and Hispanics (11.2 percent). This is an important finding, showing that major health deficits are experienced by more than one in every ten individuals in these groups. Asians and whites were less likely to report fair or poor health (5.1 percent and 9.3 percent, respectively) compared with the other racial/ethnic groups. These results are corroborated by nearly every national health survey conducted in the United States.

Similar disparities in health status have been reported for children. One seminal study that analyzed children from three consecutive years of the National Health Interview Survey (1989, 1990, and 1991) found that American Indian/ Alaskan Native and African American children were the least likely racial/ethnic groups to be rated by their parents in "excellent" or "good" health (66 percent and 68 percent, respectively). Hispanic children fared somewhat better than these

FIGURE 3.4   Self-Reported Fair or Poor Health Status among Adults Eighteen to Sixty-Four Years, 2008

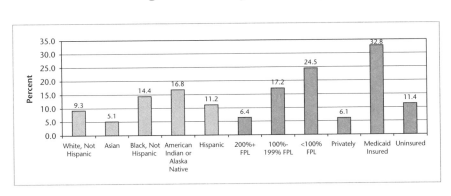

Source: New analysis of the 2008 National Health Interview Survey.

groups, with 74 percent of these children reported to be in excellent or good health, and white children had the highest rate (85 percent). In the same study, after further adjustment for SES and family demographics, the odds of being in less than excellent or good health were higher for all racial/ethnic groups compared with whites: Native American (OR = 2.12; CI: 1.85–2.43), Asian/Pacific Islander (OR = 1.32; CI: 1.18–1.47), African American (OR = 1.92; CI: 1.83–2.0), and Hispanic (OR = 1.23; CI: 1.17–1.30) (Flores, Bauchner, Feinstein, and Nguyen, 1999). These findings have been replicated in many other studies (Flores, Olson, and Tomany-Korman, 2005; Flores and Tomany-Korman, 2008; Stevens, 2006; Stevens, Seid, Mistry, and Halfon, 2006).

The poorer self-assessed health status of racial/ethnic minorities is underscored by a range of more objective measures of health. Racial/ethnic minority groups have higher rates of infant mortality (death in the first year of life), lower birth weight, and higher overall and condition-specific mortality rates than whites. In 2005, for example, African American mothers had more than twice the infant mortality rate of whites (13.6 versus 5.6 deaths per 1,000 live births). Hispanics and Asians or Pacific Islanders had low infant mortality (5.6 and 4.9 deaths per 1,000 live births) (see Figure 3.5). Perhaps even more interesting is the variation in infant mortality rates within racial/ethnic subgroups in the population. For example, Puerto Rican Hispanics have a much higher rate of infant mortality than other Hispanic groups (8.3 deaths per 1,000 live births) and Cuban Americans have the lowest rate (4.4 deaths per 1,000 live births).

One of the main contributors to infant mortality is low birth weight. For the past thirty years, infant mortality rates have been climbing steadily.

FIGURE 3.5   Infant Mortality Rates by Race
and Ethnicity, 2005

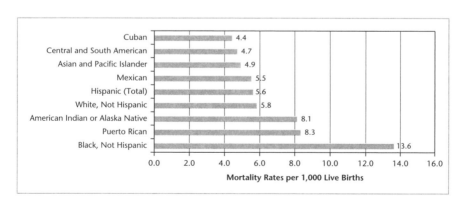

Source: National Center for Health Statistics (2009).

FIGURE 3.6 Low Birth Weight Rates by Maternal Race/Ethnicity, 1980–2006

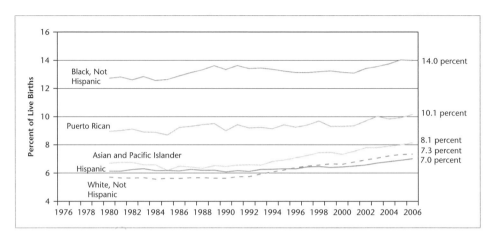

Note: Low birth weight is defined as less than 2,500 grams.
Source: National Center for Health Statistics (2009).

Across all years, African Americans have had higher rates of low birth weight than other racial/ethnic groups. In 2006, the rate was 14.0 percent compared with 10.1 percent among Puerto Ricans, 8.1 percent among Asian or Pacific Islanders, 7.3 percent among whites, and 7.0 percent among Hispanics. Figure 3.6 shows the slight upward trend in low-birth-weight rates across racial/ethnic groups over the past three decades. Not only do low-birth-weight rates contribute to higher infant mortality, but they also have been associated with increased risks of *developmental disabilities*, mental retardation, and cerebral palsy (Escobar, Littenberg, and Petitti, 1991; Horbar and others, 2002; Thompson and others, 2003).

Figure 3.7 presents several other key national mortality statistics by race and ethnicity. Exploration of mortality rates from homicide, HIV, breast cancer, prostate cancer, and diabetes reveal striking patterns of racial/ethnic disparities. For example, African Americans have mortality rates from homicide that are about seven times that of whites, mortality rates from breast cancer that are about three times higher than that of Asians, and HIV mortality rates that are about ten times higher than that of whites and nineteen times higher than that of Asians. Hispanics have the second highest mortality rates for most of these causes, and Asians have the lowest rates, followed by whites (with the exception of breast cancer, for which the rate is higher for whites than among Hispanics, American Indian or Alaska Natives, and Asians).

FIGURE 3.7   National Cause-Specific Mortality Rates by
Race and Ethnicity, 2006

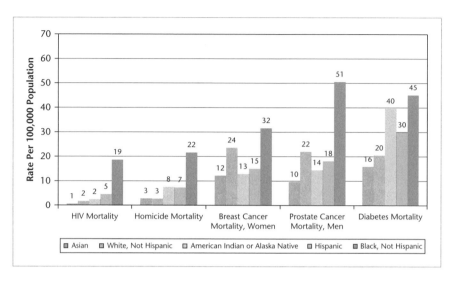

Source: National Center for Health Statistics (2009).

These racial/ethnic differences in mortality are particularly important because much of this mortality can be prevented. Homicide mortality, for example, can be reduced with stronger gun laws, reduced availability of firearms, and violence prevention interventions. Similarly, breast cancer mortality can be reduced through regular mammography screens and early detection, and HIV mortality can be reduced through health education about safer sex practices, regular testing for HIV, and access to effective medications to reduce virus growth. Diabetes mortality rates can be prevented by reducing weight gain and obesity, closer monitoring of diets, and better management of blood sugar and insulin levels.

While overall mortality rates in the United States have fallen consistently since 1930, the decreases have not been equitable for all Americans (National Center for Health Statistics, 2009). Age-adjusted mortality rates in combined data from 2004–2006 show that African American individuals had a mortality rate of 1,006 deaths per 100,000 individuals (down from 1,121 deaths in the year 2000) compared with just 789 deaths per 100,000 white individuals (down from 850 deaths in the year 2000). Interestingly, Asians, Hispanics, and American Indian and Alaska Natives all had lower overall age-adjusted mortality rates than either whites or African Americans (rates of 437, 580, and 653 deaths per 100,000 individuals, respectively), due in part to the average age of individuals in these groups skewing younger.

Heart disease ranks as the top cause of death for all racial/ethnic groups. African American adults, however, suffer from the highest mortality rates from heart disease—almost 50 percent higher than white Americans. They also suffer from higher mortality rates due to cancer (specifically breast, colon, prostate, and lung cancer) and asthma than any other ethnic group (Grant, Lyttle, and Weiss, 2000; Jones-Webb and others, 2009; Lee and others, 2009; Lillie-Blanton, Rushing, and Ruiz, 2003). Hayward and Heron have shown that these higher rates of mortality are accompanied by reduced active life expectancy rates (the number of years of life spent in good health without disability) for racial/ethnic minority groups. This study showed that at the age of twenty, the active life expectancy was about fifty-two years for Asian men, forty-five for whites, forty-two for Hispanics, thirty-nine for Native Americans, and thirty-seven for African Americans (Hayward and Heron, 1999).

McCord and Freeman published one of the most widely cited studies illustrating that general improvements in health over time have not been felt equally by all Americans (McCord and Freeman, 1990). Death certificate records from the New York City Health Department and 1980 census data were abstracted for the analysis. They examined death rates of the residents of Harlem, an inner-city neighborhood in New York City. When the 1980 census was taken, Harlem was 96 percent African American, and 40.8 percent of the families living there had incomes below the federal poverty line.

The residents of Harlem had the highest mortality rates of any area in New York City. Compared to all white men in the United States in 1980, the standardized mortality ratio (SMR) for men in Harlem was almost three times higher (SMR = 2.91), resulting in 948 per 100,000 annual excess deaths for the residents of Harlem. For Harlem women, the magnitude of excess deaths was slightly lower (SMR = 2.70), but still much higher than for white women in the United States. The disparities were so great that the rate of survival beyond age forty was actually lower in Harlem than in parts of developing Bangladesh. The authors also compared the death rates in Harlem to the remaining 342 health areas in the city of New York with a population of more than 3,000 residents. They found fifty-four additional areas of New York with mortality rates similar to those found in Harlem. In all but one of these areas, more than half of the resident population was either African American or Hispanic.

These mortality studies provide a grim picture of racial/ethnic disparities in health in the United States. As we presented earlier, these higher rates among racial/ethnic minorities may be partially attributable to differences in the quality of specific health care treatments they receive. In addition, the disparities might be partially attributed to certain greater health risk behaviors as described next.

Figure 3.8 shows several key findings in health risk behaviors by race/ethnicity. With obesity and overweight status fast becoming the leading contributors to

FIGURE 3.8   Health Risk Factors by Race and Ethnicity, 2005–2007

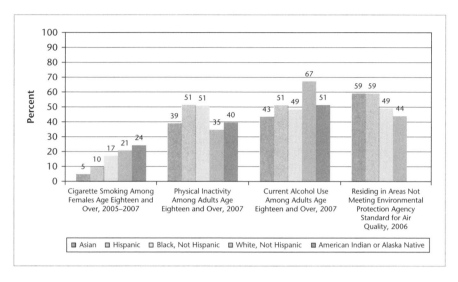

Source: National Center for Chronic Disease Prevention and Health Promotion (2006); National Center for Health Statistics (2009).

mortality in the United States, it is important to examine differences in physical inactivity rates by race/ethnicity. While Asian and white adults have similar rates of inactivity (39 percent and 35 percent, respectively), meaning that these adults engage in absolutely no leisure time physical activity during a given week, about half of all African Americans and Hispanics (51 percent each) report no physical activity (National Center for Health Statistics, 2009). Considering that obesity contributes to heart disease, stroke, diabetes, and many cancers, there is good reason to focus future efforts on reducing racial/ethnic disparities in physical activity rates.

Cigarette smoking also remains a prevalent health risk in the United States and in most developed countries. Though smoking rates among U.S. men have been leveling off or decreasing slightly, rates among female adults have been increasing. American Indian and Alaska Native females are more likely to smoke (24 percent) than females from other racial groups, putting them at increased risk of lung cancer, heart disease, stroke, and other health problems. White females are the second most likely group to smoke (21 percent) followed by African American females (17 percent), while Hispanic and Asian females smoke at low rates (10 and 5 percent, respectively). Moderate rates of smoking among African Americans in conjunction with high physical inactivity rates may contribute to the higher rates of mortality among African American adults from some of the most common health conditions.

Taking an environmental, rather than behavioral, approach to examining health risk factors, the figure also reports the percentage of each racial/ethnic minority group (except American Indian or Alaska Native individuals, for whom no data were available) residing in an area not meeting air quality standards issued by the U.S. Environmental Protection Agency (EPA). Asians and Hispanics were at least 10 percent more likely than other groups to live in these areas (59 percent each), putting them at higher risk for asthma and other respiratory problems (National Center for Health Statistics, 2009).

SOCIOECONOMIC STATUS DISPARITIES

Socioeconomic status is one of the most enduring contributors to disparities in health and health care. There have been many studies documenting the association of lower SES with poorer health status, barriers to accessing needed health services, and lower rates of using health care services. SES is defined by a combination of factors that typically include personal income, education, and occupation.

Income represents the ability to acquire material resources and the potential to access different lifestyles, and it provides a sense of security. Education reflects the potential to acquire knowledge and resources and the ability to navigate through social institutions to meet one's desired ends. It has also been found to be associated with health-related behaviors. Occupation reflects an ability to acquire resources, which influences feelings of *self-efficacy*, and comes with a societal prestige and privilege associated with one's occupation.

Despite the creation of numerous social welfare and safety net health care initiatives to compensate for lack of income, education, or occupation, the United States has not been able to effectively reduce the number of individuals experiencing low SES. For example, in 1997, 13.3 percent of (or 36 million) Americans lived below the federal poverty level. A decade later, in 2008, the estimated poverty rate was nearly unchanged at 13.2 percent (or 39.8 million people) (U.S. Census Bureau, 2009a). The proportion of Americans living in poverty has remained relatively constant since the early 1970s despite fluctuations in economic growth rates and the expansion and retraction of programs to help the poor.

Health Care Access

With regard to accessing health care, we find even greater differences associated with individual SES than with race and ethnicity. Lower income, education, and occupational status are all associated with poorer access to care. Among these factors, income appears to contribute most significantly to variations in access to care, though fewer studies have examined the effects of education and occupation on this outcome. Consequently, the following review focuses mostly on the effects of income and poverty status.

Figure 3.1 shows the likelihood of lacking an RSC according to poverty status. The data source divided income into three groups: (1) poor (below the federal poverty line), (2) near-poor (between 100 percent and 199 percent of poverty), and (3) not poor (above 200 percent poverty). The figure shows that poor adults are more than twice as likely as non-poor adults to lack an RSC (30.6 percent versus 13.9 percent). Interestingly, those in near-poverty were nearly as likely as those living in poverty to lack an RSC (28.6 percent), suggesting that the poverty line may be set too low (or rather, the eligibility criteria for assistance programs may be too narrow), at least in terms of identifying individuals at risk of not accessing needed health care.

Figure 3.9 presents the presence and type of RSC reported by adults according to educational level in California. Individuals with higher levels of education were more likely to report seeking care at a doctor's office, were less likely to report seeking care from community clinics and emergency departments, and were much less likely to not have any RSC at all. For example, only 6 percent of adults who had attended some graduate school reported not having an RSC,

FIGURE 3.9   Type of Regular Source of Care among Adults by Educational Level, 2005

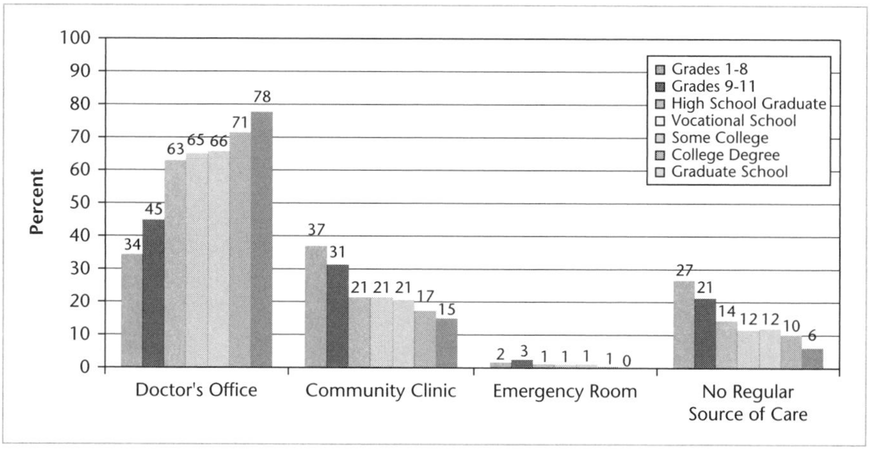

Source: New analysis of the California Health Interview Survey (2005).

and 78 percent said they sought their regular care in a doctor's office. Among those who had discontinued their education prior to entering high school (grades 1–8), more than one-quarter (27 percent) reported not having an RSC, and only 34 percent sought care in a doctor's office. They were also much more likely to seek care in a community clinic (37 percent) or emergency department (2 percent).

Individuals living at or below the federal poverty level also faced significantly more barriers to accessing their primary care site. Forrest and Starfield reviewed five barriers to access (long travel time to health center, no insurance, no after-hours care, long waiting time for scheduling an appointment, and long office wait time) and their effects on vulnerable populations (Forrest and Starfield, 1998). The most frequently reported barrier was a long wait time in the doctor's office (more than thirty minutes); 63.6 percent of the respondents to the national survey had experienced at least one of the five barriers to access. Respondents living at or below the federal poverty line faced 34.7 percent more access barriers than those living above the poverty line (1.32 versus 0.98 mean number of barriers, $p < .001$).

International data provide some interesting views of health care access related to SES. Using the 2002–2003 Joint Canada/United States Survey of Health, two studies have found major differences in access to care between the two countries (Blackwell and others, 2009; Lasser, Himmelstein, and Woolhandler, 2006). U.S. respondents were less likely to have visited a doctor in the past year, have a regular source of care, have unmet needs, and forgo needed medications than Canadian respondents. In addition, having low income and low educational attainment were strong predictors of these access measures in the United States but much less so in Canada. In Canada, there were no income effects observed at all for physician visits, which is likely explained by their universal health care system providing insurance coverage to all regardless of income. All results held after controlling for health needs.

Health Care Quality

Socioeconomic status also strongly predicts the quality of health care that people receive. To examine the link between SES and health care quality, this section reviews evidence about SES and the receipt of preventive care, preventable hospitalizations, subjective experiences in receiving health care, and satisfaction in the health care system.

The receipt of preventive services increases as SES increases. Data from *Health, United States* (National Center for Health Statistics, 2009) show the relationship between three preventive services and adult educational status (see Figure 3.10). Among women who did not complete high school, about 61 percent reported receiving a Pap smear in the past three years, compared with

FIGURE 3.10   Receipt of Preventive Care by Education
or Poverty Level, 2007–2008

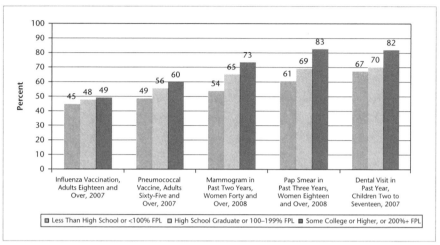

Source: Federal Interagency Forum on Child and Family Statistics (2009); National
Center for Health Statistics (2009).

69 percent of women who completed high school and 83 percent of women
who received some college education or higher. Receipt of a mammogram in
the past two years for women ages forty years and over and receipt of a Pap
smear in the past three years for women ages eighteen and over reveal similar
patterns by educational status. Mammography rates increase from 54 percent
among women with less than a high school education to 65 percent of women
who graduate from high school and 73 percent of women with some college
education. Overall, the difference in receipt of each of the services between
the highest and lowest education levels is about 20 percentage points.

A longitudinal cohort study examined the receipt of preventive health services
among roughly 6,000 elderly women who had been diagnosed with breast cancer
and the same number of matched controls without breast cancer (Earle, Burstein,
Winer, and Weeks, 2003). All of the women had Medicare health insurance,
suggesting that all had a way to pay for their health care. Reviewing health service
utilization data, the researchers examined patient characteristics (including SES)
associated with receiving influenza vaccination, lipid testing, cervical examination,
colon examination, and bone densitometry. The study found that regardless of
Medicare insurance, women with breast cancer were more likely to receive preventive services, likely due to their more frequent interaction with the health care

system due their breast cancer. Controlling for breast cancer status, the odds of receiving two or more preventive health services increased by 8 percent with each quintile of higher household income.

In a seminal study using hospital discharge data, researchers compared rates of preventable hospitalizations in both low- and high-income urban areas for those under age sixty-five years in the United States and Canada (Billings, Anderson, and Newman, 1996). Receiving high-quality primary care may prevent hospitalizations for what are known as *ambulatory care sensitive conditions (ACS)* including conditions such as asthma, diabetes, and congestive heart failure. The study found a consistent pattern of higher ACS hospitalization rates in low-income urban areas compared with high-income urban areas and a direct association between the percentage of low-income residents in a given area and admission rates for ACS conditions. In certain areas of the United States, more than 80 percent of the variation in ACS hospitalizations across zip codes could be explained solely by the percentage of low-income residents. Income differences in ACS hospitalizations were much narrower in Canada than in the United States, underscoring again the importance of universal health insurance in decreasing SES disparities. Similar findings within the United States have also been reported in other studies (Cable, 2002; Cousineau, Stevens, and Pickering, 2008; Djojonegoro, Aday, Williams, and Ford, 2000).

We further present the findings of a unique study by van Ryn and Burke (2000) of the perceived interpersonal relationships between physicians and patients according to SES. The study examined physician perceptions of patients according to patient income grouped into three strata: low, middle, and high income (see Figure 3.11). The results reveal a bias in the perceptions of physicians against patients of lower SES. In general, physicians perceive patients of lower SES to be less independent, responsible, rational, and intelligent than patients of higher SES. The gaps are greatest for perceptions of patient intelligence (17 percent), and the difference between middle- and higher-income patients is about 9 percent. These findings are important because the way physicians perceive their patients is likely to affect how physicians select and recommend treatments.

There are several examples of how these treatment recommendations may differ by patient SES. Studies have shown that physicians are much less likely to recommend mammography to patients whom they think cannot afford the service or whom they perceive will not comply (Conry and others, 1993; Grady, Lemkau, Lee, and Caddell, 1997; Urban, Anderson, and Peacock, 1994). Consequently, low-income women and those with low educational attainment are less likely to be referred by their provider for a mammogram (Meissner and others, 2007; O'Malley and others, 2001). There is a need to better understand how widespread the effects of this physician-patient dynamic are, and to what extent the bias influences recommendations for other services.

FIGURE 3.11   Physician-Reported Perceptions of Patients
According to Patient SES

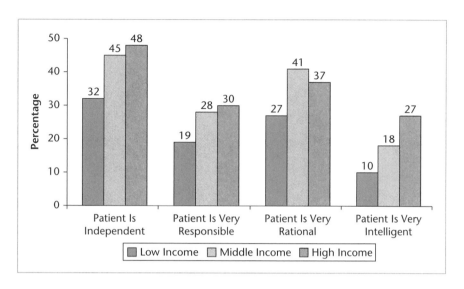

Source: van Ryn and Burke (2000).

A final measure of quality that is often reported according to SES is patient satisfaction. One unique international comparison study examined how SES influences satisfaction with the health care system across five countries, including the United States. Using data from the Commonwealth Fund 2001 International Health Policy Survey (Collins and others, 2002), the study showed that across all countries, individuals with incomes below the median income level in each country were less likely to be highly satisfied with health care and more likely to report that "the health system is so bad that it should be rebuilt." Perhaps the most interesting part of this study is that the differences in satisfaction between high-income and low-income individuals were greater in the United States than in other countries. A likely reason for this finding is that individuals in the other countries studied (United Kingdom, Australia, New Zealand, and Canada) are guaranteed universal coverage for health care without regard to income, whereas in the United States no such universal guarantee has existed (see Figures 3.12 and 3.13).

Additionally, a study comparing disparities in health care access, quality, and satisfaction in the United States and Canada found strong income-related differences in perceptions of overall health care quality and satisfaction with health

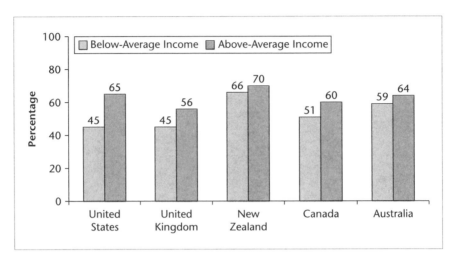

FIGURE 3.12   Percentage Reporting High Satisfaction
with the Overall Quality of Health Care
in Five Nations by Income, 2001

Source: Collins and others (2002).

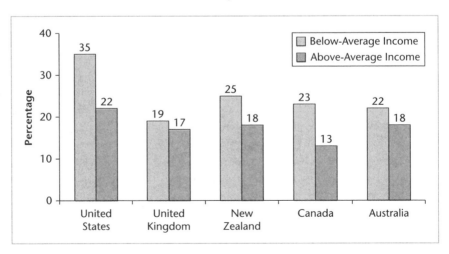

FIGURE 3.13   Percentage Reporting That the Health
System Is So Bad It Should Be Rebuilt,
in Five Nations by Income, 2001

Source: Collins and others (2002).

care in both countries (Lasser, Himmelstein, and others, 2006). For example, in both the United States and Canada, the odds of reporting that the quality of health care received was "excellent" increased with each increase in the category of income. Compared with adults with income below $20,000 (in U.S. dollars), adults with incomes from $20,000–$34,999 (in U.S. dollars) were more likely to report excellent quality (OR = 1.23 in the U.S., and OR = 1.26 in Canada). For adults earning $70,000 or more (in U.S. dollars), the odds of reporting excellent quality of care were much higher overall, albeit slightly less so in Canada (OR = 1.97 in the U.S., and 1.74 in Canada).

Health Status

Health risks and health status have been frequently compared across socioeconomic tiers. In fact, the relationship between socioeconomic status and mortality has been well documented as early as the 1960s in the United States (Antonovsky, 1967; Syme and Berkman, 1976). More recent research has shown that in addition to individuals with lower income, those with lower education and occupational status are more likely to report a range of health risks and poorer health status. In this section, we review evidence of these SES disparities in general health status, health risks, and mortality.

Figure 3.4 presents large disparities in how patients assess their own health according to poverty status. Using the same methodology as for the analysis of racial disparities in general health status, individuals in poverty report much worse health status than other income groups. The figure shows that just 6.4 percent of individuals who are not poor (incomes above 200 percent of the FPL) were reported to be in "fair" or "poor" health. However, this percentage nearly tripled (17.2 percent) for those living in near poverty (100 to 199 percent of the FPL), and nearly quadrupled (24.5 percent) for those living in poverty. This means that among those living in poverty, nearly one in every four individuals report having significantly impaired health.

New research examining SES gradients in functional limitations (long-term physical, mental, or emotional conditions that limit a person's ability walk, climb stairs, and so on) has demonstrated a large dose-response relationship between the likelihood of having a functional limitation and detailed income and education levels. For example, the percent of adults ages 55–64 years with a functional limitation decreases from about 40 percent for those with incomes below 100 percent of FPL to about 30 percent for those from 100–150 percent of FPL; about 20 percent for those from 200–299 percent of FPL; about 10 percent for those 400–499 percent of FPL; and close to 7 percent for those with income of 700 percent of FPL or higher. In short, the difference was nearly sixfold between the highest and lowest income levels (Minkler, Fuller-Thomson, and Guralnik, 2006). Earlier studies have also found a higher likelihood of severe function limiting chronic conditions for poor children compared with those in non-poor families (Newacheck, Jameson, and Halfon, 1994; Newacheck, 1994).

Socioeconomic status is also strongly associated with mental health status. Figure 3.14 combines several analyses conducted by the Centers for Disease Control and Prevention of self-reported frequent *mental distress* according to SES factors, including income, education, and employment. To present these data, we grouped the SES factors into three categories each: low, medium, and high. For income, the categories reflect incomes of less than $15,000, between $24,000 and $49,999, and $50,000 or more. For education, the categories reflect levels of less than high school, some college or technical school, and college or graduate education. For employment status, they reflect unemployment for one year or longer, unemployment less than one year, and currently employed. The analyses show that individuals with lower SES by any of these definitions are more likely to report frequent mental distress. The rates of frequent mental distress are two to three times higher for lower-SES versus higher-SES individuals.

In exploring other SES impacts on mental health, a unique longitudinal analysis of the relationship between unemployment and depression for young adults found relationships between the experience of any unemployment in young adulthood, as well as the duration of the unemployment, with depressive

FIGURE 3.14   Reported Frequent Mental Distress by Income, Education, and Employment, 2007

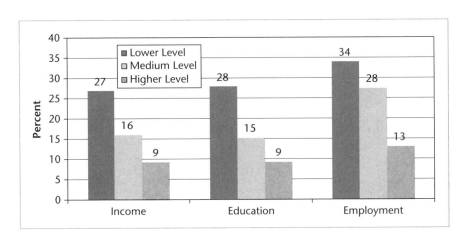

Source: Data from CDC Behavioral Risk Factor Surveillance System (2007).

symptoms in later years (Mossakowski, 2009). Following the young adults from 1979 to 1994, the study revealed that each spell of unemployment experienced was associated with a meaningful 1.2 point increase (on a 20-point scale) in total depressive symptoms at ages twenty-nine through thirty-seven years in 1994. This held irrespectively of level of education and poverty status, both of which were also associated with depressive symptoms.

Figure 3.15 demonstrates SES disparities in health risk behaviors among adults. Overall, individuals with the lowest education level (no high school diploma or General Educational Development Test, GED) compared with those with the highest education level (a bachelor's degree or higher) were more than three times as likely to report being physically inactive (43 versus 14 percent), three times more likely to be current smokers (27 versus 9 percent), and, for mothers, were five times more likely to smoke during pregnancy (18 versus 3 percent), and nearly twice as likely to breast-feed their children for less than three months (63 versus 36 percent). These gradients were apparent at each level of education in between. One major exception to this pattern was for current alcohol drinking, where the most highly educated individuals were twice as likely as those with the lowest level of education to be a current drinker (65 versus 33 percent).

International data provide a compelling picture of health of lower-income U.S. adults. Representative samples of adults ages fifty to seventy-four years

FIGURE 3.15   Health Risk Behaviors by Educational
Status, 1999–2007

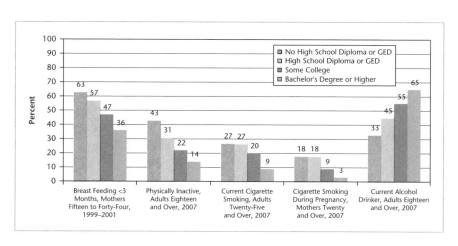

Source: New analysis of the Behavioral Risk Factor Surveillance System (2007) and National Center for Health Statistics (2009).

were interviewed in 2004 in ten European countries, England, and the United States (Avendano, Glymour, Banks, and Mackenbach, 2009). Overall, U.S. adults reported worse health statistics than did English or European adults. For example, 18 percent of U.S. adults had heart disease, compared with 12 percent of the English and 11 percent of other the European adults. This held for nearly every condition studied, including hypertension, diabetes, cancer, lung disease, and functional limitations in activity. The main contribution of this study was a revelation that income gradients in most of these conditions were significantly steeper in the United States than elsewhere, meaning that income has a bigger impact on health in this country than in England and other European countries. For example, 6 percent of the poorest adults in Europe have had a stroke, compared with about 2 percent among the wealthiest adults, reflecting a threefold difference. In this country, nearly 16 percent of the poorest adults have had a stroke compared to about 3 percent of the wealthiest adults, reflecting a fivefold difference. A larger impact of wealth was seen for lung disease, with an approximate twofold difference seen in Europe, a threefold difference seen in England, and a sevenfold difference in the United States.

The accumulation of studies documenting socioeconomic disparities in mortality and life expectancy is staggering. Income, education, and occupation are consistently correlated with higher mortality, fewer years of healthy life and lower overall life expectancy (Isaacs and Schroeder, 2004). Because of this, we highlight only a few core studies that have helped to shape our understanding of SES and U.S. mortality rates, and we include a recent international study that provides sweeping new data on income and health.

Several iterations of the Health, United States report have brought attention to SES differentials in mortality rates, particularly according to education (National Center for Health Statistics, 1998, 2003). These reports showed that infant mortality rates, mortality from *communicable diseases*, and HIV mortality rates among men are related to education level. For example, the infant mortality rate increases from 5.1 deaths per 1,000 live births for mothers with thirteen or more years of education, to 7.4 deaths per 1,000 live births for those with twelve years of education, and to 8.0 deaths per 1,000 live births for those with less than a high school education. Similarly, communicable disease mortality for women jumps from 8.6 deaths per 100,000 for mothers with thirteen years of education, to about 25.0 deaths per 100,000 for mothers with twelve years of education, and 36.0 deaths per 100,000 for those with fewer than twelve years of education. HIV mortality rates among men also show similar patterns, increasing by about 27 deaths per 100,000 (from about 37 to 64 deaths) for men with twelve years of education compared with those with thirteen years.

Using cohort data from the National Longitudinal Mortality Study in the late 1970s through 1980s, Backlund and others found that income may influence mortality differently for people at different levels of SES (Backlund, Sorlie, and Johnson, 1999). This study aimed to test the hypothesis that changes in income for low-income families would have a greater impact on mortality than changes in income among higher-income families (basically, a dollar means more to lower-income families than higher-income families). For adults with incomes at or below $22,500, the risk of mortality was found to increase by 21 percent for men and 15 percent for women per $1,000 decrease in income, after adjusting for demographic and other socioeconomic factors. For adults above this income threshold, the added risk of mortality was only 7 percent for men and 4 percent for women for each $1,000 decrease in income. This suggests that there may be a minimum material standard necessary to prevent mortality. The study also concluded that mortality might be more a function of education than income at the higher end of the SES spectrum.

The strong association of SES with overall mortality rates has also been demonstrated at the geographical level. Areas characterized by lower-SES indicators (for example, using median monthly rents of homes, median family incomes, and poverty levels of census tracts) have higher overall rates of mortality than areas characterized by higher-SES indicators. Using nine years of census data on residents (ages thirty-five and older) in Oakland, California, Haan and others found higher rates of mortality among residents of federally designated poverty areas. Adjusting for demographics, the overall mortality rates of residents in poverty areas remained 71 percent higher than those in nonpoverty areas (Haan, Kaplan, and Camacho, 1987). Even after adjusting for other determinants of mortality such as health practices, social networks, and psychological impairment, these mortality differentials remained significant.

A recent study among twenty-two European countries found that mortality rates and poorer self-assessments of health were much higher in groups of lower SES (measured by all three measures of income, education, and occupation) (Mackenbach and others, 2008). In every country, lower SES was associated with higher mortality, with relative rates of mortality ranging from about 1.5 to nearly 5.0 (meaning up to a fivefold difference in mortality between the highest- and lowest-SES classes). Education revealed similar but less striking patterns, with relative mortality rates ranging from between 1.25 and about 3.0; and occupation was associated with smaller relative mortality rates ranging from 1.25 to about 2.0. Countries in Eastern Europe, including Hungary, Czech Republic, Poland, and Lithuania, showed the greatest income differentials, suggesting that countries struggling economically are least able to guarantee the welfare of their poorest citizens, or alternately that the poorest citizens in these countries are affected more by the struggling economic situation of the country. There are potentially important lessons for the United States regarding the value of a strong welfare system during difficult social and economic times.

Front-Line Experience: Improving Primary Care Through Partnership Building

Vicki Young, the department head for clinical quality improvement, and Lathran Woodard, the chief executive officer, of the South Carolina Primary Health Care Association recount their experiences as an organization working to help vulnerable populations by connecting safety-net doctors and clinics with other major community partners. Their organization is at the core of these partnerships, and they provide some instructive lessons for others working to bring agencies together.

Improving access to quality preventive and primary health care services for all, particularly for vulnerable populations, is a national and moral imperative, one that the South Carolina Primary Health Care Association (hereafter, the Association) fully embraces and champions. Although we do not provide direct services, one of our roles as the membership organization for twenty federally qualified health centers in the state is to improve care by building and sustaining partnerships. The partnerships that we have cultivated between our member health centers and other agencies have led to valuable opportunities to really impact the provision of primary care.

Three of the Association's front-line experiences with building and sustaining partnerships have led to (1) the implementation of a state colorectal cancer screening program for the uninsured that utilizes community health centers as the entry point for patients to receive screening colonoscopies; (2) the development of a small business partnership initiative aimed at providing health care services to employees of small businesses; and (3) the formation of a coalition of stakeholders to increase the use of electronic health systems across the state.

In 2008, the South Carolina Department of Health and Environmental Control was awarded a one-time, $1 million grant from the State General Assembly to implement a colorectal cancer–screening program for the uninsured. Our organization was engaged to help develop a plan for how these funds would be spent. The plan was designed to screen uninsured and underserved adults ages fifty to sixty-four years old (ages forty-five to sixty-four for African Americans) whose income is below 200 percent of the poverty level. The program was piloted for one year with four of our member health centers and is being expanded to others in year two.

During the first year of this partnership, 656 colonoscopies were performed, exceeding our goal of 600 screenings despite a budget reduction of $200,000.

In 2005, in response to a growing number of small businesses that were unable to provide health insurance for their employees, our Association partnered with the Small Business Chamber of Commerce to develop health care service agreements, whereby our health centers would provide direct services to small business employees at discounted rates. The agreements were customizable to accommodate the needs and affordability of both the business and the employees—filling a major gap in access to care for the working poor—and provided a source of additional revenue for the health centers. Creating this partnership was mutually beneficial and increased awareness of the community health centers and the services they render.

The environment created by the American Recovery and Reinvestment Act afforded opportunities to expand health information technology. As a result, we were part of a jointly established coordinating body, known as *E-Health South Carolina*, to address this topic. The collaborative is made up of our Association, many health-related state agencies, state medical schools, and others. Its purpose is to provide a mechanism through which ideas can be shared and consensus can be achieved and provide assistance and advice to groups seeking funds to advance the use of health information technology. The collaborative first analyzed the current state of health information technology use in the state and the capability to share patient information across agencies, and then identified strategies to move the state to the next level to improve patient care.

The Association also strives to remain innovative as it works to assist its member organizations in providing quality health care to their patients. An example is supporting research in community health centers as one of our strategic priorities. We recognize the value of data as a driver of quality improvement and believe that such research helps to create an environment conducive to the reduction of health disparities.

As an advocate for safety-net primary care providers in South Carolina, our key strength is the ability to establish and bring many partners to the table. In addition to the project-specific partners we described above, we partner with many other health and non–health organizations and foundations. This diversity provides the framework to cultivate a broad impact on the lives of vulnerable populations. These partnerships have been and continue to be instrumental in improving access to health care for all in South Carolina.

We think there are many reasons that the Association is successful in building the wide range of partnerships that we have and that others might aim to replicate. First, we have built a credible reputation as an organization that assists those who directly care for the underserved at the forefront of our mission. Second, we are committed to partnering with organizations with similar missions and pursue partnerships in new and innovative areas. Third, our decision to maintain a diverse network of partners has led to the effective leveraging of resources. In these instances, the partnerships yielded a greater impact on the provision of health care services than would otherwise have been accomplished.

Although the Association has a track record of establishing effective partnerships, we face some challenges. Sustaining partnerships can be difficult as the expectations and priorities of our partnership organizations change over time, but we have tried to keep the lines of communication open in order to accommodate these changes. Building and sustaining partnerships also requires a large commitment of time and human resources, and so we often need to prioritize our levels of engagement with partners. Lastly, our potential new partners sometimes do not have a full understanding of the mission of our Association. To overcome this, we educate our potential partners about the goals of our organization and highlight how partnerships can lead to greater steps toward improving health care access for all in South Carolina.

HEALTH INSURANCE DISPARITIES

Since the mid-1960s, the U.S. government has acknowledged the vitally important role of health insurance coverage in ensuring adequate access to health care. The creation of public insurance programs like Medicare, Medicaid, and CHIP has helped millions of low- or fixed-income citizens obtain needed health care services. Because eligibility for these programs remains limited to particular citizens—primarily the elderly and the very poor—researchers and advocates have continued to document the consequences of lack of insurance for health care access, quality, and ultimately health.

Such research informs the public and provides evidence for politicians and citizens to advocate for expansions of these programs. Because these programs have previously been closely linked with social welfare programs, advocates have been concerned about the quality of care delivered in these programs, often comparing the experiences of individuals in public programs with private health insurance plans. In addition, continued expansion of managed care plans (often criticized in the past for restriction of patient and physician autonomy through extensive cost-control measures) into public programs like Medicaid has led to ongoing concern about the quality of care provided to vulnerable populations. This section reviews the evidence for disparities in health care access, quality and health outcomes among those with private insurance, public insurance, and no health insurance at all.

Health Care Access

Extensive work has been done to document the poorer access to health care experienced by people without insurance coverage. The cumulative evidence shows conclusively that people without health insurance are less likely to have an RSC, and instead seek routine care from sites such as emergency departments and delay or forgo needed health services (Institute of Medicine Committee on Health Insurance Status and Its Consequences, 2009).

Figure 3.1 demonstrated the consequences of lack of health insurance coverage on the likelihood of having an RSC for adults. Data from Health, United States, 2008 show that privately and publicly insured adults are approximately as likely to report not having an RSC (9.8 percent and 11.5 percent). Uninsured adults are five times more likely than the insured not to have an RSC (52.8 percent), a difference that is substantially greater than any disparities by race/ethnicity or poverty status. Though not shown in the figure, uninsured children are about eight times more likely than insured children to lack an RSC (4 percent versus 31 percent) (National Center for Health Statistics, 2009). Other research has shown that these differences in the likelihood of having an RSC remain even after controlling for SES factors (Stevens, Seid, and Halfon, 2006; Stevens, West-Wright, and Tsai, 2008).

Lacking insurance coverage also affects the type of RSC that individuals report having. Privately insured individuals are more likely to report a physician's office as their source of care, whereas Medicaid-insured individuals are more likely to cite a clinic or emergency department (ED) as their source of care. Cunningham and others found that even after adjustment for demographic variables and county-level use of EDs, nonurgent rates of ED use were much higher among those with Medicare, Medicaid, or other public insurance (OR 1.61, 1.47, 1.47, all $p < .01$) (Cunningham, Clancy, Cohen, and Wilets, 1995). A similar study found that uninsured adolescents were more likely than insured adolescents to use an ED as their regular source of care (9 percent versus 5 percent, respectively, $p < .01$) (Klein and others, 1999).

In a study examining the importance of health insurance coverage in meeting the health care needs of children ages birth to seventeen years (Olson, Tang, and Newacheck, 2005), using the 2000 and 2001 National Health Interview Survey, the authors showed that after adjustment for health status and family demographics, uninsured children had about 12.7 times the odds (CI: 9.5–17.0) of having delayed needed health care. Children whose health insurance coverage had been disrupted during the year (meaning they did not have coverage during the full year prior to the survey) were even more likely to report having delayed care (OR = 13.7, CI: 10.4–17.9). The authors reason that children who lose insurance coverage may require time for their families to learn ways to seek needed care, while the families of children who are uninsured during the full year may be more accustomed to seeking out and finding free or low-cost sources of health care.

Delays in obtaining health care also persist for newborns and very young children (age three and under). A study by Newacheck and others using data on children from the 1997 National Health Interview Survey revealed that uninsured young children were much more likely to experience delays in care than insured young children, despite controlling for race/ethnicity, family income, health status, and other family and community factors (Newacheck, Hung, Hochstein, and Halfon, 2002). They showed that compared to insured children, uninsured children had 9.57 times the odds of not obtaining needed medical care, 6.10 times the odds of not obtaining needed prescription medications, and 5.35 times the odds of not obtaining dental care. This study also showed that uninsured young children had nearly seven times lower odds of having an RSC ($p < .05$).

Another study sought to examine the role of health insurance coverage in differences in access to care for immigrant and nonimmigrant adults in the United States and in Canada (Siddiqi, Zuberi, and Nguyen, 2009). Analyzing data from the Joint Canada/United States Survey of Health, the authors found that in the United States, uninsured immigrant and uninsured nonimmigrant adults experienced about threefold higher odds of having an unmet health care need compared with insured nonimmigrant adults in the United States. The effects of insurance on lacking an RSC were even greater, with uninsured nonimmigrant adults having four times the odds of lacking an RSC and uninsured immigrant adults having nearly seventeen times the odds compared with insured nonimmigrants. Immigrants in Canada were also more likely than nonimmigrants to have poorer access to care, but both fared better than either uninsured U.S. group because of their universal health coverage.

A study using the 1997 Medical Expenditure Panel Survey examined the relationship between health insurance coverage type and ACS hospitalizations among adults in fourteen U.S. states (Laditka and Laditka, 2004). The study found that after adjustment for the prevalence of ACS conditions that the uninsured and those covered by Medicaid were more likely to be hospitalized for ACS conditions than the privately insured. Depending on the U.S. state, those with Medicaid were between 1.8 and 24.7 times more likely than the privately insured to have an ACS hospitalization, while the uninsured were only up to 2.8 times more likely to have an ACS hospitalization. This is notable because one would expect that adults covered by Medicaid would be less likely than the uninsured to be hospitalized, but it is important to remember that lacking health insurance prevents the uninsured to a degree from seeking needed hospital care, not just primary care. Most likely, many uninsured adults with ACS conditions simply never made it to the hospital. The study also found that among Medicare beneficiaries, those who also received Medicaid (those who are both elderly and lower income) had a higher rate of

ACS condition hospitalizations than beneficiaries with Medicare only. Many other studies have now demonstrated a relationship between health insurance coverage and preventable hospitalizations (Backus and others, 2002; Basu, Friedman, and Burstin, 2004, 2006; Billings, Anderson, and Newman, 1996; Bindman and others, 1995; DeLia, 2003; Friedman and Basu, 2001; Garg, Probst, Sease, and Samuels, 2003; Gaskin and Hoffman, 2000; Weissman, Gatsonis, and Epstein, 1992).

Health Care Quality

Much attention has been given to evaluating how the quality of health care varies according to health insurance status and type. Health care plans provide an easily accessible sampling frame for research purposes; thus, much of the work on the more detailed experiences with quality of care is often conducted among various health plan types rather than by comparing the insured and uninsured. There are, however, many studies documenting the consequences of lacking insurance coverage for the receipt of specific recommended services.

Looking again at the receipt of preventive services as an important measure of quality of care, we present our own updated analyses of an original comprehensive study that examined the lack of receiving recommended preventive care (Ayanian and others, 2000). Figure 3.16 shows a comparison of the receipt of

FIGURE 3.16   Clinically Indicated Preventive Services Not Received in the Past Year by Insurance Status, 2007

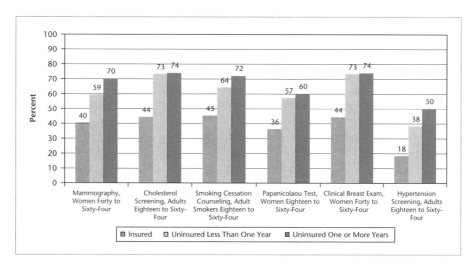

Source: New analysis of the Medical Expenditure Panel Survey, 2007 Full-Year Population Characteristics.

clinically indicated preventive services across three insurance categories: those who were currently insured, those who were uninsured for less than one year, and those who were uninsured for more than one year. The original study examined both short- and long-term lack of health insurance to reveal deficits in the receipt of preventive care associated with the duration of noncoverage, and the updated data present strikingly similar findings.

Insured women ages forty to sixty-four years, for example, failed to receive a mammogram in the past year an estimated 40 percent of the time compared with 59 percent of women who were uninsured for less than one year. Women who were uninsured for longer were almost twice as likely as insured women to not have a mammogram (70 percent). This pattern of non-receipt of preventive care associated with the duration of noncoverage holds for most of the preventive services studied, including clinical breast exams, Pap tests, hypertension screening, cholesterol screening, and receiving smoking cessation counseling.

Because uninsured individuals have substantially poorer access to primary care services, they consequently have different needs for and use of inpatient services. Researchers reviewed 1987 hospital discharge data in Massachusetts and Maryland to assess if both uninsured and Medicaid covered adults had higher rates of avoidable hospitalizations (Weissman, Gatsonis, and Epstein, 1992). A panel of physicians identified twelve avoidable hospital conditions (including asthma, congestive heart failure, diabetes, immunizable conditions, and pneumonia) that could be averted if primary care is provided in a timely and high-quality manner. After adjusting for age and gender, they found that uninsured and Medicaid patients were 71 percent more likely in Massachusetts and 49 percent more likely in Maryland than insured patients to be hospitalized for all avoidable hospital conditions combined.

In addition to disparities in the utilization and receipt of health care services, differences exist according to health insurance status in more subjective quality experiences in health care. One study used nationally representative Medical Expenditure Panel Survey data to evaluate the *primary care experiences* of adults according to health insurance status and type (Shi, 2000). The study examined the likelihood of describing a positive primary care experience (for example, appointments were made rather than simply walking in for a visit, waiting times for appointments were shorter than thirty minutes, telephone contact could be made easily, and reported satisfaction in obtaining care). The study found that most primary care quality measures were higher for insured individuals than for the uninsured and for the privately insured compared to publicly insured. For example, the odds of reporting a wait time of less than thirty minutes was 28 percent higher for the insured compared with the uninsured and 77 percent higher for the privately insured compared with those with public insurance.

Figure 3.17 presents the results of a study of health care experiences in the United States that was conducted among adults with chronic conditions to obtain the experiences among those individuals who interact with the health care system most frequently (Schoen and others, 2009). The study included those with hypertension, heart disease, diabetes, arthritis, lung problems (asthma, emphysema, or chronic lung obstruction), cancer, or depression. This study examined, in part, experiences of U.S. adults, comparing those with and without health insurance. Across the six measures studied, there were at least 10 percentage point differences between the uninsured and insured with regard to all but one of the measures. For example, uninsured adults with chronic disease were 14 percentage points more likely to report a medical, medication, or lab error; 19 percentage points more likely to wait six or more days for an appointment; and nearly twice as likely (82 versus 43 percent) to report having a problem getting any care because of the cost.

Finally, Figure 3.18 shows differences in satisfaction with care according to health plan type and changes in satisfaction over time. We compared the satisfaction of patients in Health Maintenance Organizations (HMOs) and non-HMOs on overall satisfaction, satisfaction with the choice of doctor, and whether

FIGURE 3.17   Health Care Experiences among Adults with Chronic Conditions by Insurance Status, 2008

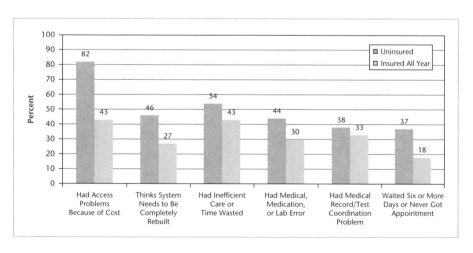

Source: Schoen and others (2009).

FIGURE 3.18   Patient Satisfaction with Health Care by Health Insurance Plan Type, 1996–1997, 2003, and 2007

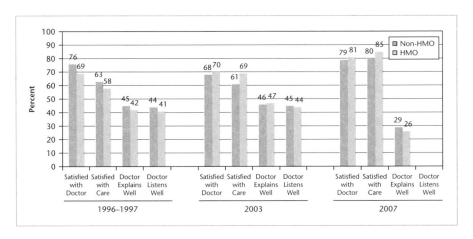

Note: Data were not available in 2007 on ratings of how well the doctor listens to patients.
Source: New analysis of the 1996 and 1997, 2003, and 2007 Community Tracking Study Household Survey.

the doctor explains and listens well. Our analysis finds that satisfaction was lower among patients in HMOs compared with those not in HMOs in 1996 and 1997. This was a period when HMOs were engaging in the most restrictive health care cost-control mechanisms (such as controls on what services patients and providers could elect to obtain or deliver) that brought a considerable amount of media backlash. Since then, HMOs have begun to loosen their grip on cost control mechanisms that patients liked the least, but they have raised their premiums in exchange (Draper, Hurley, Lesser, and Strunk, 2002; Mechanic, 2004). In 2003 and 2007, HMOs had higher ratings of satisfaction overall and became more similar to non-HMOs on ratings of how well their doctors explained things and listened to patients. These trends will need to be watched closely as major increases in health care costs may drive health plans to return to seeking strict cost-control strategies.

Health Status

Insurance coverage is closely associated with health status and health risk behaviors through a range of possible pathways described in Chapter Two. Researchers have established an association between lacking insurance and lower health care utilization and, subsequently, poorer health status (Institute of Medicine Committee on Health Insurance Status and Its Consequences, 2009; Institute of Medicine Committee on the Consequences of Uninsurance, 2002, 2003). However, most studies of insurance coverage and health rely on cross-sectional data that limit the ability to draw conclusions on whether lacking insurance causes worse health. It is still not clear, for example, whether the generally poorer health status of those in Medicaid (compared to those privately insured) is attributable to problems with accessing quality health care rather than the inherently lower SES of those using that public program. We now highlight some of the key findings regarding the association between health insurance and health.

Figure 3.4 compared the self-assessed general health status of respondents according to health insurance status and type. Using data generated directly from the 2000 MEPS, we were able to compare the health status of those insured privately, those insured by Medicaid, and the uninsured. The figure shows that adults who were uninsured were almost twice as likely to report themselves in fair or poor health compared with those who were privately insured (11.4 percent versus 6.1 percent, respectively). Individuals in Medicaid, however, were much more likely than the uninsured to report fair or poor health (32.8 percent), and this may be explained by the fact that Medicaid coverage is primarily for those living in poverty, and poverty status is associated with poorer health status. Those who are uninsured may in fact have higher incomes than those covered by Medicaid because of the program's restrictive eligibility criteria.

Not having insurance coverage is also associated with a greater likelihood of mortality in both the short and long terms. One study that was widely covered in national media during the health care reform debate of 2010 revealed the annual excess mortality in the United States associated with lacking health insurance coverage (Wilper and others, 2009). Updating a key earlier analysis, the study analyzed data on adults ages seventeen to sixty-four years in the Third National Health and Nutrition Examination Survey, exploring the relationship between uninsurance at the time of interview and predicted death in the coming year. After adjustment for age and gender only, the mortality rate of the uninsured was about 80 percent higher than the rate for insured. After additional adjustment for race/ethnicity, income, education, self- and physician-rated health status, body mass index, leisure exercise, smoking, and regular alcohol use, the uninsured were still about 40 percent more likely to die than those with insurance. It was estimated that this excess mortality translated into about 45,000 deaths each year attributable to the lack of health insurance coverage. Earlier seminal studies have also shown similar findings (Franks, Clancy, and Gold, 1993; Sorlie and others, 1994).

Children who lack health insurance coverage are also at higher risk of mortality than those who have insurance. One study examined the risk of mortality for children who had suffered trauma and entered one of the more than 900 trauma centers nationally (Rosen and others, 2009). Using data from 2002–2006 from the National Trauma Data Bank, the study found that children ages birth to seventeen years who were uninsured had nearly three times the odds of mortality (OR = 2.97, CI: 2.64–3.34) compared with insured children. The relationship only strengthened after the study adjusted for age, gender, race, injury severity and type, and hospital setting, rising to a 3.32 higher odds of mortality (CI: 2.95–3.74). When examining the type of health insurance coverage, children on Medicaid also had slightly higher odds of mortality compared to the privately insured (OR = 1.19, CI: 1.07–1.33). While the authors were not able to explain the difference in mortality, they believe that uninsured children may face delays in treatment, receive fewer diagnostic tests (since they have no insurance to cover the costs), or have greater communication barriers between physicians and family members.

Using hospital discharge data and the New Jersey Cancer Registry, researchers studied 4,675 women ages thirty-five to sixty-four diagnosed between 1985 and 1987 with invasive breast cancer (Ayanian, Kohler, Abe, and Epstein, 1993). They found that upon initial diagnosis, uninsured women had significantly more advanced breast cancer than privately insured women. The study showed that 12.3 percent of uninsured women compared to 7.3 percent of privately insured women were initially diagnosed with advanced breast cancer (or cancer that had spread beyond mammary lymph nodes, chest wall, subcutaneous tissue, or overlying skin; $p < 0.001$). Following women prospectively, the researchers compared chances of survival beyond diagnosis. After adjusting for age, race, marital status, household income, coexisting diagnoses, and disease stage, uninsured women faced a 49 percent higher risk of death than those privately insured. The results are explained by the likely greater frequency of delayed care and the associated missed opportunities for earlier detection of cancer among the uninsured.

Using a national sample of hospital discharge data for nearly 600,000 patients hospitalized in 1987, Hadley and others explored the association between insurance status and condition on admission to the hospital, inpatient resource use, and in-hospital mortality (Hadley, Steinberg, and Feder, 1991). The sample of discharged patients was divided into sixteen subsamples by age, sex, and race. In thirteen of the sixteen age-sex-race-specific cohorts, the uninsured had a 44 to 124 percent higher risk of in-hospital mortality at the time of admission than privately insured patients. When the researchers controlled for this baseline difference in mortality on admission, the in-hospital mortality remained higher for the uninsured in the majority of the cohorts. After adjustment, the actual in-hospital death rate was 1.2 to 3.2 times higher among uninsured patients in eleven of sixteen cohorts.

The effect of being uninsured on mortality is similar to its effects on morbidity. In a unique and widely referenced study by Lurie and others on the effects of cutbacks to California's Medicaid program, researchers followed all poor adults who had been receiving care from a medical group practice but who had lost their Medicaid coverage due to the cutbacks (Lurie, Ward, Shapiro, and Brook, 1984). They were compared after one year to 109 patients in the same practice whose benefits had not been terminated. Self-reported health status and blood pressure measurements were obtained for all hypertensive patients.

The data showed that the general health of the medically indigent adults had declined 10 points on a 100-point scale ($p < 0.002$) after one year of follow-up. Among hypertensive patients, those who had lost health coverage showed serious deterioration in blood pressure levels compared with those who had stayed on the Medicaid program. The proportion of hypertensive patients with blood pressure under 90 mm (a healthy level) was 75 percent at baseline but only 51 percent by the end of the follow-up. The authors suggested that the deterioration of health status among their adult indigent population is directly related to their loss of health care coverage and resulting barriers to access and use of health services. Although the county was mandated to provide care to this population, there were no stipulations to provide free care, suggesting that the patients who lost coverage were not easily finding care elsewhere.

Focus on Vulnerability in Clinical Practice

Clinicians in primary care practice are responsible for caring for the most common health problems their community experiences. If this includes an outbreak of a particular strain of the flu in their patient panel, clinicians need to be well informed about how to prevent and treat such transmissions. If the community is increasingly overweight and obese, the clinician needs to be aware of what can be done to prevent the condition in the first place and capable of caring for its consequences. If the clinician's patient panel is mostly low income and living in an economically deprived area, he/she must be aware of how living conditions create and aggravate health problems. Stressors such as poverty create levels of depression, suicide, and violence not seen in higher economic neighborhoods, and poor living conditions directly aggravate problems like asthma (from poor hygiene, home care, and air quality) and heart disease (from lack of safe neighborhood spaces for walking and other physical activity, and nutritional food sources).

Clinicians often have difficulty knowing exactly what problems their community faces and typically have to rely on memory and anecdote to gauge the prevalence of any health problems and risk factors. The same difficulty exists for health insurance plans that are aiming to understand what problems their beneficiaries are experiencing. Since most plans and medical providers continue to rely heavily on paper medical records, the ability to gather and synthesize patient information requires manual labor. The growth of electronic medical records will facilitate this process, but only if specific efforts enable the records to be integrated in ways that allow for reporting at provider, medical group, and health plan levels. Ideally, providers could search across their patient panels to know which individuals have a problem like asthma and which individuals are at higher risk for poor asthma outcomes based on any number of risk factors that can be gathered.

Although this is only beginning to occur at the individual provider level, groups that are engaged in public health or population health activities have been working to produce such information at a range of geographic levels. In the United States, data are combined to determine medically underserved areas. Indicators such as provider to patient ratios, infant mortality and poverty rates, and the proportion of elderly are used to identify these areas and provide funding to support the expansion of health services. More detailed are data on health care utilization and costs that are analyzed and compiled in the *Dartmouth Atlas of Health Care*. These data are presented as detailed geographic maps showing the frequency of certain health services and specific procedures and costs, often in combination with other data to reveal inefficiencies and even discrepancies in health care delivery.

These data only skim the surface of what is possible with regard to measuring and reporting health data to inform public health, health systems, and clinicians. One example of what is possible comes from the United Kingdom. Like the medically underserved areas in the United States, government officials there have developed a methodology to identify geographic areas in need of the greatest assistance with regard to health care, public health intervention, and social services. The technique is known as the Index of Multiple Deprivation, and separate indices exist in the four U.K. countries: England, Ireland, Scotland, and Wales. An index is created from data on levels of family income, employment, health and well-being, education, housing, access to services, and crime.

In Scotland, for example, the index uses thirty-eight indicators to create rankings of deprivation for 6,505 geographic data zones of approximately the same population size. In this way, the most deprived areas are easily identified and, based on the levels of deprivation factors that are present, can be targeted for increases in funding for services or other policies and interventions. Since these deprivation index data are available at useful geographic levels (in some cases as small as neighborhoods within a city), localities and even clinics have been able to use the data, for example, to target teenage pregnancy interventions and advise police beats to improve neighborhood safety. Perhaps the greatest strength of these indices is that they are traceable over time, since data have been collected every two to three years since 2004. This enables monitoring of patterns and trends and allows for the *evaluation* of interventions, especially since the data can be downloaded and merged with other data that local health authorities, clinics, or other health and social service organizations collect.

SUMMARY

This chapter has reviewed the extensive evidence of disparities in health care access, quality, and health status and outcomes by three major vulnerability characteristics: race and ethnicity, SES, and health insurance coverage. The literature provides abundant evidence that racial/ethnic minorities, lower-SES individuals, and the uninsured experience worse access to care, lower-quality care, and poorer health status and health outcomes than whites, higher-SES individuals, and those who are insured. Although we present only some of the highlights of the extensive research base, the comprehensiveness and consistency of the findings, using many analytic approaches, populations, and data sources, should convey a solid foundation upon which to enhance efforts to eliminate disparities and improve equity in health and health care.

KEY TERMS

Evaluation

Ambulatory care sensitive conditions

Communicable diseases

Culturally appropriate

Developmental disabilities

Healthy People initiative

Mental distress

Primary care experiences

Qualitative experiences

Self-efficacy

Unmet health care needs

Well-child care

REVIEW QUESTIONS

1. Briefly describe the relationship between race/ethnicity and mortality. Which racial/ethnic group experiences the highest rates of mortality (overall and cause specific)? Which group experiences the lowest rates of mortality? Describe one nonmedical explanation, using what you learned from Chapter Two, for why the mortality rates for these groups are higher or lower.

2. Briefly describe the relationship between education and the receipt of preventive services for women. How strong is this relationship? Using what you learned from Chapter Two, what are two possible explanations for this relationship?

3. Briefly describe the relationship between health insurance status and access to primary health care for children. Describe how Medicaid-covered children differ from the privately insured in terms of access, and explain why differences might occur.

ESSAY QUESTION

You are the director of a large managed care health insurance plan. You have a particular interest in reducing disparities in the receipt of preventive care among the large population of adults enrolled in your plan. Prepare a written presentation to the chief executives in your health plan to convince them of the importance of addressing this issue. Make sure to discuss what the benefits of preventive care are and where the disparities lie in terms of race/ethnicity and SES. Based on what you have learned from previous chapters, propose two possible courses of action for your organization that would help remedy these disparities.

CHAPTER FOUR

THE INFLUENCE OF MULTIPLE RISK FACTORS

LEARNING OBJECTIVES

- To recognize that risk factors for any range of health or health care problems tend to cluster together, such that having one risk factor increases the likelihood of having another, and that these risk factors have cumulative impacts on poor health care access, quality, and outcomes.

- To understand how research that examines the combined effects of multiple risk factors reveals new and potentially more useful information about health disparities and how and where to best intervene.

- To become aware of the rich data sources that are available for studying health disparities in more sophisticated ways and the types of reports and publications that regularly convey the data for use by public health and medical professionals.

A S shown in the previous chapter, there have been many studies exploring the independent influences of being a member of certain racial/ethnic minority groups, having low socioeconomic status (SES), and lacking health insurance coverage on health care access, quality, and health outcomes. These risk factors are closely intertwined, such that having one risk factor increases the likelihood of having another, and it is this overlap of risk factors and their cumulative impact that is the focus of this chapter.

One way to think about multiple risk factors is in terms of individual risk profiles. This approach characterizes individuals according to the presence or absence of certain risk factors for any given outcome. A risk profile can be developed for each person to describe the number and type of risk factors he or she has. In the United States, there is substantial overlap of the three key risk factors (described in the previous chapter) that are associated with a wide range of measures of access to care, quality of care, and health outcomes.

In Figure 4.1 we present the overlap of these three risk factors—minority race/ethnicity, lower SES, and lack of health insurance coverage—in the national adult and child populations using data from the 2007 National Health Interview Survey (NHIS). For both adults and children, the most common single risk factor is minority race/ethnicity, with 29.5 percent of the adult population and 26 percent of the child population being a racial/ethnic minority with no other

FIGURE 4.1   Overlap of Three Risk Factors among U.S. Adults and Children, 2007

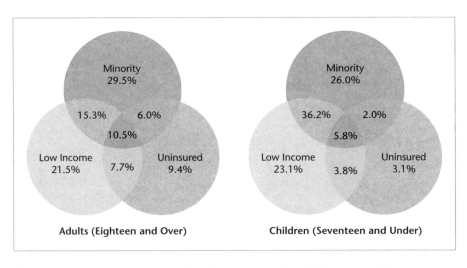

Adults (Eighteen and Over)   **Children (Seventeen and Under)**

Note: Low income is defined as families with income less than 200 percent of FPL.
Source: New analysis of the 2007 National Health Interview Survey.

risk factors. The overlap of risk factors is the focus of these diagrams and reveals that about 29 percent of the adult population has any combination of two risk factors. Comparing to equivalent data from the 2002 NHIS, where only 24 percent of adults had two risk factors, this reflects a five percentage point increase in the concentration of multiple risk factors.

Among children, the proportion with two risk factors is much higher (42 percent), as children are more than twice as likely as adults to be minority and low income (36.2 percent of children versus 15.3 percent of adults), a result that is explained by the fact that lower-income families tend to have more children. It is important to note that the percentage of the population that is minority and low income has nearly doubled since 2002, when 17.4 percent of children and 7.2 percent of adults were low income and a racial/ethnic minority. This rise can be attributed to the more than twofold increases in the percentage of low-income adults and children (10.9 percent and 11.4 percent, respectively, in 2002 versus 21.5 percent and 23.1 percent in 2007). Adults are more likely to be both minority and uninsured than are children (6.0 percent versus 2.0 percent), which is explained by the greater availability of public health insurance programs for children.

Of greatest interest is the proportion of the population sharing all three risk factors. These individuals are less prevalent in the population (10.5 percent among adults and 5.8 percent among children) but the numbers have increased since 2002 for children (from 4.2 percent) and doubled for adults (from 5.0 percent). In total, 39.5 percent of all adults and 47.8 percent of all children in the United States have any combination of multiple risk factors, up considerably from 2002, when just 29.3 percent of adults and 31.0 percent of children had multiple risk factors. This means that more than one-third of adults and nearly half of all children are at elevated risk for poor access to care, quality of care, and health outcomes. They are the focus of the data presented in this chapter.

While many studies have documented linkages of these risk factors, only recently have studies begun to look more explicitly at the combined influence of these risks on health care access, quality, and health status. There are an endless number of potential risk factors that could be studied. Many of these risk factors have a very specific or limited influence; for example, lack of transportation is directly related to the ability to attend medical visits. Although we present studies addressing many different risk factors, this chapter continues the primary focus on the interaction of race/ethnicity, SES, and health insurance coverage. Studies are beginning to document disparities using risk profiles, yet most continue to examine interactions of two risk factors at most. To add to the body of literature on combinations of risk factors, we present new analyses of the Medical Expenditure Panel Survey (MEPS), National Health Interview Survey (NHIS), and California Health Interview Survey (CHIS).

Front-Line Experience: Establishing Trust among Vulnerable Populations

Kena Burke is the executive director of The Children's Health Initiative (CHI) in San Luis Obispo County, California, an organization dedicated to ensuring that all children have access to quality health care. Through collaborative partnerships, the CHI has created a one-stop referral system for parents to find health insurance for their children. Kena recounts the story of one woman—Isabel Ruiz—who became a powerful community advocate and essential CHI partner by building trust and connections between the Latino families she worked with and the social services around them.

I used to tease Isabel that in a roomful of children, she could sniff out those who were uninsured. Trained as a physician in her native country of Peru as an OB/GYN, Isabel had followed her husband to San Luis Obispo County early in life, where they were to become stalwarts in the community. Napoleon Ruiz started his life as a farmer and later became a prominent vineyard manager; Isabel, his wife, worked with families of the farm workers to help them access the health services these families needed.

Isabel's word was golden in our county. Young Latina mothers knew that if they had questions, they could ask Isabel. One example of her role as trusted educator unfolded before me at a WIC clinic. I observed an anxious, young mother holding her newborn baby tightly as she approached Isabel. The young mom wanted to know why the doctor had bruised her baby's heel in the hospital. Isabel lovingly examined that baby's foot with both hands and explained that the doctor needed a few drops of blood from the heel prick to test for certain diseases. It was the cause of the bruise and nothing to be concerned about. I watched this young mom exhale a sigh of relief. "Even if a mother doesn't speak English, she still deserves to understand what is happening to her and her child." Isabel's goal was to be the bridge that would lead struggling families to a self-sufficient life.

Isabel's accomplishments were built on characteristics that can help all advocates in their work with at-risk populations. She uniquely understood that as an advocate for a child, she had to go where these children lived—in the schools, daycare, or the Migrant Head Starts. Isabel could be found in the fields with the families, with Human Resource directors of large employers, at Latino outreach events, and in community clinics where care was offered to those who could not afford health insurance. When low-income families wanted to give up trying to get their children covered with Medicaid or CHIP because of the paperwork burden, Isabel would help families understand the process, bridging the gap between them and social services.

Isabel had a dogged determination about her that was assuring to families— particularly those in crisis: she never gave up. If they needed a dentist, insurance, or a mammogram, Isabel made it happen. Isabel established a free mammogram program for the uninsured and health screenings for seniors in our community. She never accepted anything less than a "yes," preferably along with the date and time she could expect to see the results.

At the CHI, we screen families for eligibility for health insurance. We discovered early on that more families were seeking Isabel for help in completing applications for health insurance than any Certified Application Assistors or Family Resource Center in our county put together! Therefore, as a standing rule in our office, if Isabel called, we put her requests first. We respected how busy she was and knew that by supporting her needs, more of our county's children would gain access to our program. I believed it was by Isabel's nod of approval that so many families began transitioning to my staff at the Children's Health Initiative for aid in getting health insurance for their children. Almost 30 percent of the referrals that we receive now come from word-of-mouth: a family member telling another family member, a neighbor speaking to another neighbor. I now understand, though, that she was building a different bridge.

Diagnosed with breast cancer in 1987 and again in 2000, Isabel considered each day and each encounter a gift. On July 2, 2009, our county lost one of its most tireless humanitarians and the children of our community lost a fervent advocate. The lessons from Isabel's life will continue to provide guidance to the children's advocates throughout our community as we begin to implement national health care reform. In the spirit of Isabel, we will maintain our own dogged determination, our respect for the communities we serve, and have immense hope that all children will have access to quality health care so they may grow up healthy and wise.

HEALTH CARE ACCESS

Poverty compounds the problems that minorities face in securing a regular source of health care. Figure 4.2 presents the combined effects of poverty status and race/ethnicity on the likelihood of having a regular source of care. This figure confirms the association between race/ethnicity and access, and it shows that the likelihood of lacking a regular source of care increases for each racial/ethnic group living in poverty. For example, Hispanics who have incomes at less than 100 percent of the federal poverty level (FPL) are nearly twice as likely as Hispanics who are not living in poverty (200 percent of the FPL or higher) to report no regular source of care (47 percent versus 24 percent, respectively). Hispanics living in near-poverty (100 to 199 percent of the FPL) are about 18 percent more likely than the

FIGURE 4.2   No Regular Source of Care among Adults Eighteen to Sixty-Four Years by Race/Ethnicity and Insurance Coverage by Poverty Status, 2006–2007

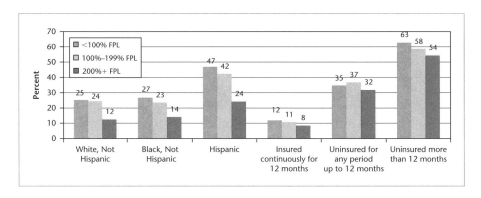

Source: National Center for Health Statistics (2009).

non-poor to lack a regular source of care. For African Americans and whites, however, living in near-poverty is similar to living in poverty with regard to lacking a regular source of care.

This figure also presents the combined influences of poverty status and continuity of health insurance coverage on the likelihood of having a regular source of care (RSC). It demonstrates that the likelihood of lacking a regular source of care increases for individuals in poverty. While poverty has only a small impact on the likelihood of having a regular source of care among those who are insured, it plays a larger role among the uninsured. For example, among the insured, there is only a 4 percent difference in having a regular source of care among adults living in poverty and those with incomes greater than 200 percent FPL. The difference is 3 percent among adults who were uninsured sporadically in the past year, but among adults who were uninsured for at least one year, the difference is 9 percent.

Vulnerable populations often rely on emergency departments for basic care. Although it is difficult to identify from national surveys whether visits to an emergency department are due to true emergencies, patterns vary by combinations of race/ethnicity, insurance coverage, and poverty status. Figure 4.3 shows that use of emergency departments increases for those living in poverty or in near-poverty, but income seems to affect emergency department use more so for whites than for other groups. For example, the difference between those who are poor and who have an income of 200 percent of FPL or more is 15 percent for whites, but

FIGURE 4.3   Emergency Department Visit in the Past Year Among Adults Eighteen to Sixty-Four Years by Race/Ethnicity and Insurance Coverage, by Poverty Status, 2007

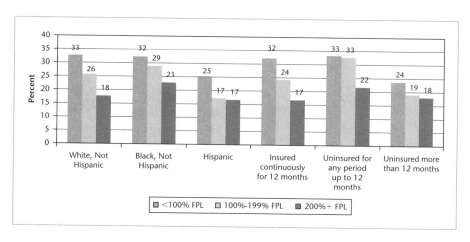

Source: National Center for Health Statistics (2009).

only 9 percent for African Americans and 8 percent for Hispanics. Income also affects emergency department use more for insured adults than for the uninsured. Differences by poverty status were as much as 15 percent for insured adults compared with 11 percent for those uninsured for one year or less, and 6 percent for those insured longer than one year.

A discussion of socioeconomic risk factors inhibiting health care access would be incomplete if the only indicator considered was household income. The 2008 National Healthcare Disparities Report, a yearly publication prepared by the Agency for Healthcare Research and Quality of the United States Department of Health and Human Services, used the 2006 National Health Interview Survey, to examine health insurance coverage for people under age sixty-five by race/ethnicity, in combination with income and highest level of education. The report found that Hispanic adults were less likely than non-Hispanic white adults to have health insurance at all income and education levels, but that the gap widened as education level decreased. The difference among Hispanics and non-Hispanic whites was about 18 percent among those who had a college education (78 percent versus 96 percent) but about 37 percent among those who had less than a high school education (77 percent versus 40 percent) (Agency for Healthcare Research and Quality, 2009).

Zuckerman and others compared access and use of health care services among American Indians/Alaska Natives (AIANs) and whites using data from the

1997 and 1999 National Survey of America's Families, a nationally representative survey of the nonelderly civilian population (Zuckerman, Haley, Roubideaux, and Lillie-Blanton, 2004). The study focused on differences in access to care across combinations of race/ethnicity and health insurance coverage, with an emphasis on the Indian Health Service, a system of hospitals and clinics established in 1955 for federally recognized AIANs, primarily on or near Native American reservations. The study classified coverage into the following: employer, public, Indian Health Service, and uninsured. Access to health care was quantified using various indicators.

After controlling for socioeconomic and demographic characteristics, the study found that insured whites and insured AIANs were similar in terms of health care services access and utilization. A significant difference was found, however, in the probability of having an emergency room visit in the past year, which was 29 percent for insured whites and 36 percent for insured AIANs. Rates of reported unmet health needs were the same among insured whites, insured AIANs, AIANs with Indian Health Service coverage and uninsured AIANs, but uninsured whites reported two-to-three times higher rates of unmet health needs (about 18 percent versus 9 percent of uninsured AIANs, and 6 percent of AIANs covered by the Indian Health Service). This suggests a protective effect of Indian Health Service coverage, although AIANs with Indian Health Service coverage did not always have the same rates of utilization as insured whites. The study found that AIAN women were less likely to have had a breast physical examination, a preventive service, in the last year.

Similar findings regarding multiple risk factors and access to care have been reported for children. Young minority children are as likely or more likely than white children to report having no health care visits to an office or clinic in the past twelve months (see Figure 4.4). With regard to health visits, white and African American children are about equally likely to be impacted by poverty. For African American children living in poverty, 11 percent report no health care visit, compared with 10 percent of those living at 200 percent of the FPL or higher. The difference for white children is slightly different (11 percent versus 9 percent). The effect of poverty is greater, however, for Hispanic children, with more than one in five (21 percent) of all poor Hispanic children having no health care visit, compared with about one in ten (13 percent) of those living at 200 percent of the FPL or higher.

A similar story exists for the combinations of insurance coverage, continuity of coverage, and poverty status. For children insured continuously for one year, there is little difference in lack of a health care visit between those living in poverty and those not (10 percent versus 9 percent among non-poor children). Among uninsured children, the effect of poverty is more striking: For children

FIGURE 4.4   No Health Care Visits in the Past Year Among
Children Under Eighteen Years of Age by Race/Ethnicity
and Insurance Coverage, by Poverty Status, 2006–2007

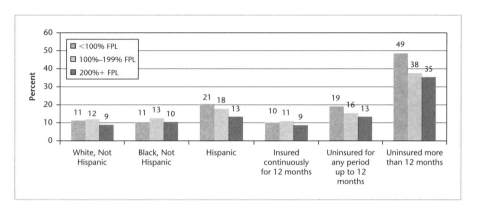

Source: National Center for Health Statistics (2009).

living in poverty and uninsured for one year or less, 19 percent lacked a health care visit, while only 13 percent of their non-poor counterparts lacked a health care visit. This difference increased dramatically for children uninsured for more than one year, with 35 percent of non-poor children lacking a health care visit, increasing to 38 percent for children living in near-poverty and 49 percent for those living in poverty.

Lacking health insurance also has a differential impact by race/ethnicity on health care visits. Researchers used data from the 2003 and 2004 MEPS to compare differences in access to health care for children aged one to eighteen years with private insurance, Medicaid, and no insurance coverage. The study found that across the board, having health insurance improved children's access to health care, though it did not eliminate disparities across racial/ethnic groups. White children with private insurance were 25.9 percentage points more likely than the uninsured to have a physician visit, compared with a difference of 16.6 percentage points for African Americans and 34.5 percentage points for Hispanics. Lacking health insurance also most strongly affected Hispanics in terms of having a regular source of care, with 50.3 percent of uninsured Hispanics lacking a regular source of care, compared with about 7.5 percent of privately and Medicaid-insured Hispanics (a difference of 42.8 percentage points). The difference was 23.6 percentage points for African Americans and only 14.4 percentage points for whites (Lillie-Blanton and others, 2009).

Employing a more complex model of multiple risk factors, a study examined the potential benefit to children ages birth to eighteen years of enrolling those who were currently uninsured but eligible for public health insurance (Stevens, Seid, and Halfon, 2006). Using the 2001 CHIS, the study examined three measures of access to care and health status for children who were insured by public insurance and those children who were uninsured but estimated to be eligible, based on family income, family size, and immigration status. The study made these comparisons at all levels of vulnerability, defined as the number of risk factors that children had, with the hypothesis that higher-risk children may gain the most from insurance. A risk profile was based on the following risk factors: nonwhite race/ethnicity, living in poverty, and having parents who did not graduate from high school and did not speak English.

The study found that uninsured but eligible children were less likely than publicly enrolled children to have a physician visit in the past year, a dental visit in the past year, and a regular source of care. Uninsured but eligible children with multiple risk factors experienced greater disparities than children with one or no risk factors. For example, enrollees were more likely than uninsured but eligible children to have a regular source of care among children with two, three, or four risk factors (differences of 26, 26, and 25 percentage points) compared with one risk factor (19 percentage points) and zero risk factors (12 percentage points). A similar pattern was found for dental visits and health status but not for physician visits. The study concluded that providing health insurance to children with the highest level of risk would lead to the greatest improvements in access to care.

Because the number of studies using risk profile type analyses in relation to health care access is limited, we conducted new analyses to examine the combined effects of three risk factors (race/ethnicity, income, and education level) on adults' access to care using the 2006 MEPS. The model we present reveals clear gradients associated with multiple risk factors in having a regular source of care and any health care visit in the past year (see Table 4.1). The table, ordered from top to bottom based on increasing risk profiles, shows that adult minorities, low-income adults, and those with less than a high school education (and particularly those with combinations of the risk factors) more often lack a regular source of care and a health care visit in the past year. While this pattern does not hold in every instance, a pattern is clearly identified.

In another new analysis of the 2007 NHIS, we assembled even more detailed models of vulnerability. We created risk profiles for adults based on income, health insurance, and regular source of care and examined them by race/ethnicity so that differences in the influences of risk factors across racial/ethnic

TABLE 4.1 National Risk Factors and Access to Health Care, Adults Eighteen and Over, 2006

Risk Factors				
Race/Ethnicity	Income	Education	No regular source of care (percent)	No health care visit in past year (percent)
White	High income	College and higher	15.1	17.4
		High school and less than college	14.8	21.8
		Less than high school	13.2	24.1
	Middle income	College and higher	19.1	18.3
		High school and less than college	19.0	24.2
		Less than high school	20.2	24.4
	Low income	College and higher	23.1	22.3
		High school and less than college	23.2	24.7
		Less than high school	21.2	25.2
Minority	High income	College and higher	25.0	25.7
		High school and less than college	26.9	35.2
		Less than high school	23.5	31.2
	Middle income	College and higher	29.8	34.5
		High school and less than college	33.8	41.3
		Less than high school	40.4	48.4
	Low income	College and higher	38.0	43.4
		High school and less than college	37.5	42.1
		Less than high school	40.3	45.3

Notes: Total sample size is 21,851 adults ages eighteen and over.

Source: New analysis of the 2006 Medical Expenditure Panel Survey Full-Year Consolidated Data File.

groups could be readily detected. The profiles were examined in relation to reports of delaying or missing medical care, prescriptions, mental health care, and dental care when they thought that it was needed. The analyses reveal that regardless of race/ethnicity, having low income, lacking insurance coverage, and not having a regular source of care combine to create substantial barriers to care (see Tables 4.2 to 4.4).

A substantial proportion of U.S. adults (about one in five) has multiple risk factors for unmet health care needs, and these combined risk factors create up to fivefold differences in reported rates of delayed or forgone care between the most vulnerable and least vulnerable profiles. Whites and African Americans (versus Asians and Hispanics) appeared most likely to be impacted by the combination of risk factors. This can be seen by examining the odds of forgone care for

TABLE 4.2   National Risk Factor Prevalence by Race/
Ethnicity, Adults Eighteen and Over, 2007

Risk Factors	Asian (percent)	Black (percent)	Hispanic (percent)	White (percent)
Low income (<200% FPL)*	25.1	42.1	51.4	19.5
Health insurance				
Private coverage	68.8	54.7	40.9	74.1
Public coverage	15.7	26.4	19.4	14.6
Uninsured*	15.5	18.9	39.7	11.3
No regular source of care*	17.1	13.8	27.6	12.0
Vulnerability risk profiles**				
0 risk factors	57.4	42.7	31.7	64.1
1 risk factor	28.8	39.0	33.9	26.0
2 risk factors	9.9	13.1	19.3	7.2
3 risk factors	3.9	5.2	15.1	2.8

Notes: Total sample size is 54,595 adults ages eighteen and over.

FPL = Federal poverty level.

*Denotes the category of the variable that was considered a risk factor and included in the risk profile.

**Risk profile is a count of the number of risk factors a person has based on being of low income, uninsured, and no regular source of care.

All risk factors and risk profiles for each racial/ethnic group were statistically different from those of whites by at least a significance level of $p<.001$.

Source: New analysis of the 2007 National Health Interview Survey.

TABLE 4.3   Risk Factors Predicting Unmet Needs, Adults Eighteen and Over, 2007
(Odds Ratios and 95 Percent Confidence Intervals)

	Delayed needed medical care	Did not get needed medical care	Delayed filing a prescription	Delayed mental health care	Delayed dental health care
Race/Ethnicity (versus white)					
Asian	**0.46**	**0.47**	**0.44**	**0.50**	**0.48**
	(0.34–0.63)	(0.32–0.68)	(0.31–0.64)	(0.29–0.85)	(0.36–0.64)
Black	**0.62**	**0.75**	0.89	**0.40**	**0.72**
	(0.54–0.73)	(0.64–0.89)	(0.76–1.04)	(0.30–0.54)	(0.62–0.83)
Hispanic	**0.54**	**0.56**	0.73	**0.47**	**0.64**
	(0.46–0.63)	(0.46–0.67)	(0.61–0.86)	(0.35–0.63)	(0.55–0.75)
Low income (versus higher)*	**1.69**	**1.86**	**1.76**	**2.09**	**1.79**
	(1.47–1.95)	(1.59–2.19)	(1.51–2.05)	(1.57–2.80)	(1.57–2.04)
Health insurance (versus private)					
Public coverage	1.03	**1.25**	**1.32**	**1.55**	**1.58**
	(0.87–1.23)	(1.03–1.51)	(1.10–1.58)	(1.12–2.14)	(1.35–1.86)
Uninsured*	**5.89**	**6.58**	**5.04**	**4.36**	**5.14**
	(5.07–6.84)	(5.55–7.80)	(4.28–5.94)	(3.27–5.81)	(4.46–5.92)
No regular source of care*	**1.38**	**1.46**	1.15	1.09	**1.26**
	(1.19–1.60)	(1.24–1.73)	(0.98–1.35)	(0.82–1.43)	(1.10–1.45)

Notes: Total sample size is 54,045 adults ages eighteen and over.

Models are adjusted for age, gender, marital status, education, employment, health status, and geographical region.

*Denotes the category of the variable that was considered a risk factor and included in the risk profile in Table 4.4.

Statistically significant results (at least $p < .05$) are bolded.

Source: New analysis of the 2007 National Health Interview Survey.

TABLE 4.4   Risk Profiles Predicting Unmet Needs, Adults Eighteen and Over, 2007 (Odds Ratios and 95 Percent Confidence Intervals)

	Delayed needed medical care	Did not get needed medical care	Delayed filing a prescription	Delayed mental health care	Delayed dental health care
White (versus zero)					
1 risk factor	2.44	3.22	2.61	2.85	2.71
	(2.06–2.90)	(2.61–3.98)	(2.13–3.21)	(1.99–4.07)	(2.28–3.22)
2 risk factors	7.80	10.71	6.69	6.01	6.68
	(6.29–9.67)	(8.38–13.69)	(5.24–8.54)	(4.07–8.88)	(5.42–8.23)
3 risk factors	13.97	20.56	10.93	8.41	11.78
	(10.37–18.83)	(15.01–28.16)	(7.99–14.96)	(5.22–13.55)	(8.90–15.59)
Black (versus zero)					
1 risk factor	2.56	2.97	2.21	3.42	2.28
	(1.72–3.81)	(1.90–4.64)	(1.49–3.27)	(1.02–11.46)	(1.59–3.26)
2 risk factors	10.58	11.16	7.04	12.58	7.35
	(7.09–15.80)	(7.10–17.54)	(4.68–10.60)	(3.93–40.19)	(4.95–10.92)
3 risk factors	17.60	19.66	9.75	20.46	12.48
	(10.65–29.07)	(11.48–33.66)	(5.86–16.21)	(5.84–71.68)	(7.70–20.24)
Hispanic (versus zero)					
1 risk factor	2.12	2.05	2.49	2.34	2.39
	(1.40–3.19)	(1.29–3.25)	(1.65–3.76)	(0.94–5.82)	(1.66–3.46)
2 risk factors	6.93	6.14	6.37	7.91	4.93
	(4.61–10.43)	(3.91–9.65)	(4.20–9.66)	(3.20–19.56)	(3.34–7.27)
3 risk factors	7.84	7.74	6.98	10.75	6.82
	(5.10–12.04)	(4.75–12.61)	(4.39–11.10)	(4.26–27.08)	(4.48–10.37)
Asian (versus zero)					
1 risk factor	2.91	3.82	1.70	4.59	4.50
	(1.25–6.75)	(1.23–11.89)	(0.47–6.14)	(0.85–24.70)	(2.20–9.22)
2 risk factors	10.15	11.84	7.66	8.77	8.15
	(4.17–24.70)	(3.85–36.39)	(2.57–22.88)	(2.18–35.25)	(3.51–18.91)
3 risk factors*	9.87	14.16	19.24	29.13	14.61
	(3.16–30.81)	(3.93–50.99)	(6.03–61.34)	(3.22–263.43)	(5.96–35.81)

Notes: Total sample size is 54,045 adults ages eighteen and over.

Models are adjusted for age, gender, marital status, education, employment, health status, and geographical region.

individuals with three risk factors versus zero risk factors. The odds of not getting medical care when it was needed, for example, was about twenty times higher for whites and African Americans and about fourteen times higher for Asians and seven times higher for Hispanics. This can also be graphically seen by looking at how the number of risk factors influences unmet needs for dental care (see Figure 4.5) for each racial/ethnic group.

Interestingly, our analyses show that whites were more likely than other racial and ethnic groups studied to report delayed or missed care for each type of health service. After controlling for other risk factors, minorities had 23 percent to 51 percent lower odds of reporting delayed or missed care than whites. Since minorities tend to have lower income, are more likely to be uninsured, are less likely to have a regular source of care, and have poorer health status than whites, it is difficult to believe that whites are truly more likely to have delayed or missed needed care. One possible explanation for this finding is that whites may have different ideas or perceptions of health needs or a greater belief in their ability to access care than other groups. Thus whites may feel more empowered to speak up or report problems when their perceived health needs are not being met. Whites might be over-reporting unmet needs, but given that many minorities tend to have poorer health, it may be that minorities are actually under-reporting unmet needs.

FIGURE 4.5   Risk Profiles and Delayed Dental Care in the Past Year, Adults Eighteen and Over, 2007

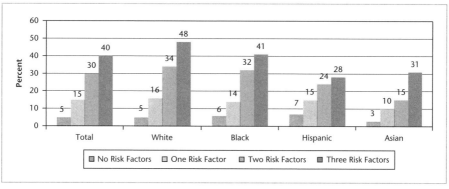

Source: New analysis of the 2007 National Interview Survey.

QUALITY OF HEALTH CARE

As for access to care, studies of multiple risk factors have also shown clear associations with the quality of health care that is received. While there are still a small number of analyses of health care quality that explore disparities using risk profiles or other methods to account for the interactions of risk factors, the studies that do exist provide some exceptional information about where and how those interested in improving health care quality might intervene.

One of the most commonly reported quality measures is the receipt of recommended preventive health care services. In one study, researchers examined the receipt of adult preventive services associated with combinations of health insurance coverage and the presence of a regular source of care (DeVoe, Fryer, Phillips, and Green, 2003). The study used nationally representative data to show that individuals with both insurance and a regular source of care were more likely to receive each service, compared with those without insurance and a regular source of care. For example, 85 percent of adults who had both insurance and a regular source received a blood pressure check in the past year versus only 46 percent of those without either insurance or a regular source. While 57 percent of women aged forty to sixty-nine years with both insurance and a regular source of care received a mammogram in the past year, just 16 percent of uninsured women without a regular source did so. Those with either a regular source or insurance but not both had intermediate levels of preventive services. This pattern was the same for all the services studied, including cholesterol screening, physical exam, dental checkup, a Pap test, and breast exam.

Poor preventive care may result in the advancement of undiagnosed disease. One key study examined the influence of community income levels, education levels, and race on diagnoses of advanced-stage breast cancer among 38,000 breast cancer patients in New York City (Merkin, Stevenson, and Powe, 2002). The study demonstrated that though lower community income and education levels were associated with late-stage diagnoses of breast cancer, the combination of the SES measures with race/ethnicity was associated with much higher rates. For white women living in areas with the lowest education levels and lowest income levels, the rates of advanced-stage breast cancer diagnoses were 10.6 percent and 11.2 percent. For African American women with the lowest education and in the lowest income areas, however, the rates were 34.8 percent and 43.8 percent.

A key component of getting good quality primary and preventive care is receiving the services in a timely way. Lack of timeliness can exacerbate illness or injury, result in emotional distress, or contribute to higher costs of care. The 2008 NHDR examined timeliness in the receipt of health services by combinations of race/ethnicity with income and with education, using the 2005 MEPS (Agency for Healthcare Research and Quality, 2009). The study showed the among adults who said they needed care right away for an illness, injury, or other condition in the past twelve months, high-income African Americans and whites had similar rates of not receiving the care as soon as they wanted or needed it (10 percent versus 8 percent). But as income decreased, the gap between African Americans and whites widened. For middle-income adults, the difference was six percentage points (18 percent versus 12 percent), and for adults living in poverty, the difference was nine percentage points (30 percent versus 21 percent). The effect of education was quite different, with African American and white adults who were lacking a high school education experiencing a smaller gap (23 percent versus 19 percent) than African American and white adults with a high school education (22 percent versus 11 percent) and some college education (20 percent versus 13 percent). The difference of effects between income and education suggest that higher education does not improve the ability of African American adults to obtain timely care the way that income does, and that education helps to increase awareness of (or expectations for) the need for medical care among African Americans (but not whites), or perhaps some combination of both.

To expand existing analyses of preventive care using more complex risk profiles, we conducted our own analyses of the 2006 MEPS. Risk factors in these analyses were based on educational status, income, health insurance, and regular source of care. Risk profiles were created from these risk factors and examined by race/ethnicity, so differences in the influence of risk factors across racial/ethnic groups could be detected. We examined five key preventive services recommended by the U.S. Preventive Services Task Force for appropriate age and gender groups: receipt of blood pressure and cholesterol screening, flu shot, Pap smear, mammogram, and dental check.

These analyses confirm the results of other studies demonstrating the independent associations of these key risk factors with lower receipt of preventive services. In contrast to other studies (Doty and Weech-Maldonado, 2003; Hegarty, Burchett, Gold, and Cohen, 2000; Stewart and Silverstein, 2002; Williams, Flocke, and Stange, 2001), our analyses suggest that racial/ethnic disparities in some preventive services are not fully explained by SES and access to care factors. Most important, this study demonstrates that a substantial proportion of adults have multiple risk factors (see Table 4.5) and that these risk factors create up to tenfold differences in preventive services received between the highest and lowest profiles, regardless of race/ethnicity (see Tables 4.6 and 4.7). Clear gradients were also seen when examining the various combinations that were used to create the profiles (see Figure 4.6).

TABLE 4.5   National Risk Factor Prevalence by Race/Ethnicity,
Adults Eighteen and Over, 2006

Risk Factors and Profiles	Asian (percent)	Black (percent)	Hispanic (percent)	White (percent)
Low income (<200% FPL)*	21.7	43.2	46.2	21.5
Education level				
Less than high school*	12.6	21.6	43.0	11.0
High school	32.1	55.8	40.9	50.6
College degree or higher	55.3	22.6	16.1	38.4
Health insurance				
Private	75.1	61.6	48.2	78.4
Medicaid	3.5	10.4	8.4	2.8
Medicare	7.3	10.7	7.5	8.4
Uninsured*	14.1	17.3	36.0	10.4
No regular source of care*	32.7	26.6	41.1	17.9
Vulnerability risk profile**				
0 risk factors	47.5	35.6	22.2	58.1
1 risk factor	32.2	32.8	25.8	28.1
2 risk factors	13.9	22.5	25.3	10.3
3 risk factors	5.3	7.6	18.7	3.1
4 risk factors	1.1	1.5	8.0	0.6

Notes: Total sample size is 21,362 adults ages eighteen and over.

FPL = Federal poverty level.

*Denotes the category of the variable that was considered a risk factor and included in the risk profile.

**Risk profile is a count of the number of risk factors based on low income, less than high school education, uninsured, and no regular source of care.

All risk factors and risk profiles for each racial/ethnic group were statistically different from those of whites by at least a significance level of $p<.01$.

Source: New analysis of the 2006 Medical Expenditure Panel Survey, Full-Year Consolidated Data File.

These findings are particularly salient when we consider that multiple risk factors are disproportionately found in African American and Hispanic populations. Approximately 78 percent of Hispanics and 64 percent of African Americans have one or more other risk factors, compared with about 50 percent of Asians and whites. Perhaps even more striking is that Hispanics are seven times and African Americans are three times more likely than whites to have the maximum risk factors (three or more) in this analysis. This suggests that addressing multiple risk factors will be essential to reducing the prevalence of racial/ethnic disparities in mortality associated with preventable diseases.

TABLE 4.6   Risk Factors and Preventive Services in the Past Year, Adults Eighteen and Over, 2006 (Odds Ratios and 95 Percent Confidence Intervals)

Risk Factors	Dental checkup	Flu shot	Blood pressure screening	Cholesterol screening	Pap smear	Mammogram
Race/Ethnicity (versus white)						
Asian	**0.72**	1.25	**0.52**	1.11	0.79	0.86
	(0.58–0.90)	(0.99–1.58)	(0.42–0.64)	(0.82–1.48)	(0.60–1.03)	(0.61–1.20)
Black	0.95	**0.69**	1.20	**1.71**	**1.51**	**1.38**
	(0.83–1.091)	(0.61–0.78)	(1.03–1.40)	(1.46–2.00)	(1.30–1.76)	(1.15–1.66)
Hispanic	**0.85**	0.87	0.90	**1.41**	1.06	**1.25**
	(0.74–0.98)	(0.74–1.01)	(0.78–1.03)	(1.17–1.70)	(0.90–1.26)	(1.00–1.55)
Low income (versus higher)*	**0.53**	**0.90**	**0.86**	**0.71**	0.86	**0.71**
	(0.47–0.59)	(0.82–0.99)	(0.76–0.98)	(0.60–0.85)	(0.74–1.00)	(0.58–0.85)
Education less than high school* (versus high school graduate or higher)	**0.53**	**0.76**	**0.65**	**0.66**	**0.71**	**0.74**
	(0.47–0.59)	(0.67–0.85)	(0.55–0.76)	(0.55–0.80)	(0.61–0.83)	(0.59–0.93)
Health insurance (versus private)						
Medicaid	**0.66**	0.94	1.15	1.30	**1.35**	0.95
	(0.53–0.81)	(0.76–1.16)	(0.90–1.48)	(0.96–1.77)	(1.10–1.65)	(0.69–1.29)
Medicare	**0.54**	1.03	**1.33**	**1.57**	0.87	0.80
	(0.46–0.63)	(0.88–1.20)	(1.02–1.73)	(1.09– 2.25)	(0.62–1.23)	(0.60–1.08)

(Continued)

TABLE 4.6 (Continued)

Risk Factors	Dental checkup	Flu shot	Blood pressure screening	Cholesterol screening	Pap smear	Mammogram
Uninsured*	**0.37**	**0.41**	**0.45**	**0.51**	**0.53**	**0.44**
	(0.32–0.42)	(0.35–0.49)	(0.39–0.53)	(0.42–0.63)	(0.44–0.63)	(0.35–0.56)
No regular source of care*	**0.55**	**0.52**	**0.34**	**0.32**	**0.53**	**0.37**
	(0.50–0.60)	(0.45–0.59)	(0.31–0.39)	(0.28–0.36)	(0.46–0.61)	(0.30–0.46)

Notes: Total sample size is 21,362 adults ages eighteen and over.

Blood pressure screening is limited to ages twenty-one and over.

Cholesterol screening is limited to women ages forty-five to sixty-four and men ages thirty-five to sixty-four.

Pap smear is limited to women ages eighteen to sixty-four.

Mammogram is limited to women ages forty to sixty-nine.

The model is adjusted for age and gender (when appropriate), health status, marital status, employment status, and managed care enrollment.

*Denotes the category of the variable that was considered a risk factor and included in the risk profile in Table 4.8.

Statistically significant results (at least $p<.05$) are bolded.

Source: New analysis of the 2006 Medical Expenditure Panel Survey, Full-Year Consolidated Data File.

Risk Profiles	Dental checkup	Flu shot	Blood pressure screening	Cholesterol screening	Pap smear	Mammogram
White (versus zero)						
1 risk factor	0.43	0.67	0.52	0.52	0.58	0.48
	(0.38–0.48)	(0.59–0.75)	(0.44–0.61)	(0.44–0.62)	(0.49–0.68)	(0.39–0.59)
2 risk factors	0.18	0.42	0.25	0.24	0.39	0.27
	(0.15–0.21)	(0.35–0.51)	(0.21–0.31)	(0.18–0.31)	(0.31–0.49)	(0.20–0.37)
3 or more risk factors	0.11	0.17	0.12	0.09	0.17	0.09
	(0.08–0.15)	(0.12–0.26)	(0.09–0.17)	(0.05–0.14)	(0.12–0.24)	(0.04–0.19)
Black (versus zero)						
1 risk factor	0.54	0.64	0.53	0.51	0.66	0.43
	(0.44–0.65)	(0.50–0.82)	(0.39–0.71)	(0.39–0.66)	(0.49–0.89)	(0.31–0.60)
2 risk factors	0.34	0.62	0.33	0.41	0.42	0.33
	(0.27–0.42)	(0.49–0.79)	(0.24–0.46)	(0.27–0.63)	(0.28–0.61)	(0.23–0.47)
3 or more risk factors	0.18	0.38	0.11	0.06	0.24	0.16
	(0.13–0.26)	(0.24–0.60)	(0.08–0.15)	(0.03–0.11)	(0.16–0.36)	(0.09–0.27)
Hispanic (versus zero)						
1 risk factor	0.60	0.59	0.57	0.57	1.15	0.60
	(0.48–0.75)	(0.46–0.75)	(0.40–0.80)	(0.39–0.83)	(0.83–1.57)	(0.42–0.85)
2 risk factors	0.33	0.45	0.32	0.39	0.92	0.58
	(0.26–0.42)	(0.34–0.60)	(0.23–0.44)	(0.27–0.58)	(0.66–1.28)	(0.39–0.85)

(Continued)

TABLE 4.7   (Continued)

Risk Profiles	Dental checkup	Flu shot	Blood pressure screening	Cholesterol screening	Pap smear	Mammogram
3 or more risk factors	**0.18**	**0.20**	**0.18**	**0.18**	**0.57**	**0.35**
	(0.13–0.24)	(0.14–0.28)	(0.13–0.26)	(0.11–0.27)	(0.40–0.82)	(0.22–0.58)
Asian (versus zero)						
1 risk factor	**0.41**	1.02	**0.53**	**0.36**	**0.61**	**0.35**
	(0.30–0.56)	(0.68–1.54)	(0.35–0.80)	(0.23–0.56)	(0.39–0.96)	(0.23–0.54)
2 risk factors	**0.16**	0.85	**0.21**	**0.19**	**0.48**	**0.27**
	(0.09–0.27)	(0.45–1.57)	(0.12–0.37)	(0.07–0.49)	(0.24–0.97)	(0.13–0.53)
3 or more risk factors	**0.10**	0.76	**0.11**	**0.04**	**0.25**	**0.11**
	(0.05–0.20)	(0.29–1.98)	(0.04–0.33)	(0.01–0.13)	(0.14–0.44)	(0.05–0.24)

Notes: Total sample size is 21,362 adults ages eighteen and over.

Blood pressure screening is limited to ages twenty-one and over.

Cholesterol screening is limited to women ages forty-five to sixty-four and men ages thirty-five to sixty-four.

Pap smear is limited to women ages eighteen to sixty-four.

Mammogram is limited to women ages forty to sixty-nine.

The model is adjusted for age and gender (when appropriate), health status, marital status, employment status, and managed care enrollment.

Statistically significant results (at least $p < .05$) are bolded.

Source: New analysis of the 2006 Medical Expenditure Panel Survey, Full-Year Consolidated Data File.

FIGURE 4.6   Combinations of Risk Factors and Receipt of a Flu Shot in the Past Year, Adults Eighteen and Over, 2006

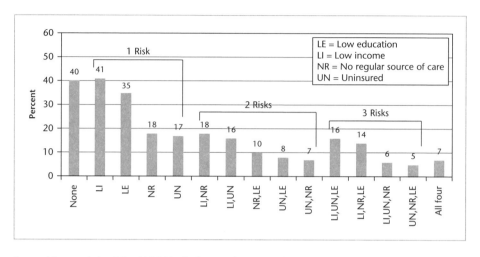

Source: New analysis of the 2006 Medical Expenditure Panel Survey, Full-Year Consolidated Data File.

Suggestive of some improvement is the finding that before and after adjustment for SES and potential access factors, African Americans and Hispanics were as or more likely than whites to report having a cholesterol screening, and African American women were more likely to receive a Pap smear. These findings are corroborated by other research (Jones, Caplan, and Davis, 2003; Martin, Calle, Wingo, and Heath, 1996; Sambamoorthi and McAlpine, 2003) that shows higher Pap smear screening and mammography rates among African American and Hispanic women. In these studies, the higher rates have been attributed to the effectiveness of targeted education and screening programs or to perceived higher risk for disease among these groups, creating a greater awareness among providers of the need for screening this population. Similar to other studies (Calle, Flanders, Thun, and Martin, 1993; Goel and others, 2003; Tu, Taplin, Barlow, and Boyko, 1999), Asians were least likely to report receiving most preventive services despite fewer risk factors. This has been attributed to low perceived risk of disease, language issues, and acculturation (Han, Williams, and Harrison, 2000; Tang, Solomon, and McCracken, 2000; Yu, Hong, and Seetoo, 2003).

Similar results are seen in studies associating sociodemographic risks with preventive care for children. Researchers used the general vulnerability model to study the relationship of multiple risk factors with measures of health care access and quality for children ages birth to eighteen years (Stevens, Seid, Mistry, and Halfon, 2006). Using the 2001 CHIS, the study counted non-white race/ethnicity, living in poverty, having parents who did not graduate from high school, being uninsured, and not speaking English as risk factors, which were examined individually and as a risk profile.

The study showed that a striking 43 percent of children in California had two or more risk factors for poor access and quality. A higher number of risk factors was associated with poorer access (such as a lower likelihood of a physician and dental visit in the past year and a lower likelihood of lacking a regular source of care) but with the receipt of more *preventive counseling* on a range of health risk behaviors. For example, compared with children with no risks, those with two risk factors were 23 percent more likely than those with zero risk factors to lack a regular source of care, but 24 percent more likely to be counseled on STDs, 27 percent more likely to be counseled on smoking, 45 percent more likely to be counseled on alcohol and marijuana use, 59 percent more likely to be counseled on use of seatbelts, and 85 percent more likely to be counseled on violence. These patterns were even greater for children with three or more risk factors. From this analysis, it seems that physicians are correctly targeting preventive counseling to children perceived as higher risk, though all children and their families should certainly be counseled on these topics.

Studies have explored the impact of multiple risk factors on other types of health care quality, including more qualitative, interpersonal aspects of care. The 2008 National Health Care Disparities Report examined patient-provider communication as a reflection of patient-centered care, examining patients who said their provider only sometimes or never does one or more of the following: carefully listens to them, communicates clearly, has respect for what they say, or spends enough time with them (Agency for Healthcare Research and Quality, 2009). Across all education levels, African Americans, Hispanics, and Asians were more likely to report poor communication with health care providers than whites. The gap in quality of communication between whites and other groups was predictably smallest among the most highly educated adults and largest among those with the least education. Comparing African Americans and whites that did not graduate from high school, the difference in reporting communication problems was about 6 percent (18 percent versus 12 percent). The difference between African Americans and whites was 4 percent (13 percent versus 9 percent) for those who graduated from high school and just 1 percent (9 percent versus 8 percent) for those with some college education. The 2008 NHDR reported similar patterns in communication by race/ethnicity and income for children.

In a classic study, Shi and others, using data from the 1996–1997 Community Tracking Study Household Survey, examined the influence of race/ethnicity, poverty status, and health status on the reported quality of adult interpersonal relationships with their health care providers (Shi, Forrest, Von Schrader, and Ng, 2003). The interpersonal patient-provider relationship was based on responses to questions about interpersonal trust, communication, and competence. The researchers grouped individuals into profiles of risk and demonstrated reductions in patient-provider relationship ratings associated with increasing vulnerability profiles (see Figure 4.7). The study also demonstrated gradients in office wait times by number of risks, such that 73 percent of whites with high income and good health waited thirty minutes or less to be seen, compared with the worst rate of 41 percent among Hispanics with low income and poor health.

To further explore more complex models of risk, we conducted new analyses of the 2007 CHIS to examine three risk factors (English language ability, income, and education level) in relation to health literacy measures. The analyses demonstrate gradients associated with multiple risk factors in adult reports of having difficulty in understanding literature from a doctor and in understanding prescription bottle instructions (see Table 4.8). Not surprisingly, problems with health literacy are particularly pronounced for adults who speak English poorly. For example, those who speak English very well, have high income, and graduated high school reported low rates of having difficulty understanding literature and prescription bottle instructions (9.7 percent and 2.6 percent, respectively), compared with those who do not speak English very well, have low income, and did not graduate from

FIGURE 4.7   Ratings of Interpersonal Patient-Provider Relationships among Adults, by Race/Ethnicity, Income, and Health Status

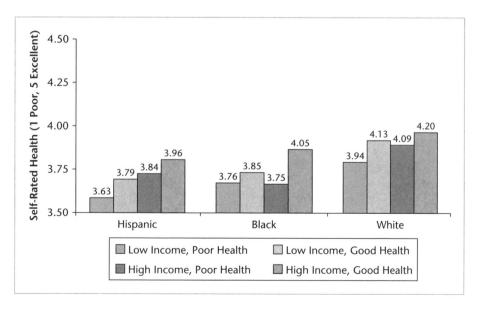

Source: Shi and others (2003).

TABLE 4.8   Risk Factors and Health Literacy in California,
Adults Eighteen and Over, 2007

| Risk Factors | | | | |
English Language Speaking Ability	Income	Education	Difficulty Understanding Literature from Doctor (percent)	Difficulty Understanding Prescription Bottles (percent)
Very well	Higher income	High school graduate or higher	9.5	2.6
		Less than high school	11.5	3.5
	Lower income	High school graduate or higher	12.5	4.3
		Less than high school	23.6	10.2
Well	Higher income	High school graduate or higher	13.9	8.5
		Less than high school	19.2	7.9
	Lower income	High school graduate or higher	15.3	11.5
		Less than high school	27.3	12.6
Not very well	Higher income	High school graduate or higher	25.7	19.3
		Less than high school	33.8	18.4
	Lower income	High school graduate or higher	33.5	21.7
		Less than high school	43.7	26.3

Notes: Total sample size is 51,048 adults ages eighteen and over.
English language speaking ability is among adults who report speaking a language other than (or in addition to) English at home.

Source: New analysis of the 2007 California Health Interview Survey.

high school (43.7 percent and 26.3 percent, respectively). These results suggest that providers need to be concerned about how well people with these risk factors are able to understand their treatment recommendations and should adjust their communication appropriately. For these higher-risk individuals, simply handing out literature and stating instructions for medication use once are probably not enough to ensure that families adhere to their therapies.

Another study of a range of more qualitative measures of health care quality used the 2003 National Survey of Children's Health to examine how the quality of a primary care medical home for children ages birth to seventeen years varied according risk profiles (Stevens, Seid, Pickering, and Tsai, 2009). The study created risk profiles based on non-white race/ethnicity, income below 200 percent of FPL, parent education less than high school, and non-English-language usage. Medical home quality was measured according to five dimensions: accessibility, *continuity of care*, comprehensiveness of the services received, the degree of *family-centered care*, and how well coordinated care was between primary and specialty care for children who needed such care. A total medical home quality score was also created.

The study found that all of the studied risk factors were associated with poorer quality medical home dimensions and a lower total medical home score. Summarized through *risk profiles*, children who experienced all five risk factors had 93 percent lower odds of a quality medical home, compared with children without any risk factors. Interestingly, using the median score as a cut-off to define higher quality versus lower quality, the study found that only about 64 percent of children with no risk factors had a higher-quality medical home, which suggests that there is room for improvement in delivering high-quality primary care even for children who are traditionally not considered vulnerable. By comparison, just 8 percent of children with all five risk factors had a higher-quality medical home. The risk factors most strongly associated with poor quality were lacking health insurance coverage and living in or near poverty, and particularly the combination of both risks. This suggests that reforms to increase coverage and to help families out of poverty can make the greatest improvements in gaining access to a quality medical home.

Overall, improving the quality of care for vulnerable populations will require multifaceted clinical and policy interventions. While research is needed to determine how to intervene for particular risk groups most effectively, a range of efforts that might be adopted could simultaneously include identifying the risk groups, providing education about how to best use health services and what to expect, linking vulnerable populations with accessible providers who are experienced in serving these populations and who serve as a quality medical home, and potentially reducing cost sharing for these services. Such multifaceted approaches address these interactive influences of multiple risks and may better help reduce disparities.

HEALTH STATUS

The cumulative impact of multiple risk factors can also be seen on health status and other measures of health. Using data from the 2006 MEPS, we assessed differences in perceived health status by race and ethnicity and income. The impact of income on health status was found to be very different across racial/ethnic groups (Figure 4.8). For example, having lower income (defined as below 200 percent of FPL) created a gap in adults reporting fair or poor health status of fourteen percentage points for both African Americans and whites (24 percent versus 10 percent for African Americans and 21 percent versus 7 percent for whites). Income only created gaps of six percentage points for American Indians and Alaska Natives and Hispanics. Asians, who were least likely to report fair or poor health status, had only one percentage point difference between those with higher and lower incomes (6 percent versus 7 percent).

We also conducted two new analyses to include more complex risk profiles in understanding health status. In the first new analysis, we used data from the 2006 MEPS to analyze the relationship between multiple risk factors and self-perceived physical and mental health status among adults (see Table 4.9). We examined combinations of income, education, and race/ethnicity and found that physical health status and mental health status declined for those with low education and to a lesser extent for low-income individuals. Combinations of these risk factors

FIGURE 4.8   Fair or Poor Health Status by Race and Ethnicity and Income, Adults Eighteen to Sixty-Four, 2006

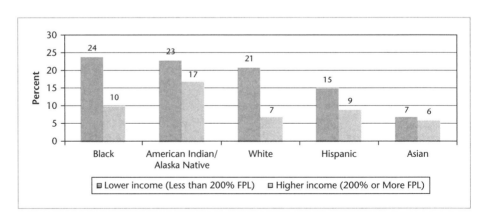

Source: New analysis of the 2006 Medical Expenditure Panel Survey, Full-Year Consolidated Data File.

TABLE 4.9   National Risk Factors and Self-Reported Health Status,
Adults Eighteen and Over, 2006

Risk Factors				
Income	Education	Race/ethnicity	Poor Physical Health Status (percent)	Poor Mental Health Status (percent)
High income	College and higher	Minority	5.1	2.0
		White	5.7	3.3
	High school and less than college	Minority	7.4	4.6
		White	9.0	4.9
	Less than high school	Minority	15.1	6.0
		White	13.3	9.1
Middle income	College and higher	Minority	9.4	2.6
		White	7.1	4.2
	High school and less than college	Minority	10.6	5.8
		White	12.2	5.9
	Less than high school	Minority	17.2	8.8
		White	17.1	8.5
Low income	College and higher	Minority	9.2	5.3
		White	17.2	11.8
	High school and less than college	Minority	18.0	11.6
		White	22.4	14.0
	Less than high school	Minority	26.0	13.4
		White	31.3	17.8

Notes: Total sample size is 22,058 adults ages eighteen and over.

Source: New analysis of the 2006 Medical Expenditure Panel Survey, Full-Year Consolidated Data File.

were associated with increases in poor physical and mental health statuses, though adults who were of minority background seemed to do slightly better than whites at most levels of income and education.

Our second new analysis compiled risk profiles to examine the health status of children, using data from California. The analyses used parent-reported data on 9,913 children from birth to eleven years of age from the 2007 CHIS. Each risk factor was examined alone and as a risk profile constructed as a count of six risk factors: minority race/ethnicity, family income less than 200 percent of the FPL, parent education less than high school, child uninsured status, noncitizenship, and language other than English. The results (see Table 4.10) suggest that

TABLE 4.10   Risk Factors and Health Status, Children Eleven Years and Under, 2007

	Frequency Among the Child Population (percent)	Excellent or Very Good Health Status (percent)	Excellent or Very Good Health Status** (odds ratio)
Child race/ethnicity			
White	30.1	90.9	(ref)
Asian/Pacific Islander*	9.9	77.3	0.34
African American*	5.5	75.5	0.31
Latino*	49.6	67.3	0.20
Other*	4.9	85.8	0.60
Poverty level			
Less than 100% FPL*	21.0	54.8	0.15
100-199% of FPL*	20.6	68.0	0.26
200-299% of FPL	13.1	83.4	0.62
300% or more	45.3	89.1	(ref)
Insurance coverage			
Private	4.4	91.1	(ref)
Uninsured*	5.1	73.9	0.23
Medi-Cal	28.5	58.3	0.13
Healthy Families	6.5	65.6	0.19
Other	55.6	86.7	0.63
Education of respondent			
Less than high school*	18.4	51.0	0.13
High school graduate*	22.4	73.4	0.34
Some college*	23.1	81.4	0.55
College graduate	36.1	89.1	(ref)
Citizenship status			
Child and parent both citizens	65.9	85.4	(ref)
Parent noncitizen*	30.6	60.4	0.25
Child and parent both noncitizens*	3.5	58.1	0.26
Only English language at home			
Yes	50.1	87.5	(ref)
No*	49.9	65.7	0.27
Vulnerability risk profiles			
0 risk factors	20.5	92.2	(ref)
1 risk factor	21.2	89.1	0.69

(Continued)

TABLE 4.10   (Continued)

	Frequency Among the Child Population (percent)	Excellent or Very Good Health Status (percent)	Excellent or Very Good Health Status** (odds ratio)
2 risk factors	18.7	81.7	0.37
3 risk factors	12.4	75.9	0.26
4 risk factors	12.3	57.3	0.11
5+ risk factors	14.8	48.7	0.08

Notes: Total sample size is 9,913 children ages eleven years and under.

*Indicates the risk factors included in the combined vulnerability risk profile.

**Model was adjusted for child age and gender.

All results were statistically significantly different from the reference group at $p < .01$ or greater.

Source: New analysis of the 2007 California Health Interview Survey.

a considerable proportion of all children in California (40 percent) have three or more of these risk factors for poor health. Each risk factor was independently associated with poorer child health status, and the risk profile revealed a strong association between the number of risk factors and reported child health status. The odds of being in excellent or very good health compared to good, fair, or poor health decreased for each additional risk: one risk (31 percent lower odds), two risks (63 percent lower odds), three risks (74 percent lower odds), four risks (89 percent lower odds), and five or more risks (92 percent lower odds) compared to no risks.

A number of multiple risk factor studies have also been conducted for measures of mortality. Figure 4.9 shows the combined effects of race/ethnicity and maternal education on infant mortality rates. The figure reveals large disparities in infant mortality across racial and ethnic groups and shows the added effects of low maternal education. For example, the African American infant mortality rate increase is the highest among racial/ethnic groups, but education level contributes to a 30 percent difference of 3.4 deaths per 1,000 live births between mothers with less than a high school education compared with those with some college education (thirteen or more years of education). Whites tend to have lower infant mortality rates than African Americans, but the impact of maternal education appears to be greater, more than doubling the mortality rate (from 4.1 to 9.3) as maternal education decreases. Hispanics and Asians have the lowest rates of infant mortality, but their rates are not as strongly affected by maternal education as whites, with differences of 13 and 18 percent, respectively.

FIGURE 4.9   Infant Mortality by Race/Ethnicity and Maternal Education, 2005

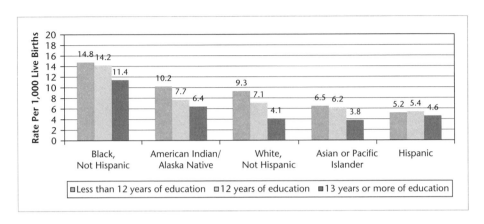

Source: National Center for Health Statistics (2009).

To better understand the effects of race and poverty on patterns of mortality, a classic study conducted by Geronimus and others analyzed 1990 standardized mortality rates for African Americans and white, poor and non-poor adults, ages fifteen to sixty-four, living in eight geographic areas in the United States (Geronimus and others, 1996). In each geographic area, data were analyzed from residents of an area of persistent poverty and residents from another of higher income. The mortality rates for each of the eight groups were compared to national standardized 1990 death rates for whites; the results for men and women are shown in Table 4.9. *Multivariate analysis* of the data showed that the likelihood of a fifteen-year-old African American girl in Harlem surviving to forty-five years of age was the same as a typical white girl anywhere in the United States surviving to sixty-five years. For African American boys in Harlem, the likelihood of surviving to age forty-five was even lower.

Several studies have shown that when SES is taken into account, the disparities between African Americans and whites for various health measures may diminish but are not eliminated. Researchers examined the association of race and social class with stroke mortality among a ten-year cohort of North Carolina men ages thirty-five to eighty-four (Casper and others, 1997). They defined social class by occupation in four categories: primary white collar (executive, managerial, administrative), secondary white collar (sales and clerical), primary blue collar (production, craft, and repair), and secondary blue collar (services, machine operators, transportation, and farming). The researchers concluded that both lower social class and

TABLE 4.11   Mortality Rates Among Black and White Populations in Selected Geographic Areas, 1989–1990 (per 100,000 Resident Population)

	Annual Male Death Rates	Annual Female Death Rates	Male SMR (95% CI)	Female SMR (95% CI)
Whites	417	225	1.00	1.00
Low-income area				
Lower East Side	625	250	1.50(1.40–1.61)	1.11(0.99–1.26)
Detroit	838	428	2.01(1.88–2.15)	1.90(1.73–2.09)
Appalachia	574	311	1.38(1.27–1.49)	1.39(1.24–1.55)
High-income area				
Queens	363	190	0.87(0.80–0.95)	0.84(0.76–0.94)
Sterling Heights	172	121	0.41(0.36–0.47)	0.54(0.45–0.64)
West Kentucky	360	203	0.86(0.78–0.95)	0.91(0.80–1.03)
Blacks	791	439	1.90	1.95
Low-income area				
Harlem	1,713	759	4.11(3.91–4.32)	3.38(3.15–3.62)
Central Detroit	1,163	580	2.79(2.67–2.92)	2.58(2.42–2.75)
Watts	1,216	584	2.92(2.77–3.07)	2.60(2.43–2.79)
High-income area				
Queens-Bronx	491	242	1.18(1.10–1.26)	1.08(0.98–1.26)
Northwest Detroit	691	335	1.66(1.56–1.76)	1.49(1.37–1.62)
Crenshaw	781	347	1.87(1.75–2.00)	1.87(1.75–2.00)

Note: SMR is standardized mortality ratio.

Source: Geronimus and others (1996).

being a minority placed individuals at greater risk for premature stroke mortality. For all races, the highest rates of premature stroke mortality occurred among the lowest social classes. African American men in the lowest social class were 2.6 times more likely to die than African American men in the highest social class, and for whites this risk was about 2.3 times higher. Illustrating the influence of multiple risk factors even further, the study showed that within each social class group, there were significant differences in rates of premature stroke mortality between African American and white men: the stroke mortality ratio ranged from 4.0 in the highest social class to 4.9 in the lowest social class. This increasing mortality ratio across social classes suggests that race, ethnicity, and social class combine to influence rates of mortality above and beyond the effects of either race or social class alone.

Using the same population, researchers also found that an observed decrease in mortality from coronary heart disease seen over time has not benefited African

American men of lower social class to the same degree as white and African American men of higher social classes, controlling for age. For all social classes, the age-adjusted mortality rates from coronary heart disease were higher for African American men compared with white men. Although there was a clear decline in heart disease mortality rates for white men across all social classes, only African American men in the highest social class had any decline. The researchers point to the importance of targeting public health efforts to vulnerable subgroups and highlight the needs of addressing multiple risk factors (Barnett, Armstrong, and Casper, 1999). Similar findings regarding social class and race/ethnicity have been reported with regard to asthma prevalence among adults and children (Grant, Lyttle, and Weiss, 2000; Miller, 2000).

Several previous studies among children have shown that the accumulation of risk factors influences health status and child development. They demonstrate an association between higher social class (measured as a combination of parent education and employment levels) and several domains of both child and adolescent health status (Starfield, Riley, Witt, and Robertson, 2002; Starfield, Robertson, and Riley, 2002). In addition, Sameroff and others (1987) and later Furstenberg and others (1999) demonstrated strong associations of the number of risks and adolescent social-emotional health, psychological adjustment, academic performance, and even IQ scores. The selected risk factors were chosen to reflect risks related to family processes (parent investment and discipline), parent characteristics (education, mental health), family structure (marital status, welfare receipt), community factors (social resources and neighborhood SES), and peer networks (antisocial versus prosocial). These studies showed that it is not only family risk factors that have an influence on child health but also peer, neighborhood, and community risk factors.

A more recent study used the 2003 National Survey of Children's Health to examine the association of multiple social risk factors with four child health outcomes: overall health status, dental health, socioemotional health, and overweight status (Larson, Russ, Crall, and Halfon, 2008). Parents of children aged seventeen and younger were interviewed. Risk factors for poor child health outcomes included parent education of less than high school, family income less than 200 percent of FPL, not a two-parent household, African American/Hispanic race/ethnicity, uninsured status, family conflict, low maternal mental health, and living in an unsafe neighborhood. Each risk factor was independently tested as a predictor of child health outcomes, and the risk factors were summed to create a social risk index.

The study found that nearly every risk factor was independently associated with poor health outcomes. In analyzing the social risk indices, the study found that an increasing number of social risk factors saw concomitant worsening of child health across all health outcomes. For example, 5 percent of children with zero risk factors were reported to have suboptimal health status compared with 26 percent with four risk factors and 46 percent of children with six or more risk factors. An even steeper gradient was found for dental health (measured as the condition of the child's teeth): 14 percent of children with zero risk factors had suboptimal condition of teeth, while this was true for 64 percent of children with six or more risk factors. The gradients are less dramatic for child socioemotional health and overweight, with about a threefold and twofold increase, respectively, for children with six or more risk factors, compared with zero risk factors.

The multiple risk factor approach is also increasingly seen in studies of mental health. For example, researchers sought to examine multiple risk factors as predictors for psychiatric disorders among adolescents in a prospective study of households in the Houston metropolitan area (Roberts, Roberts, and Chan, 2009). Psychiatric disorders included anxiety, mood, eating and disruptive disorders, substance abuse, and attention deficit hyperactivity disorder. Risk factors included demographics and social status (age, gender, total family income, perceived socioeconomic status), personal resources (self-esteem, coping, mastery), social resources (social support, family functioning), and stressors (neighborhood stress, school stress, economic strain, family stress). Each risk factor was independently tested for association with psychiatric disorder prevalence and incidence. The number of risk factors was then added to estimate the cumulative effects of multiple risk factors.

The study found that the specific predictors varied by psychiatric disorder. Although there was much variation among the disorders, at least six and as many as thirteen of the nineteen measured risk factors were associated with each of the psychiatric disorders. The presence of multiple risk factors increased the risk for psychiatric disorders. For example, compared to adolescents with no risk factors, those with three or more risk factors had more than sixteen times the odds of having an anxiety disorder, and those with eight risk factors had more than forty-seven times the odds. The odds of having a mood disorder with ten risk factors versus none was more than fiftyfold. Finally, the most pronounced increase was seen in the odds of having two or more psychiatric disorders diagnosed in the past year: adolescents with seven risk factors had about sixty-seven times the odds as those with zero or one risk factor.

Maternal mental health is the focus of several studies using a multiple risk factor approach (Mistry and others, 2007; Popp, Spinrad, and Smith, 2008). One study examined cumulative risk as a predictor of depression in mothers of infants born preterm or at a low birth weight (Poehlmann, Schwichtenberg, Bolt, and Dilworth-Bart, 2009). In this longitudinal study, families were assessed immediately prior to hospital discharge and then at four, nine, sixteen, and twenty-four months. A cumulative risk index was created based on maternal sociodemographic and infant risk factors. Sociodemographic risks were based on maternal age and years of education, family income, number of dependents, and maternal race. Infant risks were determined by whether or not the infant experienced ventilation, was born at less than 1000 grams, was part of a multiple birth, and spent more than thirty days in the hospital. At each time point, mothers were assessed for depressive symptoms. The study found that mothers with high sociodemographic and infant risk indices experienced more depressive symptoms in the first two years of their child's lives than mothers with lower risk indices.

In another new analysis (see Table 4.12), substantial gradients were found in health status and *developmental risk* for young children according to risk profiles.

TABLE 4.12   Association of Risk Factors and Profiles with Health Status and Developmental Risk, Children Under Three Years, 2000 and 2007 (Odds Ratios and 95 Percent Confidence Intervals)

Risk Factors and Profiles	Excellent or Very Good Health Status 2007	At Risk for Developmental Delay 2000
Child race/ethnicity (ref: white)		
Black*	0.61	1.22
	(0.43–0.88)	(0.81–1.85)
Latino*	0.33	1.53
	(0.25–0.45)	(1.08–2.19)
Other*	0.66	1.46
	(0.37–1.16)	(0.69–3.06)
Family social class** (versus Higher)		
Lower social class*	0.29	1.53
	(0.21–0.39)	(0.94–2.48)
Middle social class*	0.53	1.19
	(0.38–0.74)	(0.81–1.74)
Insurance coverage (ref: private)		
Uninsured*	0.48	1.05
	(0.30–0.77)	(0.68–1.64)
Public (Medicaid/CHIP)	0.35	1.37
	(0.27–0.46)	(0.87–2.16)
Other	0.34	2.75
	(0.19–0.63)	(1.59–4.74)

(Continued)

TABLE 4.12   (Continued)

Risk Factors and Profiles	Excellent or Very Good Health Status 2007	At Risk for Developmental Delay 2000
Maternal mental health (ref. Good health)		
Moderate mental health	—	**1.77** (1.23–2.54)
Poor mental health*	—	**1.47** (1.04–2.09)
Risk profiles** (ref: zero)		
1 risk factor	**0.52** (0.38–0.71)	1.08 (0.65–1.76)
2 risk factors	**0.25** (0.17–0.35)	**1.95** (1.18–3.20)
3 risk factors	**0.18** (0.09–0.37)	**2.86** (1.66–4.94)
4 risk factors	—	**8.56** (3.95–18.59)

Notes: Total sample size is 2,962 children ages 0–35 months for health status and 2,068 children ages 0–35 months for developmental risk.

*Indicates the risk factors included in the combined vulnerability risk profile.

**Social class was measured by parent education alone for health status, and was measured using a combination of income and education for developmental delay.

***Maternal mental health was included in the risk profile for developmental delay only.

Both models were adjusted for child age and gender; the developmental risk model was additionally adjusted for maternal age and employment status and single-parent household.

Statistically significant results (at least $p < .05$) are bolded.

Source: New analysis of the 2007 California Health Interview Survey for health status and Stevens (2006) for developmental risk.

Data on health status were analyzed from the 2007 CHIS and data on developmental risk are reported from a study that analyzed the 2000 National Survey of Early Childhood Health conducted by the National Center for Health Statistics (Stevens, 2006). The risk profile in these analyses encompasses four risk factors: non-white child race/ethnicity, lower family social class (composed of parent education alone for health status and a combination of income and education for developmental delay), lack of child health insurance, and poor maternal mental health. General health status was measured with a five-point Likert-type scale (from poor to excellent). Risk for developmental problems was measured with an instrument that assesses parent concerns regarding child development and accurately identifies children at risk of developmental delays (Glascoe, 2003). Logistic regressions predicting these outcomes are presented, adjusting for child age and gender, maternal age and employment, and single parent household.

These analyses suggest that child minority race/ethnicity, lower and middle social class, being uninsured or having public insurance, and poor maternal mental health were independently associated with the outcomes. Young children with two risk factors had 52 percent lower odds of being in excellent or very good health status than children with zero risk factors. Children with three risk factors were even less likely to be in excellent or very good health with 82 percent lower odds. The results for being at risk for developmental delays are similar to those for health status and are presented in Figure 4.10. This figure shows the percentage of children with each combination of risk factors who are at higher risk for developmental delays. The gradients found in these analyses are particularly important because they are evident in the first few years of life and threaten how children develop, how well they make friends, whether they succeed in school, and whether they mature successfully.

FIGURE 4.10   Risk Factor Combinations and Proportion At Risk for Developmental Delay, Children Under Three, 2001

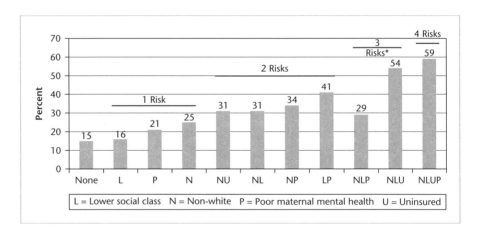

Notes: $p < .01$ for the difference among the risk factor combinations within the three risk factor categories. No other differences within risk factor categories were statistically significant.

Source: Stevens (2006).

Focus on Vulnerability in Clinical Practice

Clinicians of all types commonly assess the likelihood of disease or outcome of a disease based on a number of different risk factors. To assess the chances of adverse outcomes associated with heart disease, for example, they monitor patients for a range of clinical risk factors including high blood pressure, unusual heart rhythms, poor blood flow, and high cholesterol levels. Clinicians also know which individuals are at a higher risk based on their case histories: those who smoke, eat poorly, exercise less, are overweight or obese, and those who have diabetes. For women, taking certain oral contraceptives (especially in conjunction with smoking) may also heighten the risk of heart disease. Often, doctors take these risk factors into account informally, intuitively knowing that individuals who report more of these risk factors are at higher risk of a heart attack, heart failure, stroke, and other outcomes.

It has become more common (albeit still not a regular occurrence in the United States) for clinicians to use checklists and guidelines in caring for patients. These instruments and tools can be helpful to clinicians in formalizing the process of assessing risk and providing the appropriate level of care. Checklists or guidelines often make the process of risk assessment explicit and, by doing so, tend to remind providers to assess all the relevant risk factors and to formally account for the contribution of each to the chances of an illness or a poor outcome. Instruments can range from questionnaires that can tell a clinician when to provide counseling on a particular issue (for example, screening for sexual activity and at-risk behaviors, and providing guidance on preventing pregnancy and sexually transmitted infections), when to refer to other clinicians or educators (for example, screening for poor nutrition and exercise patterns and referrals to nutritionists and/or health and fitness classes), or even how to prioritize limited resources (for example, screening for risk factors for noncompliance with therapy for tuberculosis and assigning case managers for individuals at highest risk).

There are now many great examples of such guidelines. One tool was developed to know when to look for depression among women with breast cancer, as clinicians were finding that some women with breast cancer were having difficulty adhering to their treatment regimens, and that depression was a likely (and predictable) contributor to this difficulty. The tool, known as the Breast Cancer Vulnerability Index, was designed to assess nine risk factors for depression among women with early stage breast cancer (Patel and others, 2010). The risk factors included the following: (1) age less than forty-five years old, (2) not being married, (3) having children younger than age twenty-one, (4) economic adversity, (5) perceived poor social support, (6) poor marital or family functioning, (7) history of psychiatric problems, (8) stressful life events in the past year, and (9) history of alcohol or other substance abuse. The tool uses a count of the number of risk factors, and using a given cut-off (either one or two risk factors, depending on the user) it can correctly predict future depression during the course of treatment about 90 percent of the time.

Another example is a screening instrument that can be used in a variety of health care and even non–health care settings such as schools and child care centers to identify children at higher risk of developmental delays and other problems such as autism. The instrument, known as the Parents' Evaluation of Developmental Status, was designed to elicit concerns that parents have about their child's development, including behaviors, fine and gross motor skills, language use and understanding, and early social skills (Glascoe, 2003). The instrument was designed because many clinicians had tended to only informally observe a child's communication, motor skills, and behavior during typical fifteen-minute well-child visits. Clearly this was not enough time to detect abnormalities, and parents were better observers and reporters of specific developmental issues, although they need some prompting by clinicians. The instrument requires just a couple of minutes to complete, can be self-administered or administered by professionals, and requires a simple algorithm to determine a child's level of risk and what course of action should be taken, such as screen as usual for low-risk children, monitor closely for those at moderate risk, conduct further testing for those at higher risk, or refer for special testing and intervention for the highest-risk children.

SUMMARY

This chapter has reviewed the existing evidence and presented new data regarding the markedly negative influence of multiple co-occurring risk factors on health care access, quality of care, and health status. Once we acknowledge that vulnerable individuals with multiple risk factors are common in the population (and would be even more common if we could account for all of the known risk factors in existence) and recognize the synergistic influences of these co-occurring risk factors on health and health care experiences, there is a clear call for assisting these vulnerable populations in more comprehensive ways.

KEY TERMS

Continuity of care

Developmental risk

Family-centered care

Multivariate analysis

Preventive counseling

Risk profiles

REVIEW QUESTIONS

1. Describe the distribution of multiple risk factors (using race/ethnicity, income, and health insurance coverage) within the national population. How does this distribution vary between adults and children? Based on what you have learned so far, why does this distribution vary?

2. When considering other risk factors such as income, insurance, education, and having a regular source of care, how does the distribution of multiple risks vary by race/ethnicity? Which groups are most at risk, and which are least at risk?

3. Briefly describe how race/ethnicity, SES, and health insurance profiles are associated with health care access, quality of care, and health status. If you were asked to present some of these data to a group concerned with children's health, what would you say are the biggest gaps in knowledge about multiple risks?

ESSAY QUESTIONS

1. Why do risk factors tend to cluster within groups of individuals? Select three risk factors in addition to non-English language, and describe how they are related and how they increase the likelihood of each other. Draw a model with arrows linking these risks. How do these risk factors have the potential to be replicated across generations? Where are the most and least feasible places to intervene to interrupt these relationships? What would likely happen to each of the risk factors once the pathways were disrupted?

2. You have been awarded a large research grant to study the implications of multiple risk factors on access to care, quality, or health status. What three risk factors would you study, and in relation to what outcomes? Justify your decision by considering the previous research on the risk factors and outcomes you select, the feasibility of collecting and measuring this information, and what gaps in knowledge this research will fill. What are the results you would expect to find?

CHAPTER FIVE

CURRENT STRATEGIES TO SERVE VULNERABLE POPULATIONS

LEARNING OBJECTIVES

- To become familiar with major health programs and policies to address health and health care disparities.

- To compare the roles of the federal government, state and local governments, and private interests in addressing health and health care disparities.

- To understand the strengths and weaknesses of these programs, including their effectiveness and sustainability.

THE previous two chapters have presented a range of evidence showing the relationships of individual and multiple risk factors with poor access to care, poor quality of care, and poor health outcomes. Government agencies and private organizations have developed a variety of policies and programs to help mitigate the adverse consequences of vulnerability. This chapter reviews the most widely recognized and successful programs currently in place, discusses the mechanisms of vulnerability addressed by each, and systematically critiques their potential to improve the health of vulnerable populations.

The programs are organized according to the vulnerability factor addressed. A growing number of programs now address multiple risk factors, in which case we categorize those programs according to the risk factor most explicitly targeted by the program. Within these large categories, the programs are further grouped according to financial sponsorship: federal government, state and local government, or private agency. We review the history, purpose, current activities, and budget (if available) of each program.

Programs were identified through correspondence with and from the Web sites of many sources, including government agencies, national associations for legislators and health care professionals, and private health policy organizations. We supplemented our discussion with information gathered from the peer-reviewed literature. Our review of existing programs is again not intended to be exhaustive but rather illustrative of the major successful programs available to vulnerable populations. A complete listing of the program Web sites and contact information is provided in Exhibit 5.1.

We critique the potential impact of the programs according to four criteria. First, we examine the validity of the programs and whether they address the most appropriate mechanisms (discussed in Chapter Two) contributing to the disparities targeted by the programs. Second, we examine the scope of the programs, including the number of vulnerable people served and whether the programs reach their intended populations. Third, we explore the sustainability of the endeavors, including the stability of their funding sources and revenues and the ability of the programs to adapt to and integrate changes in financing of the health care system. Fourth, we examine the effectiveness of the programs and, when possible, incorporate into our analyses the findings of published evaluations. The chapter concludes with a summary of the major strengths and weaknesses of existing programs and identifies gaps in serving vulnerable populations.

Exhibit 5.1   Contact Information for Current Major Programs to Serve Vulnerable Populations

The program name, in italics, is followed by the address, telephone number, and URL.

Association of Schools of Public Health/Kellogg Taskforce
Health Disparities Research & Diversity Resource Center
Association of Schools of Public Health
1101 15th Street NW, Suite 910
Washington, DC 20005
202–296–1099, diversity.asph.org

California Children's Health Initiatives
1017 L Street, #289
Sacramento, CA 95814
707–527–9213, www.cchi4kids.org

California Department of Public Health Strategic Plan
California Department of Public Health
616 Capitol Avenue
Sacramento, CA 95814
916–558–1784, www.cdph.ca.gov

California Endowment's Building Healthy Communities Initiative
The California Endowment
1000 North Alameda Street
Los Angeles, CA 90012
800–449–4149, www.calendow.org

Center for Health and Health Care in Schools
School of Public Health and Health Services
The George Washington University
2121 K Street NW, Suite 250
Washington DC 20037
202–466–3396, www.healthinschools.org

Community and Migrant Health Centers
Bureau of Primary Health Care
Health Resources and Services Administration
5600 Fishers Lane
Rockville, MD 20857
301–594–4300, www.bphc.hrsa.gov/chc

Head Start
Office of Head Start
Administration for Children and Families
1250 Maryland Avenue, S.W.
Washington, D.C. 20024
202–205–8573, www.acf.hhs.gov/programs/ohs/index.html

Health Care for the Homeless
Office of Minority and Special Populations
Bureau of Primary Health Care
Health Resources and Services Administration
5600 Fishers Lane
Rockville, MD 20857
301–594–4303, www.bphc.hrsa.gov

Healthcare Group of Arizona
701 E. Jefferson St, MD 1400
Phoenix, AZ 85034
800–247–2289, www.healthcaregroupaz.com

Healthy Howard Health Plan
P.O. Box 2275
Columbia, Maryland 21045
410–988–3737, www.healthyhowardplan.org

Healthy Start

Health Resources and Services Administration

Maternal and Child Health Bureau

Parklawn Building Room 18–05

5600 Fishers Lane, Rockville, Maryland 20857

301–443–7678, mchb.hrsa.gov/programs

Indian Health Services

Indian Health Services Headquarters

801 Thompson Ave., Suite 400

Rockville, MD 20852–1627

301–443–1083, www.ihs.gov

Johnson & Johnson Community Health Care Program

Johns Hopkins Bloomberg School of Public Health

624 N. Broadway, Room 261

Baltimore, MD 21205

443–287–5138, www.jhsph.edu/johnsonandjohnson

Kansas City TeleKidcare

Center for TeleMedicine and TeleHealth

University of Kansas Medical Center

2012 Wahl Annex, 3901 Rainbow Blvd.

Kansas City, KS 66160–7171

913–588–2226, www2.kumc.edu/telemedicine/Programs/TKC.htm

Massachusetts Commonwealth Health Insurance Connector Authority

877–623–6765, www.mahealthconnector.org

Minnesota's Eliminating Health Disparities Initiative

Office of Minority and Multicultural Health

Freeman Building, 5C

PO Box 64975

St. Paul, MN 55164

651–201–5813, www.health.state.mn.us/ommh/grants

National Center on Minority Health and Health Disparities

National Institutes of Health

6707 Democracy Boulevard, Suite 800

Bethesda, MD 20892–5465

301–402–1366, ncmhd.nih.gov

National Health Service Corps

Bureau of Health Professions

Health Resources and Services Administration

5600 Fishers Lane

Rockville, MD 20857

800–221–9393, nhsc.hrsa.gov

Office of Minority Health

Office of Minority Health Resource Center

P.O. Box 37337

Washington, DC 20013

800–444–6472, minorityhealth.hhs.gov

Project HEALTH

Boston Medical Center

88 E. Newton Street, Vose 522

Boston, MA 02118

617–502–3294, www.projecthealth.org

Public Housing Primary Care Program

Office of Minority and Special Populations

Bureau of Primary Health Care

Health Resources and Services Administration

5600 Fishers Lane

Rockville, MD 20857

301–594–4303, www.bphc.hrsa.gov

Racial and Ethnic Approaches to Community Health Across the United States

Centers for Disease Control and Prevention

Mail Stop K-30

4770 Buford Highway, N.E.

Atlanta, GA 30341–3717

404–639–3534, www.cdc.gov/reach

Robert Wood Johnson Foundation Aligning Forces for Quality Project

School of Public Health and Health Services

The George Washington University

2021 K Street, N.W., Suite 800

Washington, DC 20052–0015

202–994–8659, www.rwjf.org

South Carolina Welvista Program

2700 Middleburg Drive, Suite 104

Columbia, SC 29204

803–933–9183, www.welvista.org

Strengthening Primary Care Providers for the Poor

Health Foundation of Greater Cincinnati

Rookwood Tower

3805 Edwards Rd., Suite 500

Cincinnati, OH 45209

888–310–4904, www.healthfoundation.org

PROGRAMS TO ELIMINATE RACIAL AND ETHNIC DISPARITIES

It is now widely accepted that race and ethnicity are determinants of health and health care experiences. Seminal reports on racial/ethnic disparities issued by the Agency for Healthcare Research and Quality and the Institute of Medicine have brought national attention to the importance of these issues among health policy professionals and call for the development and expansion of initiatives to eliminate these disparities (Agency for Healthcare Research and Quality, 2003, 2009; Smedley, Stith, and Nelson, 2002). Programs to address racial disparities have been in place for many years, but only recently has an extensive effort been made to address non-socioeconomic pathways.

Federal Initiatives

The federal government has implemented several broad-sweeping programs that include the development of national governmental agencies, offices, task forces, and health provider recruitment and training programs. These federal initiatives have generally served to bring attention to racial disparities in health, centralized efforts to monitor and reduce these disparities, and provided health services to underserved minority communities.

U.S. Office of Minority Health   The Office of Minority Health (OMH) was created within the Department of Health and Human Services (DHHS) in 1986. It was proposed as part of the Report of the Secretary's Task Force on Black and Minority Health (Task Force on Black and Minority Health, 1985), and its stated mission is "to improve and protect the health of racial and ethnic minority populations through the development of health policies and programs that will eliminate health disparities." Under the direct supervision of the deputy assistant secretary for minority health, OMH advises the secretary of the DHHS on public health issues affecting minorities.

The OMH plays an important role in the development and coordination of federal health policy by promoting minority health issues in Congress and ensuring that the government is actively accountable to the needs of disadvantaged and minority populations. Specifically, the OMH continues to collect and analyze data on the health of racial and ethnic minority populations and monitors national efforts to achieve the goals in Healthy People 2020, which will continue to prioritize equity in all aspects of health and health care. The OMH also continues to regularly fund cooperative agreements and grants that support many research and demonstration programs.

In addition, the OMH has a history of coordinating large national and state initiatives to address health disparities, beginning with its role in designing and carrying out the DHHS Initiative to Eliminate Racial and Ethnic Disparities in Health that began in 1998. The OMH assisted the surgeon general in identifying and promoting six minority health target areas and collaborated with the Centers for Disease Control and Prevention to award and monitor grants supporting initiatives to reduce racial disparities in community health. The Initiative no longer formally exists, but the legacy of the initiative can be seen in the National Partnership for Action (NPA) to End Health Disparities that aims to create a national strategy for OMH and its partners to address disparities. The NPA was formed out of the 2006 National Leadership Summit on Eliminating Racial and Ethnic Disparities in Health that brought together 2,000 experts and community leaders, and was furthered by a similar summit in 2009 that created the national blueprint for action.

In 1987, OMH established the Office of Minority Health Resource Center to meet the public's need for timely information and technical assistance on issues affecting the health of minority populations. Since that time, the resource center has become one of the nation's largest repositories of minority health information. Some of its services are referrals to minority providers and programs, publications on minority health issues, and publication of a newsletter, "Healthy Minorities, Healthier America," which reports on national, state, and local activities related to minority health.

Racial and Ethnic Approaches to Community Health Across the United States   Originally known as Racial and Ethnic Approaches to Community Health (REACH 2010), the program was launched by the Centers for Disease Control in 1999 to support the goals of Healthy People 2010 in eliminating racial and ethnic disparities in health and health care. REACH 2010 was a demonstration grant program that supported community coalitions in designing, implementing, and evaluating efforts to eliminate health disparities. Each coalition comprises a community-based organization and three other organizations, such as local or state health departments, a research university, or a research organization. These programs addressed one or more of the six target topics identified as part of the presidential initiative.

In late 2005, CDC went through a strategic planning initiative to prepare for a reincarnation of REACH 2010 that resulted in REACH U.S. in 2007. By building upon the body of knowledge produced by REACH 2010, REACH U.S. shares promising interventions nationwide by disseminating effective strategies, lessons learned, and best practices. REACH U.S. continues to prioritize projects that focus on breast and cervical cancer, cardiovascular disease, diabetes, adult immunization, and infant mortality, and also added three new areas: hepatitis B, tuberculosis, and asthma.

The program appropriated $35.5 million for 2009 to support forty partners, some of which are existing partners funded through REACH 2010. Supported projects are eighteen Centers of Excellence in the Elimination of Disparities (CEEDs) and twenty-two Action Communities. CEEDs are national expert centers that implement, coordinate, refine, and disseminate intervention programs. They also provide pilot funding, support, and local training to encourage the initiation of new projects to eliminate health disparities. Action Communities are local organizations funded to carry out specific interventions. One example is the Community Health Councils of Los Angeles, which was funded to engage a consortium of groups to promote better land use and urban policy to improve physical activity opportunities and improve existing food venues through regulation and policy development.

National Center on Minority Health and Health Disparities   In 1990, the National Institutes of Health (NIH) formed the Office for Research on Minority Health to improve the national research agenda on minority health and the national commitment and responsiveness to the health and training needs of minorities. A standout activity of the office was the Minority Health Initiative, started in 1992, which took major steps to increase participation of minorities in clinical trials and other research studies by improving community outreach, improving provider communication with minority patients about participation in clinical trials, and developing a recruitment and referral center for minority patients. In 2000, the office was congressionally expanded and renamed the National Center on Minority Health and Health Disparities, and funding was increased from about $80 million in 1999 to $200 million in 2008.

The center focuses on minority health research and promoting the development of minority researchers but explicitly recognizes the multi-factorial basis of disparities, by including work on genetics, SES, health insurance coverage, and access and quality of care. There are several key initiatives of the Center, including the Centers of Excellence Programs (totaling eighty-eight Centers in 2009), a research endowment program to increase the capacity of academic institutions to train under-represented individuals in health research, a minority loan repayment program for individuals with doctorate degrees, and a community-based participatory research initiative to foster ongoing research at the community level in order to advance the health of minority and socioeconomically deprived populations.

Indian Health Service   The Indian Health Service (IHS) is an agency within the DHHS with the mission to "ensure that comprehensive, culturally acceptable personal and public health services are available and accessible to all American Indian and Alaska Native people" and to "raise the physical, mental, social, and spiritual health of American Indians and Alaska Natives to the highest level." These populations have higher rates of death from accidents, homicides, suicide, and alcoholism than the general U.S. population. Tribes also often lack an adequate public health infrastructure, including safe water supplies and adequate waste disposal. To compound the problem, these communities also are often located in isolated areas, making it difficult to access health services.

The IHS currently provides health services to about 1.9 million American Indians and Alaska Natives (up from 1.5 million in 2001). There are more than 560 federally recognized tribes in the United States, and their members live mainly on reservations and in rural communities in thirty-five states, mostly in the western United States and Alaska. Federal recognition is reserved for tribes that signed treaties with the federal government between 1787 and the late 1800s. Not all tribes are federally recognized and therefore are not included in the IHS.

The IHS provides tribes with comprehensive health services and helps them develop their own health programs, coordinate health planning, and obtain available health resources. Comprehensive medical care is provided in 45 hospitals, 132 health stations, 15 school health centers, and 166 Alaskan village clinics owned and operated by the IHS. In locations where the IHS does not have its own facilities, it contracts with local hospitals, state and local health agencies, Veterans Administration facilities (as of 2003), tribal health institutions, and individual health care providers to deliver needed care. Services provided include preventive, acute, and emergency medical services; environmental health and engineering; mental health services; and pharmacy, dental, and laboratory services. It also has special health education initiatives in chronic disease prevention and management, methamphetamine and alcohol use reduction, maternal and child health, and mental health.

The IHS was part of the Bureau of Indian Affairs from 1924 to 1955, after which it was transferred from the Department of the Interior to the DHHS. In 1975, Congress passed the Indian Self-Determination and Education Assistance Act, giving tribes the option of staffing and managing the health services in their communities and providing funding for training tribe members to do so. Tribes can decide whether to provide all of their own health care, only a portion of it, or none at all, with the IHS remaining their provider of choice. Almost 60 percent of the IHS clinics are now administered and operated by tribes. The IHS has appropriated about $4 billion for 2010, up significantly from $3.4 billion in 2008.

Migrant Health Center Program *Migrant and seasonal farm workers*, who are primarily Hispanic and very low income, face a number of health risks due to poverty and poor living and working conditions. Problems including malnutrition, tuberculosis and other infectious diseases, and exposure to pesticides are compounded by nearly universal lack of insurance coverage and poor access to health care. The Migrant Health Act of 1962 established the migrant health program, which provides medical and support services to migrant farm workers and their families.

Within the program, migrant health centers (MHCs) have become the main health care delivery mechanism, helping more than 157 nonprofit organizations to deliver comprehensive and culturally competent primary care services in more than 500 clinic sites (up from about 400 in 2001). Since 1996, the MHC program has been administered in coordination with the Community Health Center program by the Bureau of Primary Health Care (BPHC) within the DHHS's Health Resources and Services Administration (HRSA). In 2007, the MHC program served more than 826,000 patients, up from about 600,000 in 2001.

As with all community health centers, MHCs offer primary care and preventive services, transportation, patient outreach, pharmaceutical services, dental care, occupational health and safety, and environmental health. To ensure comprehensive access to health services, MHCs also partner with state and local health departments, hospitals, specialty providers, social service agencies, and other providers. In order to tailor the services to migrant farm workers, the MHCs rely on bilingual and bicultural outreach workers and health personnel and emphasize culturally sensitive protocols.

Healthy Start   In response to high infant mortality rates among vulnerable populations, the Healthy Start program was launched in 1991 by HRSA. The goal of the program is to reduce disparities in infant mortality rates and improve maternal and early childhood health by funding community-driven interventions. Local organizations are funded to design and implement interventions that include outreach and case management for pregnant women and infants, broad-based public information campaigns, support services, individual and classroom-based health education, co-location of prenatal care services, and enhanced clinical services for women and infants. Healthy Start, now administered by the Maternal and Child Health Bureau in HRSA, originally funded fifteen communities with very high infant mortality rates in 1991. This has grown significantly to serve hundreds of thousands of individuals in ninety-eight communities in thirty-eight states and territories in 2008, supported with a total budget of about $100 million annually.

More than 90 percent of Healthy Start participants are African American, Hispanic, or Native American, and most interventions focus on using community outreach workers to bring pregnant women into prenatal care as early as possible. Mothers and their children are also linked with a medical home through the first two years after child delivery to ensure that families have continuous health services through the highest risk periods. Most programs also provide health education, transportation assistance, child care support, and substance abuse counseling and treatment.

State and Local Initiatives

States and counties have independently established programs to address the needs of racial and ethnic minorities. Initiatives established in each state and county reflect the differing racial/ethnic composition, needs, and resources of their areas. States tend to intervene in problems that federal programs fail to address adequately, and these state programs often become models and prototypes for future federal efforts. Because of the vast number of programs operating at the state and local levels, we highlight and discuss two key examples that are reflective of the types of investments of other states. More comprehensive listings of these programs are available in compilation documents produced by organizations such as the National Conference of State Legislators, the Association of State and Territorial Health Officials, and the National Association of City and County Health Officials.

Minnesota's Eliminating Health Disparities Initiative   With a history of tracking the health of minority residents reaching back to the late 1980s, and a series of state reports on health disparities throughout the 1990s, the Minnesota Department of Health (MDH) added the reduction of health disparities as one of its three strategic priorities in 1999. The MDH, state legislators, and community partners began work on a legislative proposal that built on the work of the national REACH 2010 program to provide funding for local communities to establish local interventions to address particular disparities topics. Legislation passed in 2001 providing $9.5 million every two years for a ten-year period to community projects focused on disparities. Seven priority areas were identified, including breast and cervical cancer, cardiovascular disease, diabetes, HIV/AIDS and sexually transmitted infections, violence, and unintended injuries. The legislation established a goal of reducing these disparities by 50 percent by 2010. A portion of the funds was also set aside for state activities to address infant mortality, immunizations, healthy youth development, and tuberculosis screening and treatment.

As of 2008, the initiative has funded fifty-two grantees, the majority of which focus on prevention activities and a smaller proportion of which focus on prevention and support for people with priority health conditions. Most programs focused on health education and behavior changing activities, and many encouraged preventive health contacts in primary care settings. By 2008, the programs had reached 59,200 individuals, the vast majority of whom were African American, Latino, or American Indian. An example of a funded program includes St. Mary's Health Clinics that work with Latino parishes to provide culturally appropriate health education and screening. In a ten-month period, the program reported a 75 percent increase in Latina parish members who received a Pap smear and a 73 percent increase in mammograms.

California Department of Public Health Strategic Plan   As of 2009, thirty-five states have developed specific strategic plans to reduce racial and ethnic health disparities. Of the state plans, eighteen are legislative initiatives and sixteen are plans of the state departments of public health. The plan in Pennsylvania was created by a task force of the governor (National Conference of State Legislators, 2009). Several states had such plans in place as early as 2005, but most released their plans between 2008 and 2010. Such plans are important because they set the vision for the state health activities and its funding priorities. One example is the 2008–2010 strategic plan released by the California Department of Public Health, which states as its first public health goal to "increase quality and years of healthy life, reduce disparities and promote health equity" (2008, page 13). The department identifies thirteen health objectives based on Healthy People 2010 that include topics for which disparities are widely known, including infant mortality rates, elevated blood lead levels in children, adult physical activity levels, and adult smoking. The plan also includes a goal of increasing the number of health objectives for which California data are available for all population groups in order to better monitor trends and disparities (California Department of Public Health, 2008).

Private Initiatives

A number of philanthropies and nonprofit collaboratives have developed innovative strategies or programs to address problems that are overlooked or not addressed by federal, state, and local initiatives. Often these organizations are capable of providing substantial funding to develop demonstration programs that may become models for state governments. Because of the large number of such programs, we present only a few examples.

Robert Wood Johnson Foundation Aligning Forces for Quality Project   In 2006, the Robert Wood Johnson Foundation (RWJF) launched its Quality/Equality strategy, which includes the Aligning Forces for Quality initiative to improve the quality of health care that Americans receive by lifting the quality of care overall and by targeting at-risk communities across the country. The first phase of Aligning Forces provided grants and technical assistance to community leader teams to assist them in working with physicians to raise the quality of care and to measure and publicly report quality data. The program expanded in 2008 to include hospital care and a specific focus on reducing gaps in quality for racial and ethnic minorities. The national program office is at the George Washington University School of Public Health and Health Services. This office works with fifteen grantees across the country who work on quality reporting, increasing consumer involvement in quality, engaging in quality improvement activities, and addressing language issues. One example of a funded project is the Puget Sound Health Alliance in Seattle. The alliance focuses in part on improving health literacy to ensure consumers can understand and use health care quality information, and it has released its first two public "community check-up" reports that detail twenty-one health care quality measures for 170 medical groups and forty hospitals in five higher-risk counties. The results are available online, are searchable, and are updated annually.

Association of Schools of Public Health/Kellogg Taskforce on Disparities   Effective intervention in health disparities is necessarily preceded by awareness, knowledge, and capacity to develop effective programs and policies. In support of this, a taskforce was formed in 2005 to expand the national training of health professionals to get involved in racial/ethnic health disparities research, intervention, and policy. The taskforce was formed by the Association of Schools of Public Health with support from the W.K. Kellogg Foundation. Its mission was to "engage accredited schools and programs of public health, in partnership with communities, as leaders in teaching, research, practice, service, and advocacy related to achieving the elimination of racial and ethnic disparities and their root cause—social injustice" (Association of Schools of Public Health, 2006).

After multiple meetings and a minority faculty member retreat, the taskforce released a report with recommendations for how schools of public health could address health disparities by improving their recruitment and training of health professionals. The recommendations include expanding public health training core competencies to include courses on racial/ethnic health disparities, producing more practicum placements in activities for disparities work, and disseminating best practices for minority faculty and student recruitment in public health professions. The association also currently maintains an online diversity resource center that serves as an information hub for students, faculty, and professionals on health disparities.

California Endowment's Building Health Communities Initiative   Created in 1996, the California Endowment is the state's largest health care foundation, with nearly $4 billion in assets. Since its inception, the organization has awarded more than 9,000 grants, totaling over $1.7 billion, to community-based organizations throughout the state (up from 2,800 grants totaling $900 million in 2001). The endowment has had a long-term interest in caring for minority populations, having implemented a multiyear focus on multicultural health. The ten-year Building Healthy Communities initiative that begins in 2010 expands this focus to more comprehensively address the needs of fourteen underserved communities that were picked by analyzing the accumulation of social risk factors for poor health, including poverty and uninsured rates, measures of diversity and demographic risk factors, and other community-level risk factors.

The organization plans to invest broadly in social, environmental, and medical interventions to address four "big results" areas: (1) providing a health home for all children, (2) reversing the childhood obesity epidemic, (3) increasing school attendance, and (4) reducing youth violence. The focus on youth reflects the interest of the endowment in promoting long-term changes, and the organization expects each community to address not only health care services but the availability of healthy foods, public safety, access to parks and recreation for families, air quality, and transportation issues, among others. This approach to addressing the health problems of vulnerable populations most closely reflects the general model of vulnerability described in this book and is highlighted in the front-line experience that follows.

Front-Line Experience: Dependence Is the Tip of the Iceberg for Vulnerable Seniors

Jane Marks, associate director of the Johns Hopkins Geriatrics Education Center, and Lynda Burton, associate professor of the Johns Hopkins Bloomberg School of Public Health, remind us that many of the difficulties created by the vulnerabilities discussed in this book are compounded for older patients due to a lack of mobility and transportation, unavailable family support, and a complex array of health conditions that require vigilant monitoring.

When caring for older patients, health care professionals are aware that a relatively small change in a person's health can trigger a major cascade of changes in his or her life. Nurses in our geriatrics practice, located in a primarily low-income, urban community, are trained to closely monitor these changes in health and work closely with patients and family members, if present, to address their health needs early.

In our geriatrics practice, we have recognized the need to make house calls as a strategy to serve our vulnerable older patients better. House calls are convenient for homebound patients who have limited physical mobility or transportation problems. They also help us to assess living arrangements and how they may support or hinder our patients' continued independence.

Physicians and nurses make home visits to our patients frequently. Nurses visit the homes first to assess the situation, involve the physician when necessary, and then follow up with regular phone calls. Even with this frequent follow-up, nurses still cannot reduce all of the risks that the most vulnerable patients encounter. The effect of even minor events on health and independence is enormous and is often compounded by mobility problems, lack of family support, and co-occurring health conditions, including such problems as depression. One patient served by our practice provides an example of the compounding influence of these overlapping health and social risk factors.

Helen (this is a pseudonym) is eighty-seven years old and was widowed fifteen years ago, but she has been able to care for herself while living alone in her small apartment. She has no family living in the area but does have friends in the neighborhood. Over the past five years, her congestive heart failure, hypertension, and arthritis have gradually worsened, making it difficult for her to get around. She also has macular degeneration and with her worsening eyesight was forced to give up driving, an important avenue of independence for her. She now depends entirely on her friends to help her with groceries, shopping, other errands, and, most important for her, getting to church.

Helen developed a rather serious cough, and during one of our phone conversations we recommended that she get a chest x-ray at the local hospital. She asked a friend to drive her, and while she was getting into the car, her feet got tangled and she had a minor fall. Her very worried friend helped her up and into her home, and then called us for help. Our nurses went out to the home to examine her that day and found that she did not seem to have a fracture. She was bruised but not in discomfort, and she could walk without pain. When the nurses phoned her each of the next two days, she said she was still doing fine.

Later that week, however, Helen developed some stiffness and began to have difficulty walking. Nurses made another home visit after receiving a phone call and found her near tears because she had become so stiff that she had extreme difficulty getting up from her bed. Her friends were not around enough to be able to help her move to the bathroom in time, so she chose to stop taking her diuretic (used to treat congestive heart failure) to prevent incontinence. Because she had stopped the medication, her congestive heart failure had worsened, and a hospital stay was required to get this back in control. Her evaluation showed only soft tissue injury in addition to the congestive heart failure. But her immobility had the cumulative effect of deconditioning her muscles, making it more and more difficult for her to get around.

Helen did not have sufficient income to hire a caregiver to assist her full time during her recovery once she returned home. She also had difficulty affording and maintaining her ongoing and new medications. Without physical or financial assistance, we determined that she could not independently maintain herself at home. She was admitted to a rehabilitation center, where professionals worked to help restore her mobility. Even with this rehabilitation, the minor fall that she had and the cascade of events that followed prevented her from returning to her home and living an independent life.

Since cases like Helen's are not uncommon, comprehensive assistance programs have been developed to intervene in the cascade of health deterioration. The Program for All Inclusive Care of the Elderly (PACE), for example, is available to certain older patients who are eligible for nursing home care but instead provides nursing assistance at home or in adult day care centers. PACE services would have greatly helped Helen during her recovery by providing her with a nursing assistant at home for a few days, keeping her moving to prevent immobilization, and maintaining her prescribed medications. However, PACE eligibility required that she be a Medicaid recipient and that she meet criteria for nursing home admission. Her income was above the Medicaid eligibility level, and prior to her fall, she would not have met criteria for nursing home admission. Given that the population of older patients is increasing, programs like PACE or others that afford home visits by health professionals can have a dramatic effect on reducing the burden of illness and, ultimately, the costs of care for vulnerable populations.

Strengths and Weaknesses of Programs Addressing Racial Disparities

Addressing racial/ethnic disparities in health and health care is no easy task. The success of programs and initiatives that have been developed is based on many factors, among them validity, scope and reach, sustainability, and effectiveness. Here, we review some of the major strengths and weaknesses of these programs.

Validity   The majority of federal initiatives have served primarily to generate national attention on racial disparities. The presence of OMH is particularly important because it plays a coordinating role for other federal agencies and the minority health initiatives they support. The programs presented address some key pathways leading to disparities by improving access to care through low-cost services and ensuring that individuals obtain high quality of health services (including prenatal care in Healthy Start and primary care quality in Aligning Forces for Quality). Many programs also address cultural barriers by making services and outreach available in a culturally and *linguistically appropriate* manner. The National Center on Minority Health and Health Disparities and the Association of Schools of Public Health tackle fundamental issues of capacity in research and training of minority individuals to engage in health disparities research and intervention, though future efforts might consider broader training of doctors and other health care professionals in methods to improve *cultural competence* and in caring for vulnerable populations. The California Endowment Building Healthy Communities initiative has perhaps the greatest potential to address health disparities because it tackles health issues from many angles simultaneously, focusing on health care, environmental health, violence prevention, and other issues. This initiative is only in the very early stages, and the ways in which counties design and implement their efforts will be very important.

Scope and Reach   The programs we have presented address a broad range of issues and serve extensive populations. The federal Indian Health Service and Migrant Health Center programs alone reach well over 2.5 million minorities (and about 75 percent of the entire Native American population), and the combinations of the various state and local programs serve tens of thousands more. While these service programs are designed to address specific needs of the minorities in their target populations, they continue to reflect a somewhat fragmented approach to addressing disparities in minority health and health care. The federal OMH has a major role to play in coordinating future efforts to eliminate health disparities. Yet it will remain important to balance national efforts to improve racial/ethnic equity in health and health services delivery with the ability to address the specific cultural barriers and unique needs of each minority group.

Sustainability   Most federal programs addressing racial disparities in health have been well funded to meet the aims of Healthy People 2020 to eliminate racial and socioeconomic disparities in health. The Indian Health Service and migrant health centers (as part of the CHC program) have been expanded recently and have received additional funding for a two-year period through a federal economic stimulus to revive the economy. State, local, and private initiatives are generally financially dependent on grants and reimbursements by enrolling clients in programs like Medicaid, but the sustainability of each is dependent on local supporters, federal and state policies to expand insurance coverage for the indigent, and the economy. Intervention grants such as REACH U.S. and Minnesota's Eliminating Health Disparities Initiative appear to have good funding prospects in the near future.

Effectiveness   Relatively few evaluations have been completed on national efforts to reduce racial disparities in health care. Migrant health centers are likely providing an effective safety net to migrant farm workers. A study by the National Association of Community Health Centers showed that 63 percent of farm workers had a regular source of care and that 95 percent of those workers reported health centers as that source of care. Patient experience has been positive in the health centers, with almost 100 percent of farm workers responding to a questionnaire by expressing that they were satisfied with the quality of their care at their center. Because community health centers were included in the study in addition to MHCs, it is difficult to isolate the exact benefit from the MHCs (Zuvekas, 2002). In general, the MHC program has not been well studied in comparison to the larger sister community health center program.

Studies of the IHS suggest that it has had a drastic impact on the health of Native Americans and Alaska Natives. The program is reported to have contributed to a life expectancy increase of 12.2 years, and a decrease in infant mortality by 50 percent, tuberculosis mortality by 74 percent, and gastrointestinal mortality by 81 percent among Native Americans since 1973 (Brenneman, Rhoades, and Chilton, 2006; Rhoades, D'Angelo, and Hurlburt, 1987). Healthy Start has been well studied and has been associated with mixed outcomes. The program seems to boost prenatal care utilization and healthy behaviors during and after pregnancy, but the impact on actually reducing infant mortality has tended to be mixed, suggesting that other factors may need to be addressed in these programs (Badura, Johnson, Hench, and Reyes, 2008; Rosenbach and others, 2009; Salihu and others, 2009).

Though still evaluating many new initiatives, the REACH 2010 program has demonstrated some success (Centers for Disease Control and Prevention, 2003). A REACH-sponsored South Carolina coalition to improve diabetes outcomes in the state's African American population increased the number of African American men receiving regular blood sugar testing, virtually eliminating the disparity with whites in those communities. The project also strikingly reduced amputations due to poorly controlled diabetes among African American males by between 36 and 44 percent. A REACH program in Lawrence, Massachusetts, to improve the health of Latinos reported improvements of 9 percent in blood sugar levels, 14 percent in diastolic blood pressure, and 18 percent in systolic blood pressure. In California, a REACH project helped to increase the proportion of Vietnamese women who had received a Pap test by 15 percent (Giles, 2007). The other programs we presented have not been as rigorously evaluated to date.

PROGRAMS TO ELIMINATE SOCIOECONOMIC DISPARITIES

Many programs have also been developed to address SES disparities in health and health care experiences. Most of these have focused on income-related factors, such as providing free or low-cost health services to lower-income individuals, but few have focused on other aspects of SES, such as education and occupation. We review these programs next.

Federal Initiatives

An equally large number of federal initiatives have been created specifically to assist low-income individuals and families to access high-quality health services. These programs are generally what health policymakers consider to be the nation's health care safety net and range from programs targeted to low-income populations broadly defined to specific groups of vulnerable populations, such as homeless individuals.

Community Health Centers   The federal community health center (CHC) program was established by the federal government to improve access to health care for low-income families. CHCs were created under the Economic Opportunity Act of 1964 as part of President Johnson's War on Poverty, and the first two health centers were created in 1965 in Boston. The program is now administered by the Bureau of Primary Health Care in HRSA. To qualify for federal funds under the CHC program, a health center must be located in a medically underserved area, operate as a nonprofit, have a board of directors consisting of a majority of health center patients, provide culturally competent and comprehensive primary care services to all age groups, offer a sliding-fee scale, and provide services regardless of ability to pay.

The CHC program provides family-oriented primary and preventive health services for people living in rural and urban underserved communities. It was designed to serve areas where economic, geographical, or cultural barriers limit access to primary care for a substantial portion of the population. Most CHC patients have either Medicaid coverage or are uninsured (about 46 percent and 39 percent, respectively) and 92 percent are below 200 percent of the FPL. The health centers tailor services to community needs and provide essential *ancillary services*, including laboratory and pharmacy services, health education, transportation for visits, and language translation services. The CHC program links clients with welfare programs, Women Infants and Children (WIC) services, mental health and substance abuse treatment centers, and a full range of specialty care services.

The program was reauthorized most recently in 2008 and received nearly $2.1 billion in 2009 (up from $1.2 billion in 2000). It will receive an additional two-year boost of $2 billion in early 2010 through the American Recovery and Reinvestment Act. The dollars are used to administer CHC grants to about 1,200 community-based nonprofit organizations that deliver health services in more than 7,000 sites (up from 3,000 sites in 2001). A pivotal point for the program was the addition of $165 million to the CHC budget in 2002 to expand health care services to an additional 260 clinical sites, which enabled CHCs to serve 1.25 million more people annually. In 2008, the program served about 16 million people, and this number is only expected to increase with the addition of the federal economic stimulus funds.

National Health Service Corps   More than 6,000 federally designated primary care health professional shortage areas (HPSA) exist across the nation, along with over 4,000 dental HPSA and 3,000 mental health HPSA. Individuals living in these shortage areas have little or no access to health care services because the demand for services exceeds the available resources; the services are located a great distance away; or they are inaccessible because of culture, language, and other barriers. The National Health Service Corps (NHSC) works with communities and health care facilities to provide health care to individuals living in these underserved areas. The program was originally conceived to address a severe lack of rural physicians, as many retired or moved to nonrural areas. With rural states appealing to Congress, the NHSC was created in 1972 by amendments added to the Emergency Health Personnel Act of 1970. Since then, more than 30,000 health care providers have served in the corps, and in 2009, the program appropriated $136 million to support nearly 3,800 NHSC providers. It also received an additional $300 million from the American Recovery and Reinvestment Act, which will enable the NHSC to more than double its field strength by 2010.

The NHSC assists medically underserved communities with the recruitment and retention of health care professionals, including physicians, nurse practitioners, physician assistants, dentists, and mental health professionals. It attracts providers and health professional students to serve in shortage areas for a minimum of two years by offering scholarship and loan repayment programs on a competitive basis to students and clinicians committed to serving the neediest communities. Participating providers are offered training in cultural competency to meet the particular needs of the vulnerable communities they are serving. About half of all NHSC providers work in federally qualified community health centers, but NHSC-approved sites range from Indian Health Service clinics and managed care networks to prisons and U.S. Immigration, Customs, and Enforcement sites.

Public Housing Primary Care Program   The Public Housing Primary Care (PHPC) Program was created under the Disadvantaged Minority Health Improvement Act of 1990. It was reauthorized and consolidated with other health center programs in 1996 under the Health Centers Consolidation Act and was most recently reauthorized in 2008 under the Health Care Safety Net Act. The program is currently administered by the BPHC. It supports health centers and other community providers to deliver care, either on-site or at a nearby location, to residents of public housing, low-income individuals living near public housing, and anyone benefiting from public rent subsidies. As of 2007, the program has 167 service delivery sites in twenty-four states that serve more than 134,000 clients annually.

The PHPC provides primary health care services, including direct medical care, dental and preventive care, prenatal care, health screening, health education, laboratory services, and case management. The sites conduct outreach to inform residents about services and also help residents to obtain federal assistance for health insurance coverage and social services. The PHPC programs have established partnerships with public housing authorities and resident organizations to facilitate the delivery of services. Residents are actively involved in the design and governance of PHPC programs, and they are routinely trained and employed as outreach workers, health educators, and case managers.

Health Care for the Homeless Program   The Health Care for the Homeless (HCH) Program was established by the McKinney Homeless Assistance Act of 1987 and is administered by the BPHC. The program was modeled after the successful four-year demonstration project developed and operated by the Robert Wood Johnson Foundation and the Pew Charitable Trust. The program currently supports 211 grantees (up from 135 grantees in 2001) that range from CHCs, local health departments, *community coalitions*, and other nonprofit organizations to provide services to homeless individuals. Appropriations for the HCH program grew from $65 million in 1994 to $100 million in 2001 and $191 million in 2009. It provides services to about 1 million clients annually (up from about 500,000 clients annually in 2001).

The HCH program has the sole federal responsibility for addressing the primary health care needs of homeless persons and is widely recognized as one of the most effective federal public health programs. Programs combine aggressive street outreach with integrated primary care delivery systems and substance abuse services located in places easily accessible for homeless individuals. The HCH programs can include fixed-site health clinics, services provided as homeless shelters, and mobile medical units. The sites must ensure around-the-clock access to emergency care, provide or refer clients to mental health services, conduct outreach to homeless individuals, and assist clients with obtaining health insurance coverage and assistance through social services.

Head Start   Launched in 1965, Head Start is one of the longest-running national programs to address the problems of poverty. The Head Start program is administered by the Office of Head Start within the Administration on Children and Families in the DHHS and was most recently reauthorized in 2007. The goal of the program is to prepare children for success in school by enhancing the social and cognitive development of young children through the provision of educational, health, nutritional, social, and other services to families. Head Start focuses on children from three to five years of age, while Early Head Start (launched in 1995) expands services to children under the age of three.

Head Start provides grants to local public and private nonprofit and for-profit agencies to provide child development and education services to economically disadvantaged children and families, with a special focus on helping preschoolers develop the early reading and math skills they need to be successful in school. Early Head Start provides grants that promote healthy prenatal care, enhance the development of infants and toddlers, and promote healthy family functioning. Both programs engage parents in their children's development and learning. Education activities include mostly preschool education to nationally set standards. Health services include screenings and medical and dental checkups. Social services provide family advocates to work with parents and assist them in accessing community resources.

Eligibility for Head Start services is for children in families living in poverty, though grantees have the option of expanding eligibility up to 133 percent of the FPL. Up to 10 percent of enrollment can be from over-income families or families in emergency situations. All funded programs are required to provide services to children with disabilities (an estimated 10 percent of their total enrollment nationally). The program received $6.9 billion in 2008 to serve approximately 9 million children through 1,600 community-based grantees.

State and Local Initiatives

State and local health departments have implemented a vast array of initiatives, aside from health insurance programs, to address socioeconomic disparities in access to health care. These programs often receive funding as demonstrations in conjunction with private organizations. The example programs we present here have received recognition for their achievements from a number of different organizations, including the former Models That Work Campaign that was sponsored by the BPHC in the late 1990s to early 2000s, which awarded innovative programs and published them as models for reproduction elsewhere (Crump, Gaston, and Fergerson, 1999).

South Carolina Welvista Program   Launched in 1993, Welvista, a public-private nonprofit partnership based in Columbia, South Carolina, provides free prescription medication alongside free primary care, laboratory services, and pediatric dental care to low-income uninsured people (Barone and others, 1998). It provides services through a network of volunteer health professionals offering free or low-cost services in their offices and clinics during regular working hours or at local schools for pediatric dental care. Volunteers include physicians, pharmacists, pharmaceutical companies, hospitals, labs, and other providers who donate their resources to persons in need.

In 2006, there were more than 14,000 patients enrolled in the program, obtaining free health care services from a network of more than 2,500 providers.

Patients call a toll-free number to apply for the program, and operators determine if their annual income qualifies them for any other government programs, such as Medicaid. Once approved, patients can use the same toll-free number to obtain a referral to any participating provider in their area. If medications are prescribed, prescriptions are filled at no cost through its central-fill, mail order pharmacy among other participating pharmacies. An extensive list of corporate and community partners includes philanthropic foundations, hospitals, clinics, colleges, pharmaceutical companies, and many businesses. In 2008, Welvista, in partnership with twelve pharmaceutical companies, dispensed prescription medications valued at $34.5 million to more than 12,000 working, uninsured individuals.

Healthy Howard Health Plan   In response to a high number of uninsured residents of Howard County, Maryland, county officials and health advocates formed a nonprofit organization, Healthy Howard, Inc., to organize low-cost community health services for uninsured residents with income under 300 percent of the FPL. The program was launched in 2008 and has received considerable media attention for its goals, if not its actual enrollment to date. Healthy Howard Health Plan is not an insurance plan, but it provides access to low-cost medical care, including discounted prescription medication, coordinated through a local community health center. The program offers free ambulance rides, reduced prices for emergency room visits, and waived hospital fees if participants are admitted at the Howard County General Hospital. Once enrolled, each member is assigned to a primary care provider as well as a care coordinator. Members are allowed six primary care visits annually without additional costs, with women also allowed one annual gynecological examination. Care coordinators assist with proper referrals, finding prescription medication at reduced rates, and providing information on services available through the plan. In addition, members are paired with a health coach to develop goals and objectives to improve health and well-being.

The program received $2.8 million in funding, with $1.6 million coming from fees that participants pay (either $50 or $85 monthly per person, based on income), $700,000 coming from private philanthropic sources, and $500,000 coming from the county. The funding is expected to support up to 2,200 people each year, but by the end of 2009, only 1,100 individuals had applied. Interestingly, all but 20 of these individuals were actually eligible for, and then enrolled in, Medicaid or other public programs. The program has recently renewed its outreach to specific groups of people that most likely will benefit from the plan, including some state and county workers, public housing residents, community college students, small businesses, and parents of children in CHIP.

Kansas City TeleKidcare   TeleKidcare of Kansas City, Kansas, is a unique health care delivery system that has successfully removed obstacles to obtaining health care encountered by medically underserved children of Wyandotte County, Kansas. In 1998, the Kansas University Medical Center partnered with the city school system to launch the country's first *telemedicine* delivery system in school to address the lack of access to health care services. Between 1998 and 2006, the number of participating schools increased from twelve to thirty-one, but by 2009 the project limited services to just fourteen schools in response to project funding availability and the needs of schools. TeleKidcare initially received federal, state, and foundation grant funding as a demonstration program but now has contracts with and can bill health insurance companies for the delivery of telemedicine services. Due in large part to its efforts, Kansas Medicaid and other private insurance companies now reimburse for telemedicine services. The program received recognition from the Models That Work Campaign by the BPHC in 2000 as a best practice.

When a school nurse or other school professional identifies a child who needs medical assistance, the nurse schedules a telemedicine appointment. The system transmits real-time information to a physician over an encrypted Internet connection using videoconferencing technology. Electronic stethoscopes and otoscopes allow the remote physician to conduct physical exams and diagnose health problems. The program was originally designed to provide acute care for sore throats, earaches, and similar ailments but has shifted to also provide mental health care as parents and school nurses identified a gap in these services. The creators of the program have developed a training program for interested school districts and continue to develop partnerships with medical schools, school districts, and foundations.

Private Initiatives

Many of the private initiatives to address socioeconomic disparities in health are delivered through medical organizations and community organizations, but a vast majority receive their funding through national and regional philanthropies. The creation of the majority of major philanthropic health-oriented organizations occurs through the conversion of health plans from nonprofit to for-profit status. Law requires that profit from the conversion support health care initiatives consistent with the original mission of the health plan, and the assets of the newly created philanthropies are typically used to improve the health of low-income families in the community.

Project HEALTH   Founded in Boston in 1996 by a college student, the program aims to break the link between poverty and poor health by recruiting college undergraduates to volunteer in community clinics and connect patients with various local health resources. Funding is provided by philanthropic foundations, including a $2 million grant from the Robert Wood Johnson Foundation (RWJF) in 2009, and university and hospital partners. The students, who commit to at least six hours per week over a one-year period, staff family help desks in pediatric and prenatal care clinics, newborn nurseries, pediatric emergency rooms, health department clinics, and CHCs. Physicians working at these locations "prescribe" food and housing assistance, public health insurance, job training, travel assistance, child care, and other social support services. Volunteers at the help desks work with families to obtain these resources and services and coordinate efforts with physicians, social workers, and lawyers to meet the needs of patients. This contribution is believed to be successful because students are not limited by time and reimbursement constraints, as are physicians, and provide a formal infrastructure for assisting families with these SES and socially oriented services that are critical to promoting family health.

Project HEALTH operates in six cities with sixteen unique help desks staffed by 600 volunteers, dedicating 80,000 hours each year. During a six-month period in 2009, a single help desk at Boston Medical Center assisted 205 families with securing low-income housing; 154 families with obtaining spaces in low-cost child care, after school, and Head Start programs; 135 families with accessing food stamps and other food assistance programs; and many other varied services.

Center for Health and Health Care in Schools   The Center for Health and Health Care in Schools (CHHCS) is a non-partisan program resource center located at the George Washington University School of Public Health and Health Services. The center has been a leader in the development of school-based health center programs for children for more than twenty years and is the current incarnation of the Making the Grade program that began funding school-based health centers in the 1980s. The center receives the majority of its funding from RWJF to disseminate information about school-based health care programs; analyze programs and policy options to promote school health; and test new school-connected health care strategies to expand medical, dental, and mental health services.

The CHHCS also serves as a leading advocate for school-based health centers. The center analyzes options for organizing and financing health programs in schools, advises government leaders and health care institutions on how to provide cost-effective and accountable health care programs in schools, and synthesizes research on school-based health centers to inform policymakers and the public about the best approaches to delivering health care in schools. Among its priority issues are to improve the financial stability of school-based health centers by collaborating with publicly sponsored health insurance programs. CHHCS also aims to increase access to dental and mental health services through school-based health centers.

In support of these priorities, the CHHCS has served as the national program office for several major RWJF grant initiatives. This includes most recently the Caring Across Communities Initiative that started in 2007. Fifteen sites were funded over three years with $4.5 million to improve school-connected mental health services for children, particularly those who are immigrant or refugee families that are affected greatly by economic, social, and personal hardships (such as separation of family members, issues of acculturation, and so on). Grant recipients are geographically diverse and range from hospitals and medical schools to public school districts and health centers.

Strengthening Primary Care Providers for the Poor   The Health Foundation of Greater Cincinnati is a social welfare organization dedicated to improving community health and has developed, as one of its initiatives, a program of grants aimed at strengthening primary care systems for the poor in Cincinnati and twenty counties in Ohio, Kentucky, and Indiana. In 1998, an advisory group to the foundation identified two community-focused strategies to target funding toward strengthening the capacity of primary care providers. Their focus on provider support is based on the fact that primary care providers for the poor struggle to deliver care while dealing with a large volume of patients, complex financial issues, inadequate staffing, and little resource development. The first strategy is to strengthen the primary care infrastructure and improve the resources and networks of information available to primary care physicians serving the poor. The second strategy is to improve the *integration of care* among primary care providers and service providers for special needs individuals, including gerontology, mental health, substance abuse, and health literacy. The support the foundation provides is meant to increase the sustainability of these providers and create an environment where they can collaborate to share resources and best practices. The foundation has assets of nearly $260 million, and since its inception it has awarded more than 150 grants to improve primary care for the poor.

Johnson & Johnson Community Health Care Program   Founded in 1987 as part of Johnson & Johnson's corporate commitment to social responsibility, the Community Health Care Program's goal is to provide support to community-based, nonprofit organizations that propose innovative ways to improve access to quality health care for the impoverished and medically underserved.

The program's support is financial; qualifying organizations receive a two-year, nonrenewable $150,000 grant. Grants are primarily awarded to health, education, and human services organizations. Since the program's inception, $15.5 million in community health care support has been awarded to more than 100 distinguished health care organizations across the country and Puerto Rico. In 2008, Johnson & Johnson awarded $1.5 million in grants to ten community health care organizations. In 2007 and 2008, the program focused on communities affected by Hurricane Katrina.

Strengths and Weaknesses of Programs Addressing Socioeconomic Disparities

Addressing socioeconomic disparities in health is perhaps one of the most challenging health-related tasks before the United States. These programs have met with varying levels of success, and we review the strengths and weaknesses of these programs next.

Validity   Most federal safety net initiatives are administered by the BPHC. Centralizing the administration of these programs, along with legislation combining their funding in a single legislative bundle in the mid-1990s, has led to a greater capacity for coordination and cooperation among programs. The programs at the federal, state, local, and private levels generally address disparities in access to health care. The programs frequently establish or expand comprehensive health clinics or service delivery units (mobile vans and school-based health centers, for example) in underserved areas or assemble networks of providers willing to provide vulnerable populations with free or low-cost services. Although these programs address socioeconomic disparities through an access-to-care mechanism (see Chapter Two), they tend to overlook even greater (though less amenable to intervention) contributors to disparities in health, such as education, occupation, and community social cohesion factors.

One major exception is the national Head Start program, which focuses on health promotion for the youngest children with the goal of preparing them for learning in school. Because of this focus on enabling school achievement, it is possible that Head Start may be among the most effective programs at reducing SES disparities over the long term because of its investment in reducing the actual prevalence of lower SES. In this sense, we would do well to also consider policies such as Affirmative Action and programs such as the Bill and Melinda Gates Foundation college scholarships for minority students as potentially effective strategies to reduce SES disparities in health.

Scope and Reach   The safety net programs serve a large number of vulnerable individuals and address the needs of several unique populations, including children, residents of public housing, and the homeless. These programs have only increased in scope since 2001. The CHC program is by far the largest safety net program in the country. CHCs operate in nearly every state and annually serve more than 16 million low-income individuals. Another large program, Healthcare for the Homeless, now serves a million people each year. Even the smaller state and local initiatives have provided thousands of individuals with access to health care services. Moreover, national programs such as school-based health centers are expanding with increased federal funding and are gaining wider recognition among policymakers at both the state and local levels who are interested in replicating the successes of the strategy in their localities.

Sustainability   Federal safety net health centers and programs have fared well recently. Beginning with President Bush's Initiative to Expand Access to Health Care in 2004 and continuing with recent economic stimulus funding, CHCs are experiencing a renewal of interest in and financial support for their activities. There remain, however, substantial threats to the long-term financial stability of these programs, including the need to remain competitive service providers for Medicaid clients to obtain reimbursement, collaborating with managed care organizations, and adapting to changes in the financing of health care, while maintaining the financial ability to offer supportive services like transportation and case management to indigent clients. Funding for school-based health centers is on the verge of improving as well, with proposals to federally mandate their role as primary care providers in public programs (many have been excluded in prior years because they function a bit differently than a regular doctor's office) and require a higher reimbursement rate for the services they provide, since they, like CHCs, often need to provide supportive services that are not regularly reimbursed. Head Start funding has continued to grow steadily each year, although advocates argue that funding has not kept pace with the number of expansion programs, meaning less money for each program.

Effectiveness   Safety net programs have been well evaluated. CHCs are studied frequently because of their predominance in caring for vulnerable populations. Studies have revealed the cost-effectiveness of CHCs and an ability to help reduce costs to the Medicaid program. They have also been shown to reduce infant mortality, lower hospital admissions and length of stay, and deliver high-quality care for vulnerable populations (Dievler and Giovannini, 1998; Shi, Regan, Politzer, and Luo, 2001; Shi, Stevens, and Politzer, 2007; Shi and others, 2004).

School-based health centers have been similarly successful at improving access to medical and dental care, decreasing emergency room visits through access to primary care and mental health services, and leading to greater satisfaction compared with other community clinics (Kaplan and others, 1999; Lear, 2007; Lear, Barnwell, and Behrens, 2008; Terwilliger, 1994; Young, D'angelo, and Davis, 2001). Still, many school-based health centers face difficulties educating policymakers about the role of school health services, collaborating with managed care organizations, and reassuring users of the confidentiality of their services (Lear, 2007).

Head Start programs have also been well researched, with a body of evidence suggesting major impacts on the cognitive, emotional, and social development of young, vulnerable children (Administration on Children and Families, 2009; Barnett, 1998; Bierman and others, 2008; Ludwig and Phillips, 2008; Whitaker, Gooze, Hughes, and Finkelstein, 2009). While the program has been criticized for uneven quality across the programs it supports, there exists strong support for the program as a model. As a result, there is debate about the balance that should be struck between the national program encouraging programs to stick to an established model versus allowing flexibility to experiment and meet the needs and interests of local populations (Gray and Francis, 2007).

Other programs are less well studied. The Public Housing Primary Care program reported that it increased immunization rates for young children to well over 95 percent in most sites and 100 percent in some. Internal data from the South Carolina Welvista Program suggests that the program has successfully reduced emergency room visits and hospitalizations, saving an estimated $3.5 million for the state.

PROGRAMS TO ELIMINATE DISPARITIES IN HEALTH INSURANCE

Health insurance coverage is an essential enabler for individuals to obtain health care services and maintain good health. Since the mid-1960s, there have been extremely large public and private investments to provide low-income individuals, who are generally unable to obtain private insurance easily, with adequate coverage through several public insurance programs. Although these programs cover large numbers of individuals, in 2008 there remained more than 46.3 million Americans without any form of insurance coverage. Thus, there remains substantial need for greater public and private investment to ensure greater equity in coverage.

The main federal and state health insurance initiatives are Medicare, Medicaid, and the Children's Health Insurance Program (CHIP; discussed in detail in Chapter Two). Together, they cover nearly 40 percent of the U.S.

population. To assist the remaining uninsured population, states and private organizations have developed their own initiatives to provide these individuals with health insurance coverage. Because there are a large number of state programs, we will highlight and discuss only a few examples. More complete listings of state efforts are available from the National Academy for State Health Policy and the National Conference of State Legislators.

State and Local Initiatives

States are exploring ways to expand the coverage of the uninsured and underinsured while still leaving the current system of employer-based insurance intact. These programs are most often directed toward covering the working poor: individuals and families who cannot afford to purchase health insurance coverage but who earn too much to qualify for public assistance through Medicaid or CHIP.

Massachusetts Commonwealth Health Insurance Connector Authority   In 2006, the Massachusetts legislature passed a comprehensive health care bill that introduced many reforms to the state's health care system, among them an individual mandate to purchase health insurance, increased employer responsibility, Medicaid restorations and expansions, and various insurance market reforms. The bill built on the existing MassHealth Family Assistance Program that started in 1998 and provided subsidies to low-income families to purchase private insurance. The centerpiece of the new bill was the creation of the Commonwealth Health Insurance Connector. Operated by the Massachusetts Department of Administration and Finance and governed by a board of appointed private and public representatives, the Connector establishes an exchange, or marketplace, for individuals and small business employers to help acquire health insurance coverage. Initially, $25 million from state funds was used for start-up costs and operating expenses.

Because the new law requires adult residents of Massachusetts who can afford health insurance to obtain it, there was a need to define what constitutes the lowest standard of care. This responsibility was given to the Connector's board. To meet this standard, known as Minimum Creditable Coverage, insurance plans must provide a set of core services without an annual maximum benefit or per illness maximum benefit, and with a limit on annual deductibles and out-of-pocket expenses. It also puts a limit on annual deductibles for prescription medication.

The Connector also administers two programs, Commonwealth Care and Commonwealth Choice, and is currently able to generate its own revenue through premiums and administrative fees from these programs. Commonwealth Care is designed for previously uninsured or underinsured low- to middle-income residents who do not qualify for public programs. It offers health services on a sliding-fee scale through five Medicaid managed care organizations. Commonwealth Choice offers unsubsidized insurance plans to those not eligible for public programs or Commonwealth Care. It currently offers services through six private companies, each with plans that differ in premium and copayments.

Since its inception, the Connector has helped Massachusetts achieve the lowest rate of uninsured residents in the nation at 2.6 percent and has become a model for states, particularly as they implement national health care reform. The state of Washington, for example, passed a similar program in 2007 called the Health Insurance Partnership, which as of 2010 is beginning enrollment.

Healthcare Group of Arizona   In 1988, the Healthcare Group (HCG) of Arizona was established by the state legislature to offer prepaid medical coverage to small businesses and the self-employed through a group of three health maintenance organizations (HMOs). While most insurance companies market their group insurance plans only to businesses with more than five employees, this program was made available to very small firms with two or more employees and to self-employed individuals. Although the state mandates HMOs to make this option available to employers, it does not subsidize any of the costs of coverage, and employers are responsible for the entire insurance premiums. There are no income limits for employee enrollment, but an employer must not have been able to offer coverage for ninety days prior to joining this program (to prevent employers from switching from more expensive private insurance). The key to keeping costs low in this program is that the three participating health plans are required to accept all part-time or full-time workers in small firms and to charge a community rate (that is, they cannot charge a company more because someone there has a major medical problem). Also, there are no preexisting condition clauses that would allow the plans to exclude someone because of a medical condition. Although the program has undergone some difficult changes, it has stabilized while providing over 4,500 small businesses with coverage for nearly 13,000 employees in 2009 (albeit the program has steadily decreased in size from 20,000 in 2001).

Private Initiatives

While there are many foundations and other private organizations that are involved in improving access to care for vulnerable populations, relatively few directly support health insurance programs or subsidize premiums for individuals and families. We present one major example of a private initiative to cover vulnerable populations.

California Children's Health Initiatives   Children's Health Initiatives (CHIs) are nonprofit, county-based coalitions that have formed in order to increase the number of children with health insurance coverage in California. The first CHI was formed in Santa Clara County in 2001 and was made up of the board of supervisors, in partnership with several local and statewide private entities. The CHI coalition sought to make health insurance available to all children in families with incomes up to 300 percent of the FPL, including children who are undocumented immigrants, by increasing outreach efforts to enroll uninsured children who are eligible for Medicaid and CHIP and implementing a new county-based insurance program, Healthy Kids, for those not eligible for public programs (mostly undocumented families). Healthy Kids is a low-cost private health, dental, and vision insurance program with monthly premiums ranging from about five to ten dollars per child per month. CHIs and their Healthy Kids programs spread to twenty-five of the state's fifty-eight counties, with most counties launching their programs between 2004 and 2006. At its peak in late 2006, Healthy Kids programs had more than 87,000 members enrolled statewide. It was also estimated that CHIs boosted enrollment in the state's Medicaid and CHIP programs between 2001 and 2006 by another 34,000 children through its outreach efforts.

Strengths and Weaknesses of Programs Addressing Health Insurance

Programs that focus on insurance coverage have perhaps the longest legacy in the United States. These programs have been created in distinct initiatives at different levels of government and community, and often in a piecemeal fashion. Nevertheless, together they reflect a movement that is leading toward more comprehensive national coverage. We review some of the major strengths and weaknesses of these programs next.

Validity   Health insurance coverage is the single largest determinant of access to care in the United States. Although the federal government has not yet elected to provide this benefit universally, many federal and state programs like those discussed are in place to ensure that most older individuals and many low-income families and children receive some form of health insurance coverage. Even among those who have coverage, there are still financial barriers to care. In addition to restricted Medicare services such as long-term care, those eligible for Medicare under age sixty-five have a two-year waiting period before they can enroll. Privately insured individuals are often under-insured for conditions of mental illness or substance abuse and are under financial pressure to pay increasingly high premiums or copayments for care.

Of the 46.3 million U.S. residents who lacked health insurance in 2008, many can access care through grant-funded safety net health programs or in emergency departments. In a strikingly obvious way, even though the government has not funded universal insurance coverage, federal and state dollars still finance the care of uninsured individuals through the rising costs of health services to make up for the costs of uncompensated care or through these safety net programs. Until health services are available to every citizen through some form of universal coverage, which will not occur even with the health care reforms of 2010, lack of health insurance will remain an important contributing factor to disparities.

Scope and Reach   The impact of federal programs such as Medicare, Medicaid, and CHIP has been tremendous. Medicare provides insurance coverage for nearly every citizen over the age of sixty-five, and Medicaid now covers more than one of every eight individuals in the United States. Although CHIP had a relatively slow start, the program had covered more than 7.4 million children in 2008, nearly double the number in 2001. Medicaid and CHIP have helped to reduce the rate of uninsured children by well over half (from 22.3 percent in 1997 to 9.9 percent in 2008), as they now collectively cover about one in four children nationally (DeNavas-Walt, Proctor, and Lee, 2009). The creators of CHIP were cognizant of the larger role of Medicaid and included options to allow the programs to function as seamlessly as possible (including giving states the option of using CHIP funds for an expansion of Medicaid) (Dubay, Guyer, Mann, and Odeh, 2007). There have remained concerns about the effect of CHIP and Medicaid possibly drawing families away from private coverage by offering coverage at lower cost (Dubay and Kenney, 2009). However, it is likely that in many cases of private-to-public substitution, public programs are still serving the role of safety net by giving low-income families relief from the expensive premiums often paid by low-wage workers for private coverage. Nevertheless, there are still uninsured adults and children eligible for Medicaid and CHIP, and despite easing the enrollment process, organizational and social barriers to enrollment remain.

State, local, and private initiatives serve an extremely important role in filling gaps in coverage. State and local initiatives have deftly designed insurance plans to encourage the affordability of insurance coverage for the working poor. Most states have also chosen (without major federal assistance) to expand Medicaid coverage to individuals above the poverty level, and many states have expanded insurance coverage for children up to 250 percent of poverty (and some as high as 300 percent). Local and private initiatives, such as the CHIs in California, are the only sources of coverage for low-income undocumented children, since they are specifically excluded from federal programs like Medicaid and CHIP. Undocumented adults living in the United States must find their own private insurance, as they receive no assistance from government.

Sustainability   Although federal funding of Medicare, Medicaid, and CHIP is ensured for the near future, concerns about future financing of these programs continue to be a problem. Medicare relies on the contributions of today's workers to pay for the health needs of the elderly. With an aging population, the number of beneficiaries is expected to outgrow the number paying into the system, creating a funding crisis for the program as early as 2019.

In economic downturns, states have difficulty financing their share of Medicaid program costs. The federal government is allowed to run a budget deficit, but states cannot. So each year, all state expenditures must be balanced with state income. In economic recessions, such as the one in 2009, families not only earn less (and pay fewer taxes as a result), but more families also rely on public safety net programs like Medicaid. For every 1 percent increase in the national unemployment rate, states can expect a 3 to 4 percent decrease in state revenues coupled with a national increase in Medicaid and CHIP enrollees of 1 million individuals and an increase of about 1.1 million uninsured individuals. Enrollment in Medicaid grew by an average of 5.4 percent in 2009 (compared to just 3.6 percent in 2001), and Medicaid enrollments are expected to grow by an additional 6.6 percent in 2010 due to the recession (Kaiser Commission on Medicaid and the Uninsured, 2009d). Because Medicaid makes up about 15 percent of a state's total budget, it is always a target for reducing state spending. In 2009, virtually every state was forced to consider or implement spending cuts in Medicaid. In California, for example, the state ended all dental coverage for adults on Medicaid as a way to balance the state budget.

Other state-only and local initiatives for the uninsured are also facing difficult times in the current economic climate. The Massachusetts Connector has helped to enroll more than 50,000 additional individuals than originally expected, meaning a higher state expenditure on subsidies to purchase the coverage. This is particularly challenging in the economic climate of 2009 but also demonstrates the great level of need for coverage that had previously been hidden from view. The Healthcare Group of Arizona continues to struggle with potential financial losses that exceed insurance premiums because many of the enrollees were unable to obtain coverage elsewhere because of high-cost conditions. Even with help from the state, members are likely to continue to see significant increases in their premiums and copayments.

CHIs and their Healthy Kids programs are successful efforts that have not yet been able to become financially sustainability. While these programs have been widely recognized for their achievements in reaching and enrolling children and were nearly incorporated into a state program during California's health care reform debates in 2006, they have not found ways to achieve self-sufficiency. Many philanthropic sources have declined to continue funding the operation of these programs, as the CHIs were originally designed to be demonstration programs and were encouraged to find alternate sources of funding. By 2009, two of the twenty-five CHIs had closed their doors, and most of the remaining CHIs have decreased enrollments by nearly half to achieve a level of operation to match their available funding (Stevens, Rice, and Cousineau, 2009).

Effectiveness   The impact of health insurance programs has been discussed previously. A number of studies show the benefits of Medicaid to vulnerable populations, such as improved access to care and improved health status. Studies show that when Medicaid coverage is interrupted for adults, there are major impacts on health (Hall, Harman, and Zhang, 2008; Lowe, McConnell, Vogt, and Smith, 2008; Lurie, Ward, Shapiro, and Brook, 1984; Lurie and others, 1986). Evaluations of CHIP have also shown impacts on access to care, quality of care, and health status (Seid, Varni, Cummings, and Schonlau, 2006; Stevens, Seid, and Halfon, 2006; Szilagyi and others, 2006; Szilagyi and others, 2004). The CHIs in California are credited with improvements in the health status of undocumented children (Howell and Trenholm, 2007) and lower overall rates of child hospitalizations that have been prevented through access to primary care (Cousineau, Stevens, and Pickering, 2008).

Due to its success in reaching previously uninsured individuals, Massachusetts Commonwealth Connector has become a model for the health care reforms passed by Congress (Lischko, Bachman, and Vangeli, 2009). When the Massachusetts reform was first legislated, state officials estimated that some 379,000 Massachusetts residents were uninsured. But nearly 440,000 residents have become insured through the Connector since the program took effect. Estimates now suggest that as many as 97 percent of working adults in the state now have coverage. Support for the reform among political leadership remains very strong, and public surveys show that support for the reform rose in the first two years of the program from 61 percent in 2006 to 69 percent in 2008 (Kingsdale, 2009).

Focus on Vulnerability in Clinical Practice

The general model of vulnerability has been used in a number of instances as a type of triaging for the delivery of interventions and clinical services. Identifying people who are at greatest risk of a particular outcome can then be targeted for special services or they can be provided with more intensive case management services. One widely noted example of this strategy was implemented in a handful of cities beginning in 2007 to identify the most at-risk homeless individuals living on the streets. Project 50, as it was most commonly known, uses a "vulnerability index" to identify the fifty homeless individuals in each city at greatest risk of death based on eight indicators. The index, administered in the form of a survey, was created by Boston's Health Care for the Homeless organization, based on data showing that individuals with the following were at a 40 percent higher risk of premature death: (1) more than three hospitalizations or emergency department visits in the past year, (2) more than three emergency department visits in the past month, (3) age sixty or older, (4) cirrhosis of the liver, (5) end-stage renal disease, (6) a history of frostbite or hypothermia, (7) HIV or AIDS, and (8) co-occurring psychiatric, substance abuse, and chronic medical conditions. Having more of these indicators increased the likelihood of premature death, such that homeless individuals were prioritized based on the number of risk factors they had in combination with how long the person had been homeless.

The vulnerability index has been used in New York, Los Angeles, and New Orleans. For three consecutive days between 3:00 AM and 6:00 AM, volunteers in each city walked the streets where homeless individuals were residing to gather information from homeless individuals, taking digital photos (with permission) to be able to follow up with each person after the vulnerability profile was calculated. While the services for the prioritized individuals varied in each city, most included a multipronged intervention strategy, such as linking them with supportive housing, substance abuse treatment, extensive case management, and medical services. In Los Angeles's Skid Row, the selected individuals were given housing in the Housing Trust, which included a satellite medical clinic in the first floor of the building. The clinic houses a team of clinicians, case managers, and social workers who are part of a local community health center but dedicated to these highest-risk individuals.

The results of Project 50 have been impressive. In New York, homelessness was reduced by 87 percent in the 20 square blocks surrounding Times Square and by 43 percent in the surrounding 230 blocks. Housing costs $36 per person per night to operate, in comparison to $54 for a city shelter bed, $74 for a state prison cell, $164 for a city jail cell, $467 for a psychiatric bed, and $1,185 for a hospital bed (Common Ground, 2010). In Los Angeles, forty-nine individuals moved into the Housing Trust, and by 2009, forty-three remained in housing. In the year prior to participation, participants had a collective 754 days in jail, 205 inpatient hospital days, and 133 emergency department visits. After intervention, these individuals had 142 days in jail, fifty-five inpatient hospital days, and thirty-nine emergency department visits. Of the thirty-six individuals with a history of substance abuse, twenty-two had become sober by 2009 (Lopez, 2009).

SUMMARY

In this chapter, we have discussed key federal, state, and private initiatives to address racial, socioeconomic, and insurance coverage disparities in the United States. While many of the programs have made substantial contributions to reducing these disparities, there remains a great need to replicate on a larger scale many of the successful programs, as well as to develop new, more sophisticated, and creative approaches to addressing gaps in access to health care, quality of care, and health status.

Prevention may be the best, most cost-efficient way to reduce the effects of vulnerability on health status; however, health care in the United States continues to be dominated by highly technical, treatment-oriented medical care. Consequently, the majority of money spent to care for vulnerable populations goes to treatment instead of making the investment earlier with preventive services. Providers need to be better trained in prevention-oriented procedures and be appropriately reimbursed and rewarded with financial incentives for integrating them into their practice. Furthermore, the physical, psychological, and social functioning problems often associated with the poor health status of vulnerable populations are difficult to address in a treatment-oriented medical care system because these conditions and their causes can fall outside the clinical domain.

Vulnerable populations require a broad spectrum of care, from clinical to social services. However, care for vulnerable populations tends to be fragmented. Funding that targets certain illnesses or very specific subgroups of vulnerable populations contributes to this fragmentation. Programs such as Health Care for the Homeless, the Indian Health Service, and Community Health Centers offer more integrated systems of care and thus a more effective safety net.

Finally, it is important to consider the complex sociopolitical origins of vulnerability. While initiatives such as the Office of Minority Health develop health policy to promote minority health issues and strive to ensure that the federal government is accountable to the needs of minority populations, it is essential to identify and continue to address the fundamental social and political influences that allow such vulnerability to persist. As greater knowledge becomes available on the determinants of disparities, newer programs will tailor their efforts to intervene in the contributing pathways. In the final chapter, we synthesize the complexities of eliminating disparities in health care and consider the next steps to achieving this goal.

KEY TERMS

Ancillary services

Community coalitions

Cultural competence

Integration of care

Linguistically appropriate

Migrant and seasonal farm workers

Standardized mortality rates

Telemedicine

REVIEW QUESTIONS

1. Describe at least two national efforts to address racial/ethnic disparities in health. What agencies and organizations are the main participants, and which government agency provides the coordinating role? How do these initiatives support the goals of Healthy People 2020?

2. The Bureau of Primary Health Care is the home of many federal efforts to address health care disparities for lower-SES individuals and other vulnerable populations. Describe two initiatives of the BPHC, discuss their purpose and scope, and identify what level of overlap there is between these programs in terms of their design and purpose. Does either program address multiple risk factors?

3. Describe the Children's Health Insurance Program. Identify those it serves, whether the program varies by state, and its current and potential effectiveness. How is the program different from Medicaid in terms of its target population? Describe the sustainability of the program.

ESSAY QUESTIONS

1. Identify one health-related program in your community or state that is designed to address health disparities for racial/ethnic minorities, lower-SES individuals, or the uninsured. Describe the program, how and when it was started, what its target disparity is, and its current activities. Assess whether the methods by which this program is aiming to reduce disparities are valid (using what you learned in Chapter Two), whether its scope is sufficient, given the size of the problem, the current and future sustainability of the program, and its effectiveness. Describe what kinds of outcomes you would use to determine whether the program is effective, and briefly summarize what kinds of evidence of effectiveness exist and what kinds of information are still needed.

2. You are in charge of a health clinic for low-income individuals in your community. The clinic has just received a five-year grant to fund a small intervention to reduce disparities in asthma among local Hispanic and African American children and teenagers. Based on what you have learned in the previous chapters and using the programs described in this chapter as examples, design a small program or initiative to address this disparity. Examples could include some type of health education offered in local schools, free screenings, efforts to improve air quality in the area, or something more creative. For your program, make sure to describe its purpose and methods (validity), the scope of its services and who will be reached, how it will be sustained after five years, and how you will assess its effectiveness.

CHAPTER SIX

RESOLVING DISPARITIES IN THE UNITED STATES

LEARNING OBJECTIVES

- Provide examples of strategies that might be used to reduce disparities associated with vulnerability risk factors.

- Describe challenges in implementing strategies to reduce disparities.

- Introduce a course of action to implement strategies that reduce disparities.

THROUGHOUT this book, we have analyzed disparities in access to medical care, quality of care, and health status using a conceptualization of vulnerability that captures the combined influences of race/ethnicity, SES, and health insurance. We have reviewed the deep social, political, economic, and medical roots of vulnerability and presented a wealth of evidence linking vulnerability risks, both individually and in combination, to poor health care experiences and health outcomes. These relationships convey a high level of health and health care inequality within U.S. society.

These inequalities are not surface deep or easily remedied, but it is our intent in this final chapter to assemble and synthesize the most progressive theory- and evidence-based strategies for preventing, treating, and eliminating national disparities in health. We begin with an overview of the Healthy People Initiative that provides the imperative and direction to resolve these health disparities. In support of this initiative, we then present a unifying solutions-focused framework for resolving these disparities, synthesizing models presented in Chapters One and Two.

Guided by this framework, we highlight and discuss examples of strategies that have been used to reduce disparities associated with vulnerability risk factors— race/ethnicity, SES, and health insurance—individually and in combination. We discuss specific examples of interventions at the policy, community, medical care, and individual levels and explore the challenges in adopting these interventions. Finally, we propose a specific course of action, accounting for practical challenges and barriers.

THE HEALTHY PEOPLE INITIATIVE

Disparities in health have become conspicuous enough in the United States to merit placement as one of two major goals selected by the U.S. Department of Health and Human Services (DHHS) Healthy People 2010 initiative. The ongoing Healthy People Initiative has spanned the past thirty years and represents the most comprehensive national effort to improve the health of Americans in this century. The initiative has produced four reports, beginning with the original 1979 publication, *Healthy People: The Surgeon General's Report on Health Promotion and Disease Prevention*. Then came three more reports produced decennially that outlined national health objectives to be completed during the following ten-year period: *Healthy People 1990* (released in 1980), *Healthy People 2000* (released in 1990), and *Healthy People 2010* (released in 2000).

Past initiatives have made important strides toward accomplishing their stated objectives. Healthy People 2000, for example, surpassed the goals set for reducing coronary heart disease and cancer and succeeded in decreasing the incidence of AIDS and syphilis. Today, more children than ever before are receiving vaccinations in a timely and comprehensive manner, and infant mortality has declined significantly since 1979, in line with two ongoing Healthy People indicators. Many other goals, however, have been missed (examples are physical activity and obesity levels) and are of continuing concern.

Prior National Goals and Objectives Set for 2010

Healthy People 2010 had two main goals: to increase the quality and years of healthy life and to eliminate health disparities. The first goal targets the general population, noting that U.S. life expectancy is ranked just eighteenth in the world despite much higher health care spending than other developed countries. The second goal targets the disproportionate burden of poor health that exists by gender, race/ethnicity, education, income, and geographical location. Figure 6.1 presents the framework for these goals as key components in the strategy to improve the public's health by 2010.

To gauge progress toward the two main goals, Healthy People 2010 identified 28 focus areas and 467 specific measurable targets or objectives to be achieved by 2010. The objectives and focus areas address an array of influences on individual health as shown in the Healthy People initiative framework for health improvement (Figure 6.2). Identifying the determinants of health reveals opportunities for intervention, and the model depicts the influence of biology, behaviors, and environment on health and how these can be modified by public policy and access to medical care. Led by the U.S. surgeon general, experts from federal agencies used this model to select focus areas and objectives, with input from the Healthy People Consortium, state organizations, and community groups.

The resulting focus areas and objectives also reflected a changing national demographic and evolving health care system. The U.S. population is becoming older and more racially/ethnically diverse, and the resulting different health needs necessitated a reallocation of resources to provide better age-appropriate and culturally specific care. Changes in the health care system included new technologies, advanced preventive and curative care, better vaccines and pharmaceuticals, and improved health surveillance. New threats to public health, such as emerging infectious diseases and bioterrorism, have also arisen and were accounted for in Healthy People 2010. The focus areas and objectives also reflected the growing recognition of the importance of community-level health influences, and the report assigned a significant role to community partners in civic, professional, and religious organizations to care for local populations.

FIGURE 6.1   Goals of the Healthy People 2010 Initiative

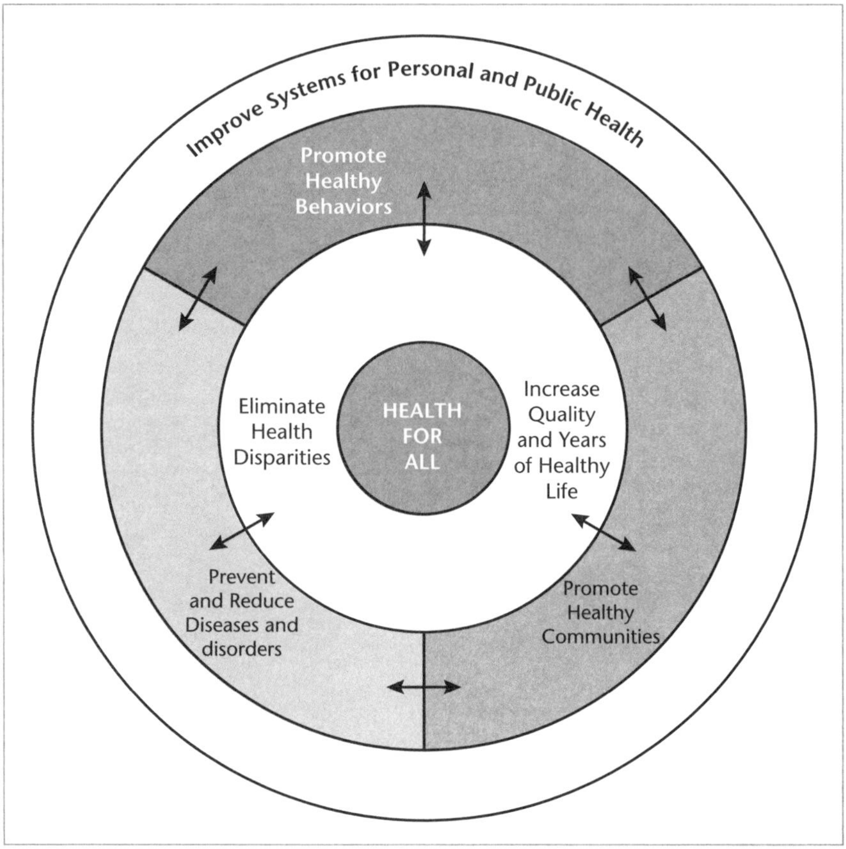

Source: U.S. Department of Health and Human Services (2002).

Healthy People 2020

The next ten-year national objectives as captured in Healthy People 2020 will reflect assessments of major risks to health and wellness, changing public health priorities, and emerging issues related to the nation's health preparedness and prevention (Secretary's Advisory Committee on National Health Promotion and Disease Prevention Objectives for 2020, 2008). The program's development is being released in two phases. The first phase, which occurred in 2009, reveals the framework, including the proposed vision, mission, and goals of Healthy People 2020, as well as the draft of objectives that may be revised based on the public input. The second

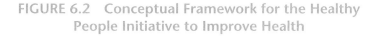

FIGURE 6.2   Conceptual Framework for the Healthy
People Initiative to Improve Health

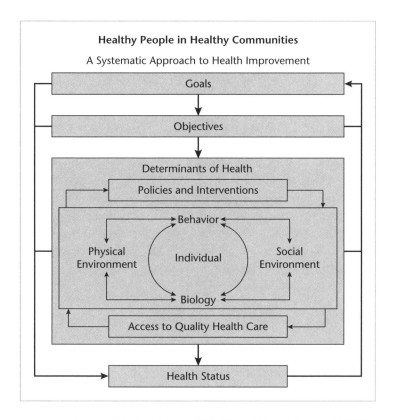

Source: U.S. Department of Health and Human Services (2000).

phase, occurring in 2010, will launch Healthy People 2020 and reveal the ten-year objectives and the guidelines for achieving these goals.

According to the released framework, Healthy People 2020 will:

■ Identify nationwide health improvement priorities
■ Increase public awareness and understanding of the determinants of health, disease, and disability and the opportunities for progress
■ Provide measurable objectives and goals that are applicable at the national, state, and local levels
■ Engage multiple sectors to take actions to strengthen policies and improve practices that are driven by the best available evidence and knowledge
■ Identify critical research, evaluation, and data collection needs

Overarching goals for both Quality of Life and Well-Being and Social Determinants of Health are being set for Healthy People 2020. One of Healthy People 2020's proposed overarching goals in its Phase I report looks to achieve health equality by eliminating health disparities and improve the health of all population groups (Secretary's Advisory Committee on National Health Promotion and Disease Prevention Objectives for 2020, 2008). Healthy People 2020 will look at all the determinants of health, including conditions of daily life, occupation, age, and environment, in addition to institutional policies and practices that may place vulnerable populations at a disadvantage. This goal essentially looks to improve the health of vulnerable populations as the advisory committee defines the term health disparity as a health difference "closely linked with social or economic disadvantage … based on their racial or ethnic group, religion, socioeconomic status, gender, mental health, cognitive, sensory, or physical disability, sexual orientation, geographic location, or other characteristics historically linked to discrimination or exclusion" (from page 46 of report). The goal is to bridge the gap of health disparities, not just in health care but in the physical and social environment that influence an individual's health status. Healthy People 2020 will measure its goal of health equity by measuring health disparities between populations. If health equity is being achieved, health disparities should be shrinking.

The released draft of the Healthy People 2020 objectives includes some objectives from Healthy People 2010 that have been kept intact or modified, as well as new additional objectives. Increasing the proportion of persons with health insurance remains one of the objectives for Access to Health Services. The draft is also looking to keep objectives aimed at reducing child, adolescent, and maternal deaths, as well as reducing complications due to pregnancy. A new topic area, older adults, has been included with objectives aimed not only to keep older populations healthy but also to protect them from abuse or neglect. In addition, the DHHS plans to develop objectives that will attain and promote a high quality of life for all people, across all life stages, and incorporate a focus on social determinants of health and on health outcomes.

Strategies and Partnerships to Achieve National Objectives

The general strategy of the Healthy People initiative is to motivate diverse groups to combine efforts in accomplishing the national objectives. The initiative's objectives are designed to be easily used and exchanged by federal and state governments and community and professional organizations to improve national health. Although the federal government maintains much of the responsibility for achieving the national goals, the initiative formed a diverse network of

FIGURE 6.3   An Action Model to Achieve Healthy People 2020 Overarching Goals

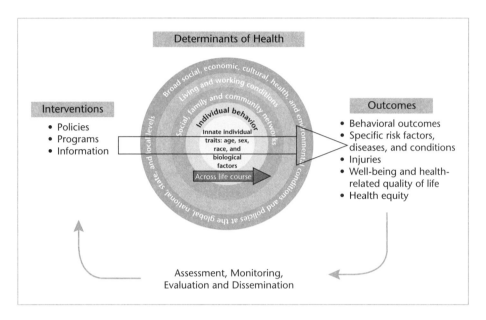

Source: Secretary's Advisory Committee on National Health Promotion and Disease Prevention Objectives for 2020, 2008; http://www.healthypeople.gov/hp2020/advisory/PhaseI/PhaseI.pdf (accessed 09-24-09).

partnerships to delegate some responsibility among state governments and interested local public and private parties. This strategic collaboration reduces redundant efforts at the national, state, and local levels and takes advantage of the unique competencies of each partner. Figure 6.3 shows the action model to achieve Healthy People 2020 overarching goals.

One of the most important Healthy People partnerships is with the Healthy People Consortium, an alliance of organizations dedicated to meeting the national goals and objectives. The Consortium's membership is an assembly of all state and territorial public health agencies and representatives from advocacy and business sectors. Members have contributed in many ways, including defining the goals and objectives of the initiative, developing national health promotion projects, and incorporating objectives into their mission statements.

Because the objectives identified in Healthy People are not necessarily relevant to every region of the country, state-specific plans were established that identify and address unique regional public health needs. In this way, objectives are accomplished more efficiently when prioritized by state or regional relevance. Historically, involvement at the state level has been impressive. Nearly all states and territories created a state-level Healthy People plan.

To facilitate the achievement of Healthy People objectives at the community level, the DHHS has established grant programs to support the efforts of local community organizations. Steps to a Healthier US program, for example, has awarded $13.7 million to communities working to combat diabetes, asthma, or obesity epidemics by promoting prevention and improving access to health care. These three conditions were identified as community targets because they have reached epidemic proportions and are generally responsive to prevention efforts. Another grant program, the Community Implementation Program, administered by the DHHS Office of Disease Prevention and Health Promotion, distributes small grants in support of health promotion pilot projects consistent with Healthy People goals and objectives.

To further encourage local Healthy People initiatives, publications were developed to aid state, community, and professional leaders in initiating health promotion programs. The Healthy People Toolkit provides guidance, technical tools, and other resources for state-specific programs. Community health endeavors are assisted by the *Healthy People in Healthy Communities* planning guide, offering information and resources on how to establish and operate community coalitions. In addition, the *Healthy Workforce* publication targets professional leaders who are well positioned to initiate health promotion efforts at their work sites. The publication explains preventive efforts (addressing Healthy People objectives) and their influence on creating a healthier workforce. A list of healthy workforce objectives and strategies is also presented to provide a road map for administering work site health promotion programs.

Private partners have also made formal agreements with federal agencies to work toward achieving the Healthy People objectives. Private partners include organizations such as the American Medical Association (AMA), the National Recreation and Parks Association, and the Academy of General Dentistry. For example, the American Heart Association and the American Stroke Association have developed a partnership to prevent cardiovascular disease through community-based health education programs; public awareness campaigns; policy, and professional development; and additional collaboration with organizations and agencies. The progress of the joint partnership is being evaluated yearly to assess its future direction.

The Healthy People Information Access Project is a strategic partnership between federal agencies, public health organizations, and health sciences libraries. The collaboration, Partners in Information Access for the Public Health Workforce, provides easy access to published research relevant to the Healthy People objectives. The National Library of Medicine and the Public Health Foundation designed a program simplifying the search engine of the PubMed database. The open door to abundant evidence-based research allows the benefits of this partnership to be realized at all levels of the health care workforce.

Tracking Progress in Achieving National Objectives

To achieve the Healthy People initiative national health objectives, it is essential to monitor improvement regularly to ensure the resources are directed appropriately and effectively. A set of ten measurable *leading health indicators (LHIs)* was developed to facilitate this monitoring progress toward achieving Healthy People objectives. The LHIs (Table 6.1) were selected from the national health objectives, emphasize high-priority public health issues, and were included based on the availability of data to measure their progress. Each LHI is tracked and reported throughout the Healthy People ten-year cycle.

For example, each of the 467 Healthy People 2010 objectives is tracked through 190 data sources to ensure that progress assessment can be made at multiple levels of the public health workforce. The National Center for Health Statistics (NCHS) has established a data surveillance system for these objectives with quarterly updates available on NCHS's DATA2010 Web site. Annual updated assessments of the nation's health are also published by the secretary of Health and Human Services in the Health, United States reports. As each initiative comes to a close, NCHS prepares a concluding review of progress made toward meeting the national objectives. The next report is due in 2010.

TABLE 6.1   Leading Health Indicators for the United States

Indicator	Priority Health Topics
1	Physical activity
2	Overweight and obesity
3	Tobacco use
4	Substance abuse
5	Responsible sexual behavior
6	Mental health
7	Injury and violence
8	Environmental quality
9	Immunization
10	Access to health care

Source: U.S. Department of Health and Human Services (2002).

FRAMEWORK TO RESOLVE DISPARITIES

In support of the Healthy People initiative and other calls to arms for eliminating disparities, we propose a single, unifying solutions-focused framework (based on models presented in Chapters One and Two) to improve the nation's health and resolve disparities for vulnerable populations. The framework focuses on both social and medical points of intervention to create a multifaceted approach to reducing disparities in health and health care by race/ethnicity, SES, and health insurance coverage. The framework is built on the ballasts of both social and medical care determinants, because the combination of these factors ultimately shapes health and well-being (see Figure 6.4). It should be noted that health in this model includes the positive concept of well-being and encompasses its physical, mental, and social components.

FIGURE 6.4   Conceptual Model of Points of Intervention for Vulnerable Populations

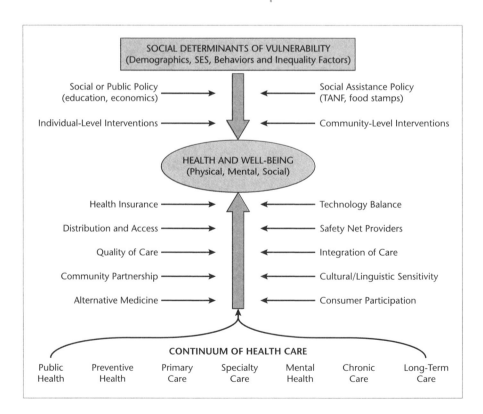

Social and Medical Influences on Vulnerability

The framework synthesizes much of what we have described in previous chapters. In this model, social determinants of vulnerability reflect personal and community-level influences, including demographics, SES factors, and aspects of social interactions. More specifically, these factors include race/ethnicity, SES (such as income, education, and occupation), behavioral factors, and social interactions (such as social networks at the individual level and social cohesion at the community level) that influence health care access and health. Behavior, it should be noted, should not be isolated from the social and environmental contexts that influence what choices are available and then made.

While social determinants influence the health and resources that patients bring to the health care system, the medical care system focuses primarily on treating poor health. The framework includes a broad range of medical services and interventions to improve health. While public health, preventive care, and primary care contribute to general health status, other services, such as specialty and long-term care, are more influential in end-of-life care services and mortality. Without access to medical care, individuals will have difficulty treating their health problems. For patients who gain access and move across the spectrum of care, they will contend with continuity and coordination of care.

In considering solutions for health disparities, policymakers should examine the balance of social and medical influences on vulnerability. Social factors are likely to have stronger influences on health than medical care (medical care typically intervenes only when a problem is identified), but there are important roles for medical care in improving health, promoting well-being, enhancing quality of life, and ultimately lengthening life expectancy. In trying to solve health disparities, one should consider the respective contributions and likely effectiveness of social and medical interventions.

Since medical care absorbs such a large proportion of national spending, special consideration should be given to where resources are directed. Should equal investments be made in all health services, or are some investments better than others? Increasing resources for primary care, for example, may make basic health services available to more individuals but would reduce the availability of specialty care. Directing resources toward specialty care (such as higher-technology services) may enhance care and extend life for people with more severe health conditions but would draw away resources from basic primary care services for all. Other considerations, such as the quality of care and access to alternative therapies, may also have an impact on health care experiences and health outcomes.

Social and Medical Points of Intervention

Considering that both social and medical determinants are responsive to numerous outside forces, our framework highlights many important intervention points. Reductions in health and health care disparities are obtainable through interventions at four levels: (1) policy interventions, (2) community-based interventions, (3) health care interventions, and (4) individual interventions. These general approaches are described below and then used to organize our discussion of intervention strategies to address vulnerability.

Policy Interventions   Social or public policy influences the health and health care of the population in many ways. Product safety regulations, screening food and water sources, and enforcing safe work environments are a few of the ways in which public policy directly guards the welfare of the nation. With fewer resources at their disposal, however, vulnerable populations are uniquely dependent on social and public policy to develop and implement programs that address basic nutritional, safety, social, and health care needs. Many of the mechanisms relating vulnerability to poor health are amenable to policy intervention, and policy initiatives can be primary prevention strategies to alter the fundamental dynamics linking social factors to poor health.

On November 7, 2009, the U.S. House of Representatives passed a health care reform bill, known as the Affordable Health Care for America Act (Kruger, 2009), by a vote of 220 to 215, taking the first step toward major health care reform. After a lengthy legislative process, on March 23, 2010, President Obama signed the Affordable Care Act to expand health insurance coverage to most Americans. The law expanded eligibility for Medicaid to increase the number of people in the program. Insurance companies would no longer be able to deny customers based on preexisting medical conditions, but nearly everyone in the country would be required to buy insurance or face a penalty, though the government would provide subsidies to help with the purchase of insurance for those families with a modest income.

Vulnerable populations will be positively affected by the bill. The increase in eligibility for Medicaid, and the mandate for nearly everyone to purchase some form of health insurance will ensure that even vulnerable populations will have the coverage they need to access health care services. The bill also focuses on bridging disparities by focusing on key vulnerable populations. For seniors who rely on Medicare, the bill seeks to improve primary care, free preventive care, lower drug costs, and safer hospital visits. For women, the bill will eliminate the power of insurance companies to deny them based on preexisting conditions, as some companies have been known to deny women insurance for domestic abuse, C-sections, and pregnancy care. In addition, deductibles and copays will be eliminated for recommended preventive services, such as mammograms and Pap smears, which can help maintain the health of women by providing more individuals access to these basic services and will facilitate catching abnormal growths during treatable stages. The law will also maintain the Children's Health Insurance Program (CHIP) and expand the age that children can remain on their parents' coverage (Kruger, 2009).

Community-Based Interventions   Disparities in health vary substantially at the community level, suggesting that some sources of health disparities may be addressed at this level. Neighborhood poverty, the presence of local social resources, and societal cohesion and support are all likely to contribute to the level of health inequalities in a community. Intervention strategies have to be tailored to address these community health risks. Because community partnerships reflect the priorities of a local population and are managed by members of the community, they minimize cultural barriers and improve community buy-in to the program.

Community-based strategies have the particular benefit of mobilizing resources at the local level to address these problems. Community resources can be applied directly to community members, providing businesses and other local organizations with greater incentives to contribute to local health causes. Community approaches also benefit from *community participatory decision making*, in which local researchers, practitioners, social services, businesses, and community members are invited to contribute to the process of designing, implementing, evaluating, and sustaining interventions. Many community programs are operated by nonprofit organizations, and in exchange for providing services, they receive subsidies through federal, state, or local funds and receive tax exemptions. Thus, they are able to offer health services at lower cost than private organizations that are obligated to earn a profit for shareholders.

Health Care Interventions   Billions of dollars are spent annually to monitor and improve facets of health care in the United States. Interventions have been designed for systems of care (such as designing integrated electronic medical record systems to better coordinate care for populations with multiple chronic and acute conditions), health care providers (such as continuing education for pediatricians to better target developmental services to children most in need), and consumers of health services (such as educating pregnant women to attend regular prenatal care visits). Health care monitoring initiatives in national, state, and local surveys have been designed to monitor the quality of care provided in health plans and can be used to examine and reduce disparities across demographic groups.

Individual-Level Interventions   While less comprehensive in scale and scope, individual-level initiatives intervene and minimize the effects of negative health-related behaviors. Altering individual behaviors that influence health, such as reducing smoking and encouraging exercise, is the focus of these individual-targeted interventions, and there are numerous theories that identify the complex pathways and barriers to elicit improvements in behavior. The integration of behavioral science into the public health field has been a valuable contribution, providing a toolbox of health-related behavior change strategies.

One of the most prominent models integrating behavioral science and public health is social action theory. Behavior in this model is described as the interaction of biology, environment, and social context, which is critical in determining the success of any health-related behavior intervention (Institute of Medicine Committee on Health and Behavior: Research Practice and Policy, 2001). Behavioral change programs can be implemented at the community level, such as in neighborhoods or in community groups, but the focus of behavior change is nonetheless on each individual.

RESOLVING DISPARITIES IN HEALTH AND HEALTH CARE

In this section, we summarize comprehensive and progressive strategies (not necessarily programs) that address racial/ethnic, SES, and health insurance disparities in health and health care. Many of the strategies stem from basic principles of epidemiology, including surveillance of the problem, examining modes of transmission, modifying or halting the process of transmission, and monitoring the problem to prevent recurrence. These concepts, which have been the foundation for many of the successes of public health (such as the displacement in the twentieth century of communicable diseases from the leading causes of morbidity and mortality), are now serving as tools for the elimination of more socially rooted health disparities. We present potential strategies for resolving disparities that focus on both individual and more integrative frameworks that address the cumulative effects of these vulnerabilities.

Strategies to Resolve Racial/Ethnic Disparities

Many promising and progressive strategies have been proposed to reduce racial/ethnic disparities in health and health care. These strategies generally target specific social or cultural factors, and many approaches overlap with those designed to address SES disparities. Examples targeting racial/ethnic disparities at the policy, community, health care, and individual levels are discussed below.

Policy Interventions   Beginning with civil rights legislation in the 1940s through the 1960s, equality has been hard won for racial/ethnic minorities in the United States. Laws mandating equal access to education and employment (such as the creation of the Equal Employment Opportunity Commission to regulate equity in employment) and prohibiting racial discrimination in public places are the foundation for major improvements in the health and health care access of minorities. Affirmative action laws were also implemented to enhance education and employment opportunities for minorities (and women and the disabled) who had suffered from discrimination.

The term affirmative action was first used by President John F. Kennedy in 1961 in a federal order requiring businesses with government contracts to hire employees without regard to race, ethnic origin, religion, or gender. Later, government contracts were awarded based on race and gender to ensure that the workforce properly reflected the actual population, and a fixed portion of contracts were set aside for minority- or women-owned businesses. Many states, communities, businesses, and schools also created their own affirmative action programs.

In 1995, the U.S. Supreme Court held that federal affirmative action programs were not constitutional unless particular programs were designed to make up for specific past instances of discrimination. This ruling opened the door widely to critics of affirmative action, and in 1996, California voters banned racial/ethnic and gender preferences in public hiring, contracting, and education. In 1998, Washington State followed suit. In 2003, the U.S. Supreme Court once again ruled in favor of affirmative action for admission into the University of Michigan's law school in the case of *Grutter v. Bollinger*, citing that the use of race in admission decisions for a more diverse student body is constitutional (see *Grutter v. Bollinger*, 539 U.S. 306, 2003). Similar to the situation in California, Michigan voters in 2006 then passed the Michigan Civil Rights Initiative, or Proposal 2, banning the use of affirmative action programs for higher education admission (Crenshaw, 2007). Rescinding affirmative action programs has caused substantial national upset, particularly with regard to opportunities for higher education in the University of California system, and recent Supreme Court decisions have ruled again for the constitutional inclusion of minority and gender status in higher education admissions.

While affirmative action policies have increased higher education enrollment rates for minorities, these rates are still not comparable to those of whites. Considering that these lower education levels lead to severe long-term financial, social, and health deficits and that affirmative action policies are constantly on the political chopping block, efforts should be made to bolster the stability of these programs. Some institutions have implemented alternate diversity programs (to replace affirmative action), but additional resources and attention should be devoted to ensuring that all vulnerable populations enter higher education at high levels. Moreover, social policies seeking to reduce broader institutionalized discrimination in higher education, the workplace, and clinical settings are helping to level the playing field for minorities and should be continued.

Social and health policies have been designed to address cultural barriers among minority populations, influencing access to and quality of medical care. In response to research illustrating negative health and health care quality for minorities associated with patient-provider language or cultural discordance, policymakers have established subsidy programs to financially support minorities entering provider-training programs. These initiatives support a racially and ethnically diverse health care workforce, mirroring the diverse American population.

The Health Careers Opportunity Program of the Health Resources and Services Administration (HRSA), for example, provides financial support and supplemental training, counseling, and stipends to help minority or underprivileged students complete a broad range of health care profession degrees. Other agencies such as the National Institutes of Health (NIH), the Agency for Healthcare Research and Quality, and the National Science Foundation are working to promote the entry of minorities in health care provider training programs (Reede, 2003).

Community-Based Interventions   An example of a successful community-based program to address racial/ethnic disparities was a Racial and Ethnic Approaches to Community Health (REACH) 2010–funded initiative in Chicago targeting diabetes outcomes (Giachello and others, 2003). The Latino Health Research Center at the University of Illinois at Chicago developed the program through a series of town meetings with interested parties and devised a new coalition of African American and Latino organizations from Chicago's diverse Southeast Side to address the well-documented disparities in diabetes outcomes. Both groups are characterized by large population size, low education levels, high levels of poverty, and poor access to care. The coalition used a process referred to as participatory action research to design the initiative, including gathering data, building community capacity, and raising the local awareness of the problem. For a comparison of community participatory action research with traditional research, see Table 6.2.

A number of factors contributed to the community's focus on diabetes, including high diabetes mortality, high diabetes-related hospitalization rates, and high gestational diabetes rates in the area. The initiative collected additional information using telephone interviews of local community residents, assessed health services capacity by conducting an inventory of all community resources ready to address diabetes, and reviewed local epidemiological health and health

TABLE 6.2   Differences between Traditional Research
and Participatory Action Research

Traditional Research	Participatory Action Research
Rigid	**Flexible**
Limited application to community problems	Aimed at solving specific community problems
Seeks limited community representation when funding	Seeks community participation/representation at all stages of the research project
Uses mainly quantitative methods	Uses both qualitative and quantitative methods
	Tends to include women and racial/ethnic minority groups
	Maximizes efforts to include groups affected by the problems
Stresses deficits and "victim" ideology	Stresses community assets and community empowerment
Research is "on" populations	Research is "with" and "by" populations
Principal investigators are in control	Shared control among principal investigator, community, and participants
Project ends when data are collected and analyzed	Real action starts when data are analyzed
Partnership is limited	Partnership is maximized
Researcher is the "expert"	Researcher is a "resource"

Source: Giachello and others (2003).

care utilization data from both state and national sources. Focus groups were conducted with health care providers and with potential clients with diabetes to help determine how best to solve the disparities.

The results of this research were presented at community forums along with a proposed action plan to address these problems. Specifically, the coalitions decided to (1) develop a centralized diabetes patient tracking information system in hospitals and clinics, (2) create a health system–based diabetes management and control educational program for people with diabetes or at risk for diabetes, and (3) establish diabetes self-care resource centers. The coalition has created two resource centers managed by lay community health workers. In addition to regular client diabetes education programs, nutrition classes, and social support, the centers help clients navigate the health care system, access medications and devices such as those for monitoring glucose, and organize community health fairs. Evaluation of the program as required by REACH 2010 is under way and was guided by the community coalitions.

The Urban League is another example of a nonprofit community-based movement with programs in over a hundred cities. The Urban League's mission is to improve the socioeconomic status of African Americans through economic self-sufficiency and educational attainment. Its programs across the country include educational support, money management skills, and professional development.

The NULITES (National Urban League Incentives to Excel and Succeed) program is one of the community-based programs sponsored by the Urban League. The NULITE youth initiative is designed to promote educational, character, and leadership qualities among local youths. Its primary strategy is a structured curriculum including required educational seminars and community service projects to enhance educational and social development. The programs are carried out in forty-nine NULITE chapters across the country and serve an estimated 8,000 youth. Each chapter is sponsored by a local Urban League affiliate. The Urban League also sponsors several community programs to teach adults how to manage their money. These Financial Literacy and Know Your Money programs are offered by community-based Urban League affiliates across the country. There are also programs for building good credit, home ownership, and professional development.

Afterschool.gov is a federal initiative that has recognized the potential of community-based programs. Among other initiatives, Afterschool.gov provides grants to community-based initiatives seeking to improve minority health. The community organizations eligible for grants explore social determinants of health, including cultural and community norms and pressures, and environmental conditions. Each community organization must demonstrate an innovative strategy to contend with these social challenges that, if successful, could be modified to help other communities. Current strategies include community outreach; improving access to health care for minorities in high-risk, low-income communities; and promoting community health coalitions involving nontraditional partners.

Health Care Interventions   Another approach to resolving racial/ethnic disparities in health and health care is to tailor health care interventions to cultural differences in health beliefs, values, preferences, and behaviors. These differences include variations in perceptions of health symptoms and health care needs; ways of communicating health needs to professionals who understand their meaning, expectations, and preferences for health care services; and differences in health behaviors and treatments for illnesses. These factors are thought to influence interpersonal interactions, including discrimination, between individuals and health professionals and to affect health care decision-making in ways that contribute to health disparities (Smedley, Stith, and Nelson, 2002).

This process has been termed cultural competence and should be distinguished from basic language competence, in which a health care system or provider ensures that its services are available and rendered in the languages spoken by their patient panels. This is infrequently, but most thoroughly, accomplished through the hiring of specialized translators trained in communicating complex medical issues. Cultural competence requires a more complex understanding of social and cultural influences on individual beliefs and expectations about health and health care, and how these may influence health behaviors and influence the delivery of health care at multiple levels of the system (Betancourt, Green, Carrillo, and Ananeh-Firempong, 2003; Carrillo, Green, and Betancourt, 1999).

Betancourt and colleagues have proposed a three-level framework for improving cultural competence in the health care system (Betancourt, Green, Carrillo, and Park, 2005). This framework consists of organizational interventions that ensure that the leadership and workforce of a health system are diverse and representative of its patient population; structural interventions to ensure that health services are accessible and of the highest quality for all patients (for example, by offering interpreter services and ensuring that health education interventions and materials are tailored to meet the needs of diverse patients); and clinical interventions that train health professionals to be effective at negotiating different styles of communication, adapting to differences in decision-making preferences, different roles of the family, sexual and gender issues, and broader issues of mistrust, prejudice, stereotyping, and racism. In order to address racial and ethnic disparities in health through mechanisms of cultural competence, strategies should be addressed at each of these levels.

A review by Brach and Fraser provides substantial conceptual and empirical support for the potential effectiveness of cultural competence strategies at reducing racial and ethnic disparities (Brach and Fraser, 2000). The authors discuss how cultural competence is likely to improve the accessibility of health care services for some minority groups, benefit interpersonal patient-provider interactions, increase the effectiveness of health education efforts, and possibly reduce misdiagnoses and improve the overall quality of care. The authors note that most cultural competence strategies have not been evaluated, and the linkages of specific strategies to improving the processes of delivering health care and patient outcomes have yet to be clearly demonstrated. This step is important, because addressing cultural competence at all organizational, structural, and clinical levels will require a substantial investment of resources.

Professional development programs in health care teach providers to deliver culturally appropriate care, and recommendations have been made to incorporate more cultural competency programs into graduate medical education (Council on Graduate Medical Education, 2005). The Cross-Cultural Health Care Program (CCHCP), for example, has developed books, resources, and training programs to improve cultural competency among health care providers, including a training program for medical interpreters called Bridging the Gap (Cross Cultural Health Care Program, 2010). Harmony in the patient-provider relationship benefits patients by improving interactions that then result in more effective communication about illness symptoms and origins and facilitates greater *continuity of care.*

Another factor to consider in the health care delivery process is the increasing use of *complementary or alternative medicine (CAM).* Complementary medicine is used in conjunction with conventional allopathic medicine, and alternative medicine is used in place of conventional medicine. Individuals tend to use CAM for its greater compatibility with their personal views on health and illness, in addition to individual dissatisfaction with conventional medicines (Council on Graduate Medical Education, 2005). In 2007, approximately 38 percent of adults and 12 percent of children used CAM in the United States (National Center for Complementary and Alternative Medicine, 2008).

With more CAM therapies, such as acupuncture and chiropractic procedures passing clinical trials, opportunities for accessing this type of care are increasing, in effect broadening the health care market to provide individuals with choices in health care they had not previously had. This addition to the care delivery system benefits the segment of the population that is skeptical of conventional medicine and those wishing to combine the two types of medicine for disease prevention and treatment. Minorities, particularly immigrants, may find themselves more familiar and comfortable with alternative care than with the conventional care more commonplace in the United States. Again, greater patient satisfaction results in higher rates of continuity with a primary source of care, which ultimately benefits the patient's health.

How accessible is alternative medicine? Interest in CAM therapies has been building during the past decade. This growing interest was officially acknowledged in 1991 when the NIH established the Office of Alternative Medicine to evaluate and identify effective CAM therapies. In 1998, the office was upgraded to a center and renamed the National Advisory Council on Complementary and Alternative Medicine (NCCAM). Since the OAM's initial budget of $2 million, the NCCAM's budget has grown to an impressive $122 million for fiscal year 2009. The NCCAM's primary focus is still to identify promising alternative therapies by using rigorous scientific methods.

Despite the federal government's effort to raise the public's awareness of CAM, patient access to CAM is often limited by the restrictions placed on CAM practitioners. Many states do not license CAM practitioners. Naturopaths are licensed in eleven states, acupuncturists in thirty-four, and chiropractors in all fifty states (National Center for Complementary and Alternative Medicine, 2008). Without a license, practitioners are limited in the types of care they can provide to the public, and they risk legal action if they practice without licensure. The CAM licensure process has been controversial, pitting allopathic practices against CAM-affiliated organizations that claim allopathic interest groups have purposefully undermined their licensure process to prevent additional competition.

Ironically, there is conflict among CAM-affiliated organizations about whether the industry is better served by state licenses. Many practitioners feel strongly that the licensure process is an expensive burden, particularly when the therapies they provide, such as massage, have little potential for harming patients. Furthermore, because some states do not offer the option for licensure, it prevents practitioners from providing and the patients from having access to these therapies in these states. Other CAM practitioners feel that the licenses lend credit to a field of medicine that has had to defend itself against insinuations of quackery from the very beginning.

A resulting Health Freedom movement has resulted in new legislation in some states that allows CAM therapists to practice without a license. Minnesota's Alternative Health Care Freedom of Access Act, for example, allows massage therapists, body workers, naturopaths, homeopaths, herbalists, and Ayurvedic healers to practice without licenses, certification, or registration in the state. The act, which went into effect in July 2000, established the state's Office of Unlicensed Complementary Health-Care Practice to oversee the industry.

Patient access to CAM therapies has been improved by other legislation protecting CAM practitioners from charges of professional misconduct. Lawsuits against CAM practitioners for providing unconventional treatment to patients bolstered suspicions of allopathic doctors, further obstructing the entry of CAM into the marketplace. The lawsuits also included allopathic doctors who had integrated components of CAM therapies into their practices. In response, Alaska, Colorado, and Georgia drafted laws to protect all CAM practitioners from professional misconduct claims.

Patient access to CAM is increasing, albeit slowly. Access has improved with some insurance companies, such as Blue Cross of Washington and Alaska, Kaiser Permanente, Prudential, and Mutual of Omaha among others, now covering these services. Access to CAM therapies can also be dictated by physician buy-in. Not all physicians feel comfortable educating their patients about alternative medicine or providing referrals to CAM practitioners. However, medical schools are now integrating more alternative medicine content into their curriculums, which should familiarize future generations of doctors with the benefits and risks of CAM. In fact, a 1998 survey of 117 medical schools found that 64 percent offered courses in CAM or courses with CAM content (Wetzel, Eisenberg, and Kaptchuk, 1998), and this number is likely to have increased.

Numerous professional organizations such as the Complementary Alternative Medical Association, the National Center for Homeopathy, and the Coalition for Natural Health are doing their best to educate consumers, practitioners, and policymakers on the benefits of CAM therapies.

Individual-Level Interventions   Many approaches have been developed to improve health at the individual level through interventions to change behaviors that influence health and well-being. Though most of these initiatives have been focused on the general population, growing recognition of the importance of cultural differences in health-related behavior has encouraged the adoption of these programs to specific populations.

Many national organizations aim to improve the health of minorities by providing education, information, training, and support for the adoption of healthier life choices. The National Rural Health Association (NRHA), for example, champions the health of rural minorities through educational interventions. NRHA has created the Contextual Community Health Profile, an intervention development tool that assists local programs in identifying demographic-specific needs of minority groups often omitted from interventions intended for the general population. This tool assists programs in constructing culturally appropriate interventions for the specific target population.

An innovative Internet-based program developed by the Black Women's Health Imperative (BWHI) is another example of an organization targeting a specific racial/ethnic population's health behaviors to address their unique health needs. The BWHI developed an educational intervention in response to data showing that heart disease was the leading cause of death among African American women and that they have particularly high levels of risk factors (such as obesity) compared with other populations of women. The BWHI created the Walking to Wellness program, which educates African American women about the risks of heart disease, develops personalized training plans, and motivates women to take steps (literally, 10,000 walking steps per day) to prevent heart disease. Another program established by BWHI was REACH 2010: At the Heart of New Orleans (though it ended in December 2007), with the goal of reducing risk factors associated with heart disease among African American women in New Orleans through self-help group sessions and educational classes (Black Women's Health Imperative, 2009).

Smoking cigarettes and abusing alcohol are two other negative health behaviors that are more prevalent among certain minority and low-income populations. For example, Native Americans have higher rates of alcohol use than other racial/ethnic groups, and African American men are more likely to smoke than white men (National Center for Health Statistics, 2009). Cigarette makers continue to target African Americans and Hispanics for promotional efforts in niche magazine advertising, strategically located billboards, and sponsorship of athletic, cultural, and entertainment events.

Interventions to reduce these disparities in smoking include mass media antismoking campaigns geared toward these populations, using a culturally appropriate message or language. The campaigns seek to raise public awareness of the addictive nature of cigarettes and the harmful long-term effects of smoking. Multifaceted cessation programs have also incorporated tax increases on cigarette products and aggressive enforcement of the 1992 law restricting tobacco sales to minors. Using these methods in statewide cessation programs in the 1990s, California, Massachusetts, and Oregon have reduced cigarette consumption.

There are also numerous resources published on the Internet to motivate individuals and guide them throughout a cessation program. The Centers for Disease Control (CDC) has published several cessation programs for individuals, such as *Pathways to Freedom: Winning the Fight Against Tobacco*, the *You Can Quit Smoking Consumer Guide*, and *Don't Let Another Year Go Up in Smoke*. Other available resources and programs include the American Legacy Foundation's Quit Plan and Smokefree.gov.

A well-known behavior change program targeting alcohol abuse is Alcoholics Anonymous. The foundation of the program is a twelve-step process that leads alcohol abusers from admitting they have a problem to acknowledging they need help for the problem and then seeking that help from the fellowship of recovered alcoholics participating in the program. The intervention has been relatively successful in changing behavior. For this success, the organization credits the twelve-step process and the unique ability of recovered alcohol abusers to reach out to the community and encourage alcoholics to seek help. The abuse of alcohol is also controlled by federal laws mandating the sale and consumption of alcoholic beverages.

Racial/ethnic minorities suffer disproportionately from AIDS. With AIDS and other sexually transmitted diseases (STDs) spreading with epidemic efficiency, particularly chlamydia in teenage populations, educating adolescents about healthy sexual decision making is essential to stemming the spread of disease as well as reducing rates of teen pregnancy. Advocates for Youth, a nonprofit organization, aims to educate adolescents about sexual health using state and community action teams, partnerships with national organizations, and community and family involvement.

The action teams promote sexual health programs focusing on the specific challenges faced by the community. Many Advocates for Youth programs target minority and gay or lesbian populations aggressively to reduce disparities. When partnering with state or national initiatives, Advocates for Youth provides technical assistance, resources, and training. Family involvement projects educate parents about their role in communicating with their children, a proven strategy to reduce unhealthy sexual behavior.

Strategies to Resolve SES Disparities

Strategies to address SES disparities in health and health care became particularly prevalent in the 1960s and have since evolved extensively. Strategies have generally focused on income, but more progressive efforts have focused on ensuring equal access to high-quality education and employment to preempt future disparities in income. One *income redistribution* program, the U.S. welfare system (now known as Temporary Assistance to Needy Families, or TANF), has been reformed to limit the amount of time families can receive benefits while remaining unemployed. These changes, which are intended to encourage self-sufficiency, have had some negative impact on insurance coverage enrollments and possibly health (Wise, Wampler, Chavkin, and Romero, 2002; Wood and others, 2002).

Policy Interventions   To reduce the rates of low SES, it is necessary to intervene in each of its antecedents: income, education, and occupation. Well-enforced social policies protect low-income families from exploitation. The Fair Labor Standards Act, for example, is a federal policy requiring employers to pay employees at least a set minimum wage. Some states have set higher minimum wage standards that companies within the state must comply with.

The act also protects vulnerable populations by regulating child labor. Children of low-income, often minority families are more likely to be employed out of necessity to contribute to the family's income. Regulations specify the maximum daily and weekly work hours for children during a school year, a minimum wage, and a nonhazardous work environment. The act further ensures that education and safety are prioritized. Employers can be heavily fined if their employees do not comply with the federal and state regulations.

Public policies also reduce poverty rates. The Earned Income Tax Credit (EITC) reduces the amount of federal tax required of lower-income families. Similar to wage regulations, some states have their own EITC programs that combine with the benefits of the federal program to offer greater tax savings to low-income families. Tax credit legislation was first passed in 1975 and has succeeded in reducing poverty. The Center on Budget and Policy Priorities published a study in 1998 reporting poverty decreases attributed to the EITC. The study found an 8 percent decrease for all Americans and a 14.5 percent decrease for children (Neumark and Wascher, 2000). The policy has succeeded in reducing poverty by helping workers increase their earnings from below-poverty level to above poverty, thereby allowing more opportunity for social and economic mobility (Smeeding, Phillips, and O'Connor, 1999).

Public policy can also influence education levels in the population. As mentioned in Chapter Three, educational opportunities are not equal for all Americans. Studies have shown public schools to be of lower quality in areas of concentrated poverty. Consequently, low-income students struggle to receive adequate education to prepare themselves for college or employment. The federal No Child Left Behind Act of 2001 works to give parents and students more of a choice in where students receive their education. This program allows students to transfer to another school in the district if their assigned school does not meet federal quality standards. If unable to transfer to a higher-performing school, students are entitled to supplemental educational services such as tutoring or remedial classes. The act empowers educational consumers by motivating schools to achieve federal quality standards and offering alternatives to students to avoid the consequences of receiving inadequate education from low-quality schools.

While in theory the program aims to improve educational quality, it places extensive and undue additional administrative pressures on schools, teachers, and students and orients teachers to train students to achieve on performance tests (without additional funds to help prepare children adequately) so that schools can maintain their already tragically low levels of funding. Moreover, federal testing results have produced inconsistent and confusing messages. For example, in Florida, nearly 75 percent of all schools failed to meet the federal testing standards despite most of them being lauded by the governor for their achievements in meeting state standards. These inconsistencies suggest trouble within the No Child Left Behind program and create difficulties with ensuring that the 75 percent of all state children who now have the option to move to "achieving" schools can be adequately accommodated. Finally, with ongoing reductions in federal funding for education, carrying out the act as intended will be difficult at best.

The federal Head Start program is another public policy program working to equalize the educational experience. The program is designed to prepare students from low-SES families for the school year. Summer classes improve school readiness for students without the same educational guidance and support as higher-income families. For example, illiterate or immigrant parents not fluent in English have difficulty helping their children develop reading, writing, and language skills, placing these children at a disadvantage before the school year begins. Head Start's services are provided outside the school curriculum and deliver additional academic support to improve learning skills. The program also offers medical, dental, and mental health services for children to ensure healthy development and reduce health disadvantages that can interfere with their school readiness.

Additional policy efforts have been made to equalize the health effects of employment disparities. As discussed in Chapter Three, vulnerable populations are more likely to hold lower-status jobs that have higher rates of injury and exposure to toxic substances. The federal government's Occupational Safety and Health Administration (OSHA), for example, ensures a certain standard of safety for every employee in the United States. In this way, employees who are not educated, organized, or powerful enough to advocate for themselves can be unconditionally protected by government regulations. The standards, which are numerous and differ by work environments, are enforced through substantial fines levied to noncompliant employers.

While these policies address root causes of vulnerable characteristics associated with low SES, the policies discussed next aim to minimize negative health behaviors, some of which are associated with lower SES. Although public policy can be very effective at protecting individuals by limiting behaviors, policymakers cannot control the individual responses to the laws and are limited in their influence. Personal safety regulations enforced by state or federal authorities, for example, include mandatory seat belt and car seat use and the regulation of alcohol use at an inappropriate age or while driving. The use and sale of drugs and prostitution are outlawed in most states in order to protect individuals from the potentially harmful side effects of these behaviors. Policies also modify behavior through disincentives. For example, alcohol and cigarette products are highly taxed to increase their retail price and discourage their purchase. Policymakers use public education to improve population health. By increasing awareness of risks and promoting healthy behaviors, public policy can instruct the general population to make healthier life choices.

Community-Based Interventions   One of the most progressive methods for resolving SES disparities in health has been to strengthen neighborhood resources through *community building*. Similar to participatory action research, community building refers to the strategic process of engaging community residents and leaders in the process of making change, building relationships, and ultimately enhancing the capacity of communities or neighborhoods to analyze and solve local problems. Prior to addressing specific racial and ethnic disparities, for example, community building strengthens the organizational assets and abilities of a community in order to identify and develop remedies for health and health care disparities. Essential to the practice of community building is a belief that communities are the foundation for the improvement of health and well-being for individuals and families.

Even groups of people that are not defined by neighborhoods or other geographical boundaries are nonetheless affected by community factors in other ways. For example, some populations, such as migrant and rural populations, may live in a dispersed network of communities but travel to obtain health care in select villages or neighborhoods. Community building in such cases involves linking them with much larger centralized resources, as well as increasing the ability of even the smallest neighborhoods to address their health issues. Community building is not limited to direct medical care issues; it also involves issues of transportation, food security, social supports, and leadership development that enhance the ability to address health issues.

One example of community building is the Harlem Children's Zone, a community-based organization that works to enhance the quality of life for children and families in a very low income area in Harlem in New York City. The program, which was founded in the 1970s, focuses not just on education, health care, and social service initiatives but also on rebuilding community life. The design of the community work was established by the community itself and includes asthma screening programs and fitness and nutrition programs; most important, it includes community-building actions such as after-school programs for children, recreational activities for families, homework assistance programs, computer training, and leadership development. These latter aspects of the program are critical to the development of future social improvements that would be expected to contribute to future capacity to address socioeconomic health disparities (Bell and others, 2002).

Vocational Foundation, Inc. (VFI) is another community-oriented nonprofit initiative, providing professional development training to economically and educationally disadvantaged young adults in New York City. The initiative's goal of economic self-sufficiency is similar to that of the Urban League, though VFI does not target any minority group in particular. The VFI program integrates academic and occupational training with counseling to address job placement and retention challenges. Since it was established in 1936, the VFI has helped 150,000 of New York City's most economically and educationally challenged residents find employment.

The Turning Point program takes a broader approach to building community partnerships. The program, supported by the Robert Wood Johnson and W.K. Kellogg foundations, is a nationwide initiative encouraging community-based and collaborative health care partnerships as a means of strengthening the country's public health infrastructure. Based on the theory that current interventions do not adequately address destructive social determinants, Turning Point hopes that uniting sectors such as education, criminal justice, and faith communities with health delivery systems will address essential needs outside the clinical domain. Nebraska, Virginia, Oklahoma, and several other states are working with Turning Point to build these partnerships among their communities.

At the Latino Center for Medical Education and Research in Fresno, California, the shortage of Latino physicians and health care professionals in California's Central Valley is addressed by an educational pipeline throughout Fresno county public schools that begins during middle school and continues into a student's undergraduate years at California State University, Fresno. It was begun by the University of California San Francisco School of Medicine in 1996 with the hope of developing young Latino students into health professionals who would one day return to the underserved area.

Health Care Interventions   As shown in Chapter Three, individuals living in *medically underserved areas (MUAs)* have poor access to health care. Federal and state governments have been trying for years to develop effective strategies to recruit more physicians to MUAs. Several states use financial incentives to attract physician practices to these areas. Maine's financial incentive strategy requires all physicians who purchase malpractice insurance to pay an additional fee that is redistributed to rural obstetricians providing care in federally designated MUAs. Alabama and Louisiana reward physicians moving to rural areas with a $5,000 state income tax credit, Oregon's rural recruitment strategy is similar and extends to other health professionals, including nurse practitioners and physician assistants. Several states also sponsor locum tenens programs that allow physicians working in MUAs temporary relief from their demanding and understaffed practices. These programs use medical school faculty and residents to rotate through designated underserved areas to relieve doctors. Locum tenens programs reduce physician burn-out and improve retention rates for medically underserved areas.

The Domestic Violence and Mental Health Policy Initiative (DVMHPI) is an impressive example of integrating fragmented services to provide better-quality care to vulnerable populations. Advocates for domestically abused women identified a glaring omission in their treatment programs. The traumatic effects of abuse render these women in dire need of significant mental health care. However, among the 1,700 domestic abuse agencies in the United States supported by public and private funds, none were redirecting resources to offer the necessary mental health support. The public mental health system could not bridge the gap because their funds were earmarked for more severe cases.

Securing additional funds from private and public sources, the DVMPHI completed a needs assessment to gauge the paucity of mental health services for domestically abused women and searched nationwide for promising models to build upon. With an initial focus on Chicago, the initiative built collaboration between fragmented providers with the help of large-scale training sessions, interagency working groups, cross-consultation, and service provider awareness campaigns to inform providers of the link between abuse and mental health (Warshaw, Gugenheim, Moroney, and Barnes, 2003).

Safety net providers offer a broad spectrum of care or services at low or no cost to patients who are underinsured or unable to afford out-of-pocket payments and private insurance premiums. Safety net programs are designed to care for the underserved in unique ways that include recruiting providers who will volunteer their services, establishing accessible and local care sites such as school clinics and mobile health vans, and reaching out to specific populations to educate them about health needs and available services.

Even after the enactment of the recent health care reform, the fact remains that a sizable number of Americans remain uninsured. One of the strategies to broaden the nation's safety net is to expand current public programs. The Children's Health Insurance Program (CHIP) has expanded the eligible population since the program's inception in 1997. Initially, children's uninsurance rates did not decrease, largely due to problems with enrollment. Since then, however, there have been dramatic increases in enrollment, with the greatest results seen in areas with high rates of uninsurance. In 2009, The Children's Health Insurance Program Reauthorization Act of 2009 reapproved CHIP through FY2013. In addition to programs such as CHIP and Medicaid, states often expand their safety-net services beyond the federal requirements (Cunningham, Reschovsky, and Hadley, 2002).

There are also numerous publicly funded safety-net programs offering prenatal and well-baby services to care for the young. For example, the CDC sponsors the Vaccines for Children program, which places a price cap on all vaccines used in federal contracts prior to 1993. As a result, providers can better afford to administer vaccines to uninsured children. Before the program's inception, vaccine prices often forced providers to refer uninsured children to public health department clinics for vaccines, resulting in lower immunization rates. Buying vaccines for participating providers affords the program enough collective purchasing power to keep vaccine costs low. In addition, the program provides free vaccines to all children who are uninsured, Medicaid recipients, and Native Americans and Alaska Natives at their doctors' offices.

In the clinical practice setting, studies have shown that the incorporating an individual's "cultural practices, products, philosophies, or environments" result in better health outcomes in ethnic minorities, such as improved behaviors when implementing interventions, and therefore providing a viable solution in bridging health disparities (Chin, Walters, Cook, and Huang, 2007). Patients responded better to more culturally appropriate care and culturally sensitive providers, though it is nonphysician health care workers, such as nurses, community health workers, and counselors, who implement most clinical interventions. Programs led by physicians were often shorter in duration and focused on educating other physicians in cultural competence or acquisition of a new language (Fisher and others, 2007).

Individual-Level Interventions   Based on a 1992 recommendation from the American Academy of Pediatrics (AAP), the U.S. Public Health Service, the AAP, the SIDS Alliance, and the Association of SIDS and Infant Mortality Program initiated a national public education campaign in 1994 to reduce the incidence of sudden infant death syndrome (SIDS), which occurs more frequently among lower-income populations. The AAP's recommendation stated that the back and side are the safest sleeping positions for infants to avoid death from SIDS. The original AAP recommendation was revised in 1996 to state that the back, not the side, is the safest sleeping position. The campaign sought to educate physicians and caregivers by distributing information to hospital nurseries, day care centers, and clinics. A public media campaign targeted parents through television commercials and other media. The campaign was a success, and by 1998, 95 percent of those surveyed had received information recommending the back or side infant sleeping position. From 1992 to 1998, the percentage of infants put to sleep on their stomachs declined from 70 to 17 percent. Concurrently, the incidence of SIDS decreased by about 40 percent (Mitchell, Hutchison, and Stewart, 2007).

Strategies to Resolve Disparities by Health Insurance

Several innovative strategies have been proposed to ensure that all individuals are financially capable of accessing health care. While the main strategies to reducing health and health care disparities according to health insurance status are typically variations on expanding coverage to the uninsured, there are several new approaches that are being proposed to ensure that everyone has financial access to medical care. Strategies include encouraging enrollment in public health insurance programs for those who are already eligible, incrementally expanding public insurance coverage's eligibility, and implementing unique state- or locally based initiatives to provide universal coverage.

Policy Interventions   There are many policy approaches for addressing disparities in health insurance coverage.

Health Care Reform Legislation   For more than seventy years, Democratic presidents and members of Congress have fought to create a comprehensive national system of health insurance; President Obama has made passing such a bill his central legislative priority. On November 7, 2009, the House approved a sweeping overhaul of the nation's health care system. The Senate passed an $871 billion bill on December 24, 2009. After a lengthy compromise process, on March 23, 2010, President Obama signed the Affordable Care Act, which will make a greater number of lower-income people eligible for Medicaid and will offer subsidies to help moderate-income people buy insurance. The law will forbid insurance companies from denying coverage of preexisting conditions, and will create insurance exchanges—new government-regulated marketplaces where individuals and small businesses can come together to buy coverage. The 160 million Americans who get their coverage through their employers will stay with that insurance. Nearly everyone will be required to get insurance or face a penalty, and businesses will be required to provide coverage or contribute to its cost. The law will allow uninsured Americans with a preexisting health condition to purchase affordable coverage, while preventing insurance companies from imposing lifetime and annual limits on care. Small business will receive tax credits to purchase coverage for their employees.

Encouraging Enrollment for Eligible Individuals   One often overlooked solution is addressing the large number of people who are eligible for, but not yet enrolled in, government-sponsored health insurance programs. According to one estimate, about 6.1 million children are uninsured but eligible for public programs such as Medicaid or CHIP (Dubay, Guyer, Mann, and Odeh, 2007). This suggests that the government is already prepared to provide financial access to health care for the majority of the uninsured. But there are substantial barriers preventing the uninsured from enrolling in these programs. Research suggests that the main barriers to enrolling are lengthy and complicated administrative procedures, lack of knowledge of the availability of the programs, and not actually wanting or needing the coverage (Holohan, Dubay, and Kenney, 2003).

Many program and administrative requirements that create these barriers were established for legitimate reasons, including ensuring that the programs serve only the children they were intended to serve. Most public assistance programs are *means tested* and require extensive documentation of income, but for many applicants, this slows the process substantially, requiring that individuals make multiple visits, complete in-person interviews, and reapply annually, if not more frequently. In some cases, potential applicants never return for a second visit, and this contributes to being eligible but still uninsured.

While a process of presumptive eligibility is already in place in fourteen states (individuals who appear to be eligible for either CHIP or Medicaid are presumed to be eligible in order to allow them to receive needed health care), this approach only temporarily covers individuals until a full eligibility determination can be made (Klein, 2003). This grace period typically lasts only one to three months; in order to maintain coverage, an individual must participate in the regular application process. This does not eliminate the barriers created by requiring people to enroll in public assistance programs separately.

An exceptional example of the efforts to improve enrollment in public health insurance programs is a process that encourages streamlining and the elimination of duplicative processes of enrolling individuals in public aid programs. Nearly 63 percent of children who are uninsured and eligible for public insurance programs are already receiving aid or benefits through programs such as food stamps, the National School Lunch Program, or the Special Supplemental Nutrition Program for Women, Infants, and Children (Horner, Lazarus, and Morrow, 2003). Because these programs frequently have tougher eligibility criteria than CHIP and Medicaid, many eligible children could be enrolled in public health insurance programs by conducting outreach to families who are enrolled in other aid programs, allowing automatic enrollment of children in health insurance programs if they are already enrolled in other aid programs, or combining enrollment processes for separate programs into a single application.

Though there are substantial challenges to coordinating enrollments across aid programs, several states have initiated creative forms of "express lane eligibility" (Horner and others, 2003). Ohio, for example, has implemented a process in its public schools to allow parents to submit a form along with their school lunch applications to obtain low-cost health care. Schools then mail these forms to the state, and application packages are mailed to interested parents for Healthy Start and the state's Medicaid and CHIP programs. In Vermont, when a family submits an application to WIC, Medicaid, or CHIP programs, the family is automatically considered for each program. In Los Angeles, the Department of Public Social Services conducted a computerized search to locate families enrolled in the school lunch program but not yet enrolled in Medicaid. These families were sent notices of their potential eligibility, and interested families returned cards that allowed food stamp information to be used to determine eligibility for Medicaid and CHIP.

Incrementally Expanding Public Insurance Coverage   In addition to enrolling individuals who are already eligible for public insurance programs, advocacy groups and politicians interested in health disparities have continued to push for the passage of legislation to expand coverage to individuals and families at even higher income levels. Until recently, attempts to pass universal health insurance coverage have largely failed in the United States. Incremental approaches to providing coverage for specific, targeted groups have been much more successful. The most recent example has been the passage of CHIP, but some states have also used funds from CHIP to cover low-income pregnant women and parents of children who are already enrolled in the program.

Numerous states have obtained approval from DHHS to provide health insurance coverage to pregnant women of potentially CHIP-eligible children. This sets a precedent for states to offer coverage for children from conception until age nineteen, the cut-off for the CHIP program (National Governors Association, 2003). While Medicaid requires states to cover pregnant women up to 133 percent of the federal poverty level, these incremental expansions provide coverage for women who do not qualify for Medicaid but who earn too little to obtain coverage through employment or through private purchase.

The most prominent incremental insurance expansion has been focused on parents of children who are enrolled in CHIP. Remarkable estimates reveal that about one-third of all children who are in Medicaid or CHIP have at least one parent who is uninsured (Davidoff, Garrett, and Yemane, 2001). There is some evidence that parents who do not have insurance coverage may be less able to manage the health care needs of their children (Hanson, 2001) and that increasing parent coverage may also help enroll more children (Selden, Banthin, and Cohen, 1999). Synthesis of these findings has encouraged some states to consider the use of CHIP funds to expand coverage to parents of children as well.

Many states have expanded coverage to low-income parents of children through Medicaid, but this allows coverage only of parents up to 100 percent of the federal poverty level (Howell, Almeida, Dubay, and Kenney, 2002). As of July 2002, only twenty states covered parents up to the federal poverty line. In 2000, states were given the option of using CHIP funds to cover parents (Ross and Cox, 2002). This required a special waiver from the secretary of the U.S. Department of Health and Human Services, and some states had used this process to cover parents at 200 percent of the poverty level or more, thus matching the eligibility levels for children in their states (Lewit, Bennett, and Behrman, 2003).

Wisconsin, for example, has used CHIP funds to expand coverage to parents. At the time that the program was enacted, 25 percent of all parents with income less than 200 percent of FPL were uninsured. In 1999, the state decided to expand coverage for parents up to 100 percent of FPL using Medicaid dollars to fund an expansion program called BadgerCare (using a waiver). This expansion began the process of ensuring coverage for parents who were not eligible for the traditional

Medicaid program, and the state further used CHIP funds (with another waiver) to cover parents up to 200 percent of FPL. The program actually enrolls only parents with incomes up to 185 percent of FPL but allows them to remain eligible until their income exceeds 200 percent of FPL. BadgerCare, and its extensive outreach and advertising campaigns, has proven to be very successful at providing families with insurance coverage.

Because many innovations in health policy begin at the state level, this approach may have become an attractive model for many states to provide insurance to many of their uninsured. Economic considerations, tightening state budgets, and the implementation of health care reform may discourage the use of these incremental approaches by states. Changes at the federal level to fund these expansions to parents in a more stable and permanent manner are likely required to keep parents enrolled for more than a few years. With the implementation of health care reform at least a few years away, some states have developed their own programs to cover parents; instead of waiting for the proverbial ship to come in, they are building the ship themselves.

Unique State Approaches to Providing Universal Coverage   States have played a remarkable role in pioneering health policies, new programs, and proposals to reduce disparities in health and health care through universal health insurance coverage at the state and local levels because of their greater *political feasibility*, relatively easier implementation, and ability to tailor innovative programs.

One example is the passage of legislation in Maine that helps ensure that every resident in the state is covered by health insurance. In June 2003 the state enacted the Dirigo Health program, which helps residents pay their health insurance premiums. Quite different from many national proposals for universal coverage, Dirigo Health acts as the sole liaison to private health insurers for low-income individuals, families, small and large employers, and the self-employed in order to obtain affordable coverage. The state pools available federal and state dollars and negotiates health insurance premiums with private plans. It then offers uninsured individuals the ability to purchase health insurance on a sliding scale, with very low payments for those with low income and slightly higher payments for those with higher incomes. Individuals and employers can all make use of this program, and providers have been asked to voluntarily limit any annual price increases to less than 3 percent, with the assurance that they will have to provide much less uncompensated care (one of the driving forces behind price increases).

While Maine is not a very large or extremely diverse state, it had the eleventh highest health care expenditures in the country and more than 180,000 uninsured individuals. The relatively homogeneous political will of Maine legislators to act as political leaders in the national health policy arena is a critical component to the passage of this program.

California also received substantial media attention in 2003 for a number of health care proposals that were targeted at ensuring universal or near-universal health insurance coverage for all state residents. Proposals ranged from establishing the state as the *single payer* (acting as the insurance provider for all residents) to a health plan called Healthy California, to which employers that do not provide health benefits to their employees would contribute in order to cover the uninsured (Sanders, 2002). Perhaps the most interesting proposal, which had gathered some national attention, is one proposed by Bruce Bodaken, the CEO of Blue Shield of California.

Bodaken's proposal is one of only a few ever to be proposed by a health insurance plan. The plan was announced at the end of 2002, to provide universal coverage to residents of California. It proposed a combination of approaches, including a mandate that all large employers offer a basic package of health benefits to its employees (preventive care, physician services, hospital care, and prescription drug coverage), an exemption for small businesses, no changes to the Medicaid or CHIP program, and a *sliding fee scale* for other individuals to purchase subsidized insurance coverage. According to the CEO, the plan would generate savings for the state by expanding preventive care, promoting earlier treatment, and offering a more secure financing system for all groups involved: patients, physicians, hospitals, and insurers.

The proposal to reform health care in California in 2002 did not pass. In 2007, another attempt to attain universal health coverage in the state was pushed by Governor Arnold Schwarzenegger. The latest plan involved employers who do not offer insurance to pay into a state fund that would cover the 6.5 million uninsured individuals of the state as well as require hospitals and physicians pay 4 percent and 2 percent of their revenues respectively to contribute to the state's Medi-Cal funds, California's Medicaid program (Steinhauer, 2007).

Community-Based Interventions   A significant challenge to these insurance programs is raising public awareness of their availability. Many underprivileged individuals do not have the resources, ability, or opportunity to research safety-net options for themselves or their families. Programs such as Washington's Children's Alliance, a nonprofit organization, help to educate the public about state-sponsored health insurance eligibility through community outreach. The alliance works closely with school districts to identify and enroll eligible children in the state's CHIP plan. Similarly, New York's Hispanic Federation works with

Latino families to boost their enrollment in health insurance programs. The fundation provides essential translation services and assistance in navigating the complex enrollment process.

INTEGRATIVE APPROACHES TO RESOLVING DISPARITIES

Although many of the potential strategies for addressing disparities in health and health care focus on single racial/ethnic, socioeconomic, or health insurance pathways, this book has highlighted the importance of addressing multiple vulnerability factors simultaneously. Without addressing the larger package of population risks, strategies to deal with these disparities may be partially effective at best and undermining at worst. Because of their relative simplicity, narrowly focused strategies and programs have the potential to direct resources away from programs, agendas, and social strategies that could more comprehensively and fundamentally address disparities. To refocus national attention on solving disparities using a broader approach, several integrative and unifying models of solving disparities are helpful. These models provide a broader view of health disparities and could serve to align and synchronize the aims of the fragmented strategies in place. In many cases, these integrative models are based on common wisdom, but they are substantiated and enlightened with modern scientific evidence.

Benzeval UK Framework for Addressing Disparities

A useful approach to addressing health and health care disparities has been proposed in the United Kingdom. In a report released by the King's Fund in the United Kingdom in 1995, Benzeval and colleagues proposed a framework for tackling inequalities in health. The framework proposed four strategies for intervention: (1) make changes to the physical environment, including ensuring adequate housing and living space, improving working conditions, and reducing pollution levels; (2) address social and economic factors, including ensuring adequate income and personal wealth, reducing unemployment, and affording individuals time and resources to develop social support systems; (3) improve access to health care and social services; and (4) reduce barriers to adopting healthy lifestyles and changing behavioral risk factors. Used as a whole, this framework can be adapted to address the combined influences of racial/ethnic disparities, disparities in SES, or health insurance status.

Enhancing Education

Education is an important contributor to health. As shown extensively in earlier chapters, educational level is strongly predictive of health status, morbidity, and mortality. Education not only influences health behaviors (for example, higher education is linked to fewer health risk behaviors), but more important, it contributes to social position, which has profound influences on health through subtle but powerful forces such as stress, life control, and political power. These nonmaterial influences of educational level have few points of intervention. Even health behaviors, which are modifiable, are harder to change among individuals with less education, who experience high levels of stressors.

Education is also an important resource for upward mobility. Chapter Two highlights the essential role of education in granting access to employment in higher-level professions. Employment in these professions helps to generate higher income and also provides access to employment-based health insurance coverage. Higher education, higher-level employment, and higher income are defining features of social position, such that individuals who attain these resources benefit not only from material improvements in life but also from the health-related benefits of higher social class. In short, education continues to be the main door opener to social and economic mobility, as well as optimal health.

Education is one of the few social resources universally available in the United States. Both primary and secondary level education is required by law for all children and adolescents. Public education is financed through taxation and is available to all families, although an increasing number of families have sought education from private schools and other alternate means, such as home schooling (Gerald and Hussar, 2003). Disparities in school resources and quality have developed based on differences in local tax bases (schools in higher-income areas derive more financial support than schools in lower-income areas), leading to concerns about the education quality provided in many public schools.

Tightening state and national budgets have also forced public schools to serve an increasing number of students with decreasing funds. Despite this, schools that have the fewest resources are being required to have their students undergo more frequent testing, which directly influences the funding the schools receive. In effect, schools that are the most financially strapped, and therefore have the fewest resources to hire high-quality teachers and provide students with good learning environments, are performing poorly on such tests and are receiving even less public funding as a result. This cycle is disproportionately affecting the lowest SES schools, schools in geographical areas with more racial/ethnic minorities, and schools serving families where other vulnerabilities are particularly concentrated, such as in medically underserved and rural areas.

These differences in school resources and school quality contribute to disparities in educational attainment among vulnerable populations. Higher dropout rates among African Americans and Hispanics are evidence of the disproportionate struggles of these schools, which are compounded by other barriers to student achievement in vulnerable communities. For example, single-parent families, parents working multiple jobs, and community violence are much more common in some of these communities and create a number of barriers to educational achievement.

Moreover, early poor educational performance in school reduces the chances that a student will choose to pursue and be admitted to higher education. These levels of education provide the most opportunity for upward social and economic mobility, and vulnerable populations still do not obtain higher education at the same rate as non-vulnerable populations. For example, only 17 percent of African Americans and 11 percent of Hispanics have a college degree, compared with 27.2 percent of whites. Though programs such as affirmative action have greatly helped improve enrollment in higher education for vulnerable groups, current rollbacks in affirmative action programs have put future college admittance for these groups on shaky ground.

Fundamentally altering how resources are allocated to primary and secondary public schools so that each school has adequate, equitable, and stable funding may be one of the most important ways to ensure equitable educational opportunities for all children. Because early success in school predicts future educational achievement, this may give vulnerable children more equal footing in obtaining higher education. While there are many other social barriers to ensure that children succeed academically, having greater funding available for all public schools may improve the chances that children will graduate from high school, obtain higher education, and enter a world of higher social position that affords many health benefits.

Community Social Cohesion

Instead of waging separate, independent battles to overcome negative social risks to individual and community health, individuals can work together in community teams to change the circumstances influencing health. Social cohesion is defined by a community's social fabric, such as the forming of associations, church groups, and advocacy organizations, as well as more subtle characteristics of social interaction, such as interpersonal trust and community norms. Research has shown that strengthening social support and cohesion helps buffer individuals from the stress of challenging social environments and other risk factors (Institute of Medicine Committee on Health and Behavior: Research Practice and Policy, 2001).

Community partnerships have particular promise for improving social cohesion by using the strengths and resources of community members to participate in and manage the initiative. Because the key players have a vested and long-term interest in the initiative's outcome and goals, there is a greater chance at sustainable success. Furthermore, a community-oriented approach sets priorities that reflect the needs of the local population. And the process of building these community partnerships, by definition, increases social cohesion.

Many American communities have realized the value of social cohesion and designed interventions to bolster it. For example, in the Bronx borough of New York City, East Side House Settlement project has established a family and community-building initiative to discourage adolescents from using alcohol or illegal drugs. The project's expectation is that by strengthening social bonds, the community will have more success in preventing negative health behaviors among community residents.

The strategies for strengthening social cohesion in this Bronx neighborhood include involving more community members in local plans and decision making, as well as creating partnerships among local agencies and organizations that share compatible community-building goals. The project reaches out to the community through its community centers, early childhood services, school-based programs, technology services, and senior citizen programs.

A similar community organization seeks to strengthen social cohesion among the Latino population in Boston. The Sociedad Latina aims to reinforce the minority community's bonds through programs promoting community leadership, educational attainment, cultural identity, and the preservation of Latino traditions. To establish a relationship with the Latino population, the organization offers assistance with minority-related challenges such as immigration issues and translation assistance, as well as short-term crisis intervention, family counseling, and referrals for food and homeless shelters.

Sociedad Latina's community-strengthening strategies include establishing the Viva La Cultura Club, which promotes and celebrates cultural pride. The Sociedad Latina sponsors a parents' support group and leadership development program, Latinos in Leadership Action and Change. In addition, there are several professional development and educational support projects offered to the local Hispanic population to enrich their individual lives and make a stronger contribution to their community.

The greatest health achievements of social cohesion are likely to be obtained when social cohesion is not limited to specific racial/ethnic groups or socioeconomic tiers. As suggested in Chapter Two, social cohesion efforts that cross these boundaries and cultivate cohesion among distinct groups are likely to have the greatest impacts on health and well-being. Interrelationships among these groups will help direct resources to needed areas, improve strategic efforts to address cross-cutting health issues, and potentially reduce relative deprivation.

Balancing Primary Care and Specialty Care

Technology has broadened the range of medical treatment options. Rapidly developing medical technology has significantly reduced the specter of infectious disease by providing vaccinations and antibiotics, thereby increasing the U.S. life expectancy. The current focus of technological innovation is on chronic, genetic, and acute disease. Technology's curative potential has become a powerful force in health care delivery, and the resulting cultural shift among patients and providers embracing technology has established its use as the norm (Patton, 2001).

Although technology has proven to be a worthwhile investment in health care (Cutler and McClellan, 2001), the overuse of technology can create negative outcomes, and it has been argued that focusing on advancing technology may not contribute as much value to society as focusing first and foremost on reducing health disparities (Satcher, 2000). Given the limited resources to invest in the American health care system, it is essential to think carefully before assuming that the best solution involves often expensive, technological innovation. Considering the broad benefits of primary care in preventing acute conditions that require technological intervention, it seems essential to strive for a balanced investment in both high- and low-technology medicine. It is also important to keep in mind the greater risks associated with technological intervention, particularly when compared with less-risky preventive interventions.

Disparity in health status could also be improved with a better-balanced investment in both high- and low-technology medicine. Studies have shown that minorities are more likely than nonminorities to experience preventable hospitalizations, which could be the result of lower-quality care or limited access to care (Gaskin and Hoffman, 2000). A similar effect was found among low-SES populations. One study that compared preventable hospitalization rates of low- and high-income cohorts in the United States and Canada found a much smaller discrepancy among low- and high-income Canadians than Americans (Billings, Anderson, and Newman, 1996). The likely explanation is that the accessible primary and preventive care available through Canada's universal health coverage provides equitable services regardless of individual wealth. Thus, the American system is more likely to spend a greater proportion of financial resources handling illness that has slipped through the cracks of cost-effective primary care and eventually requiring expensive technological intervention.

In addition, it could be argued that overuse of emergency departments for primary care or preventable care reveals the inadequate investment currently being made in the nation's primary care delivery system. Allocating more resources to provide preventive services, including primary care and chronic disease management, to underserved populations would certainly reduce costs in the health care system. Managed care organizations have sought to equalize investment in primary and specialty technological care as a cost-saving measure. However, their choices to reduce costs through restricted coverage or strategic treatment recommendations have come under scrutiny for patient negligence, as well as retarding the diffusion of medical technologies.

Administrators are using utilization management strategies to curb unnecessary visits to the emergency department. The strategies include improving same-day or next-day appointment access for primary care practices, offering telephone consultations with providers, and educating patients on the appropriate use of emergency departments. Some health insurers restricted their coverage for emergency department visits to discourage the behavior. After consumers protested these restrictions, insurers eased off and provided less-restrictive coverage. Instead of refusing to cover emergency department visits, insurers are now increasing individual copayments to control the visits (Draper, Hurley, Lesser, and Strunk, 2002; Hurley and Draper, 2002).

Some public health researchers have identified emergency department visits as primary opportunities to educate a patient population that is less likely to have a regular source of care, and with good reason: Studies have shown improved outcomes for patients who have received health education information during these emergency visits (Wei and Camargo, 2000).

Another factor affecting the health care experience of vulnerable patients is service-provider integration. Historically, health care in the United States has been hindered by a fragmented system of delivery. A categorical payment structure by payers, public payers in particular, directs funds to individual populations or individual illnesses, making it difficult for patients to experience continuity of care for a diverse range of health needs. Currently, many health care professionals advocate a removal of the restrictions placed on federal and state money that impose a fragmented delivery of care. The hope is that with fewer payment restrictions, the delivery structure can change to provide better, more integrated care.

Furthermore, with the advent of managed care in the 1990s, health care organizations sought to reduce costs by expanding the roles of lower-paid nonphysician providers, such as nurse practitioners, psychologists, and physician assistants, to include clinical responsibilities previously reserved for physicians. As a result, in the 1990s many more patients were receiving care from nonphysician providers in addition to their physician providers than they had in the 1980s (Druss and others, 2003). Under the best of circumstances, these additions to the workforce translate into benefits for patients. For example, one study has shown that integrated, multidisciplinary teams provide better care for chronic conditions (Wagner, 2000).

In response to these findings and others, clinical groups and public health care programs are working to integrate their services and better incorporate nonphysician providers, including community and lay health workers. Hospitals are now beginning to advertise the benefits of their integrated teams of physicians, nurses, community outreach coordinators, and social services staff. Training programs such as Washington, D.C.'s Area Health Education Center (AHEC) offers instruction for medical students and health professionals in providing care to underprivileged populations. AHEC discourages an autonomous practice model as incapable of meeting the health care needs of the broader community. As reflected in its curriculum, AHEC's community-oriented model depends largely on interdisciplinary team coordination and communication for success.

Life Course Health Development

A novel, unifying approach to resolving health disparities is based on the simple axiom that what happens early in life influences health and well-being later in life. This model was generated through the synthesis of empirical research from the fields of medicine, psychology, sociology, and public health. The model serves a groundbreaking role in the context of eliminating health disparities in that it provides a model of health as the cumulative result of physical, psychosocial, environmental, and historical experiences. Some of these experiences are protective of health, and others are injurious to health and well-being. It is this tug-of-war between these experiences at critical junctures or periods in life that ultimately sets the trajectory for future health and well-being across the life course (Ben-Shlomo and Kuh, 2002; Halfon and Hochstein, 2002).

According to this model, disparities in health are determined to a large extent in the early years of life. Human physiological systems, including the nervous, endocrine, and immune systems, are functionally enmeshed with one another and adapt to changes in the external environment. These systems undergo a process of embedding and programming at early ages and are susceptible to insults from environmental causes (Hertzman, 1999). For example, an infectious illness or exposure to allergens during prenatal or postnatal periods can affect the development of lungs and the responsiveness of the immune system, leading to child asthma and significant reductions in adult lung function (Holt and Sly, 1997, 2000). This early imprinting of the human physiological system is susceptible to more than biological threats. Social factors, interpersonal relationships, and family stress that infants and children experience early in life influence the development of physiological systems and contribute to health in later life. Maternal depression, for example, has been associated with poorer parenting habits, such as expressing more negative affect toward children, being less attentive to and engaged with infants, and failing to respond to the emotional signals of infants and children. These infants develop a shorter attention span, do not flourish in mastering new tasks, have elevated heart rates, and have elevated levels of cortisol (a hormone associated with stress), which have been associated with lower cognitive ability in childhood and poorer mental health in adulthood (Ashman and others, 2002; Dawson, Ashman, and Carver, 2000; Rebok and others, 2001).

Extensive evidence now links many experiences at the beginning of life with many health, disease, and functional ability outcomes later in life (Andersen and others, 2008; Ben-Shlomo and Kuh, 2002; Lemelin and others, 2009; Ramsay and others, 2008). The risk factors include low birth weight, poor weight gain during infancy, low maternal SES, parent divorce, child physical and sexual abuse, and parent smoking. These factors have been linked with poor adult cognitive functioning, diminished physical growth, high blood pressure, teen smoking, prevalence of adult STDs, psychotic illness, and many other health and mental health outcomes (Anda and others, 1999; Felitti and others, 1998; Hillis and others, 2000; Lu and Halfon, 2003).

The application of this health development model to address health disparities across the life course would suggest that interventions should be targeted to the critical period of early childhood, where lifelong *health trajectories* are set. Reducing health disparities requires reducing exposure to risk factors and promoting exposure to protective factors in order to aim and launch the life-course health trajectory as high as possible.

Consider, for example, a three-year-old child who comes from a low-income family and experiences many risk factors: having been born prematurely and with low birth weight, poor nutritional status, and a single mother who is working multiple jobs to support the family, who smokes, and who is depressed. This child may also be uninsured because the mother earns too much to qualify for Medicaid but works jobs that do not offer health insurance. Protective factors are also present for the family, including a grandmother who is available to provide a source of child care, a church program that provides social support for single mothers, and a nearby community health center that provides many free health services for her family.

According to the model, the current child health trajectory can be improved by reducing the risks and increasing the protective factors. For example, when the child reaches school age, he can be enrolled in the free or reduced-price lunch program to help him obtain better nutrition; the minimum wage could be raised to offer greater stability to families working low-wage jobs; and a primary care physician could screen the mother for depression and help her obtain appropriate treatment. Similarly, the number of protective factors could be increased. For example, the local community health center could provide outreach and enrollment services for the CHIP program to ensure that the child, and perhaps the mother, are covered

FIGURE 6.5   A Life Course View of Obesity and Health

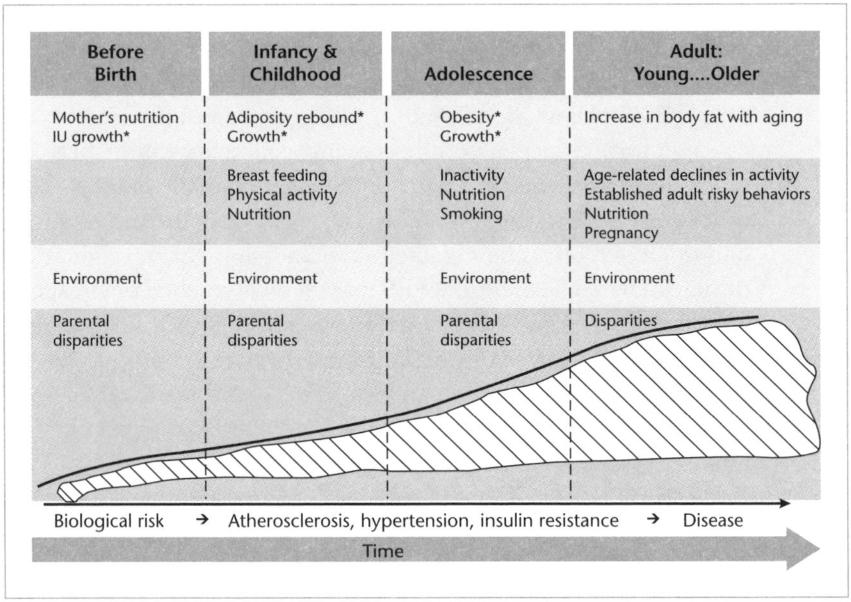

Before Birth	Infancy & Childhood	Adolescence	Adult: Young....Older
Mother's nutrition IU growth*	Adiposity rebound* Growth*	Obesity* Growth*	Increase in body fat with aging
	Breast feeding Physical activity Nutrition	Inactivity Nutrition Smoking	Age-related declines in activity Established adult risky behaviors Nutrition Pregnancy
Environment	Environment	Environment	Environment
Parental disparities	Parental disparities	Parental disparities	Disparities

Biological risk → Atherosclerosis, hypertension, insulin resistance → Disease

Time

Source: Mary Haan, University of Michigan. Adapted from World Health Organization, "Life course perspectives on coronary heart disease, stroke and diabetes: Key issues and implications for policy and research." *Summary Reports of a Meeting of Experts, 2–4 May 2001.* Available at: http://whqlibdoc.who.int/hq/2001/WHO_NMH_NPH_01.4.pdf. Accessed 10/03/08.

by insurance; the child could be enrolled in Head Start and Healthy Start programs to promote child development and early learning; and parenting support groups, such as the one at the church, could provide training sessions and children's books to help both mother and grandmother read to the child (to promote literacy) or offer literature and support to help the mother cope with stress or even quit smoking.

The life course health development model can be used at individual, community, and health and social policy levels to ensure that health trajectories are maximized early in childhood and are equivalent for all individuals in the United States. For example, Figure 6.5 shows a life course approach toward understanding obesity at different stages of human development. It identifies different contributors to obesity at different age ranges and thus suggests how interventions might vary at different ages. The role of obesity in contributing to disease is shown at the bottom of the figure. The life course approach has implications for redesigning health care systems in a way that would focus on better integrating all necessary care for a population across the life span, while making substantially greater investments in early childhood health and development (Halfon and Inkelas, 2003; Hochstein, Halfon, and Inkelas, 1998). Health systems and health plans would be rewarded for providing developmental services that prevent obesity, including pediatric services such as health supervision about parenting, such as nutrition and diet, injury prevention, literacy, and other family and psychosocial factors. Surveillance systems (that is, screening children for developmental problems such as pediatric diabetes over time) could also be instituted in a standard way across health plans and child-focused organizations, such as health clinics, preschools, and child care centers. Although the model is likely to influence thinking about the creation and persistence of health disparities, actual changes at the policy level to focus more resources on child development may be extremely difficult.

Improving National Monitoring of Disparities

Trying to equalize the quality of care for all Americans is a challenge. The American population tolerates a conspicuously high variation in health care quality—in fact, high enough that such variation in quality would be considered unacceptable in many other industries, such as travel and technology. One of the greatest obstacles for equalizing quality is the difficult task of establishing standardized methods that effectively measure quality across the health care spectrum. According to a synopsis of studies conducted by the RAND Corporation, the resources to measure quality are available, as are the distribution channels to provide information to clinicians, consumers, and policymakers (Rand Health, 1999). The problem, which continues today, is a lack of organization and oversight that prevents the systematic measurement and distribution of health care quality data. The RAND study recommends that the federal government, private sector, or an integrated partnership between the two take on the task.

The federal government does collect and distribute some data on health care quality. In a coordinated effort with other agencies such as the NIH and Food and Drug Administration, and CDC, the Agency for Healthcare Research and Quality (AHRQ) oversees much of the federal government's health care quality data collection. AHRQ is a public health service agency in the Department of Health and Human Services. One of its primary goals is to improve the quality of health care by strengthening quality measurement and improvement. The resulting information can empower patients, providers, policymakers, and administrators to make informed decisions about health care. The agency hopes to employ technology in its strategy to achieve these goals with the use of information systems to distribute performance measures and create better communication among health data organizations. In addition to quality measures, the agency conducts research on other health care outcomes, including cost, use, and access.

The Healthcare Effectiveness Data and Information Set (HEDIS) performance measures are another standardized approach to gathering data on health care quality. In addition to measuring clinical performance, HEDIS incorporates a consumer experience component to its assessments. HEDIS guidelines and assessment tools are developed by the National Committee for Quality Assurance (NCQA), an independent, nonprofit organization.

Distributing the information is essential. Only in this way can clinicians understand how their performance rates, how consumers make educated choices about their care, and how policymakers assess the health care systems' success at serving patients. Both the AHRQ and NCQA are working to make their information accessible. Currently, information for consumers is readily accessible over the Internet, though many individuals in vulnerable populations do not have the resources for access. AHRQ Web documents are also available from the DHHS by placing orders over the telephone. While some of the consumer-oriented information is available on the NCQA Web site for free, the quality assessments with information more relevant to providers and administrators must be purchased.

Consumer participation is another avenue for overcoming barriers to access. Patients are increasingly interested in educating themselves about the quality and type of care they receive and have become more assertive about receiving quality care. It is not yet clear whether patients find provider and hospital performance statistics useful in making health care decisions.

Consumer participation also offers a strategy to reduce health care costs through patient-centered improvements in health care quality. Increased communication between provider and patient will help address the broader issues of health, giving providers enough information to understand the origins of a patient's disease, in addition to managing symptoms.

Although providers must learn to encourage such a dialogue and support autonomous decision making, educating patients is the best means of empowering them and enabling a consumer-driven health care system to work. Ostensibly, patients who are educated about health, the health care system, and their choices within it could reduce emergency and acute care costs through self-care or improved personal management of their chronic illnesses (Lansky, 2003).

In an era of rapid information dissemination from the expansion of Internet use, it seems there is no better time than now to engage health care consumers. However, there are problems with relying on the Internet to educate the nation's populace on health care needs and quality services. First, the digital divide once again draws a sharp contrast between underprivileged and privileged Americans. With greater health needs and less access to care, vulnerable populations could benefit most from the Internet's accessible information but are less likely to have the means or knowledge to use it. Second, the multitude of health information Web sites disperse information ranging in accuracy from detailed and precise to misleading and vague.

Health care consumers across the nation have organized themselves effectively to better promote their empowerment movement. Organizations such as the Consumer Coalition for Quality Health Care represent a diverse patient population: the elderly, children, the disabled, and other vulnerable groups. Health care employees are also active in the organization, which works primarily through advocacy to place health care quality issues on the national agenda.

Another national nonprofit organization, Families USA, works to raise awareness among health care consumers through public information campaigns using multimedia outlets. The organization also considers itself a clearinghouse for information relevant to all consumers. Working on a more local level, Families USA offers training assistance to communities challenged by local health care issues. The Center for Health Care Rights uses similar strategies to empower consumers in the health care marketplace, with a particular focus on quality-of-care regulation in HMOs and other managed care plans.

The health care delivery strategies examined here aim to improve access to care and quality of care for vulnerable populations. We also reviewed interventions to eliminate negative social determinants contributing to poor health outcomes among vulnerable populations. The ultimate goal is to improve population health and reduce health care disparity in the United States. To achieve the desired benefit, the suggested strategies cannot be implemented in isolation but must be integrated. Only in this way can social determinant characteristics and health care delivery factors come together to create an environment harmonious for our diverse population.

CHALLENGES AND BARRIERS IN IMPLEMENTING THE STRATEGIES

Strategies and interventions to reduce health care disparity can make an impact to improve the health care experience of vulnerable populations. However, the widespread change to the American health care system that many consumers and professionals yearn for is struggling to gain momentum in our current political and cultural climate.

Instigating change in the nation's public health is consistently challenged by the conflict of long- versus short-term gains. Effective interventions may require a decade or generation before revealing a positive and sustainable outcome; however, the public prefers to see benefits in a shorter time frame. Even for policymakers, it is difficult to allocate resources to strategies that may improve health status for the next generation when the current generation still faces unmet health needs. An encouraging exception can be found in the federal Healthy People initiative, which identifies health goals to complete over a ten-year period.

As the result of political pressure to make visible changes over the short term so candidates can be reelected, investments in public health have not always been made with the population's health as the top priority. Another significant form of political pressure exerted on policymakers is that of interest groups. Buffered by influential campaign contributions and the voting power of the people they represent, interest groups can also compromise the priority of population health. To propel their agendas forward, interest groups hire professional lobbyists who are able to maneuver strategically through the nation's political labyrinth.

Minnesota witnessed this firsthand while trying to implement its first antismoking media campaign in the 1990s. The tobacco industry organized opposition to the campaign by claiming it infringed on individual rights. The industry built alliances with communities throughout the state and targeted industry groups that supported the infringement claims. The tobacco industry destabilized the political setting with influential campaign contributions to key legislators and created its own media campaign that publicly questioned the financial solvency of the antismoking program. The industry's integrated strategy was a success, leading to the defeat of the state's antismoking program and serving as a lesson to other states considering such a program of their own (Tsoukalas and Glantz, 2003).

American culture also contributes to the nation's sluggish changes in health care policy. While Americans have passionately championed many causes in the past century, a social movement for comprehensive health care benefits for underprivileged groups has not been readily cultivated by the public so as to motivate revolutionary change (Oldenburg, McGuffog, and Turrell, 2000). Instead, the changes and expansions to government-funded care for the underprivileged have been incremental and fragmented.

In lieu of a national health system, the United States has a fragmented approach in which numerous governmental agencies and congressional committees control the nation's health care budget. Public health care consumers are forced to navigate various sources of care and payment options across the health care spectrum because some services are financed differently from others. Considering that individuals over a lifetime will require most forms of care across that spectrum (preventive health, mental health, and specialty care, to name a few), fragmentation will have a negative effect on the nation's vulnerable populations by restricting access and reducing the quality of their care.

From a social determinants perspective that incorporates education, employment, behavior, and community factors into the health care paradigm, the health care delivery system is even more fragmented, making it difficult to integrate these factors into health care interventions. For example, according to Oldenburg and others (2000), behavior modification interventions are successful if they target more than just individual behavior. Local support in the form of recreational access or designated nonsmoking areas can encourage the sustainability of these interventions.

The economic repercussions of such a fragmented system have made the United States what it is: the member country of the Organisation for Economic Co-operation and Development (OECD) that spends the highest percentage of its gross domestic product on health care and yet does not offer either universal coverage or prevention-oriented care. Such a complex payment system conspicuously increases the administrative needs and costs of the health care system, creating expenditures that do not translate into benefits for patients. Our costs are also higher as a result of salaries paid to health care providers that are higher than those paid to providers in other OECD countries (Anderson, Reinhardt, Hussey, and Petrosyan, 2003).

Would expanding the role of the federal government simplify the system? Possibly, but public disdain for governmental intervention makes significant federal expansion an unlikely option. Although health care concerns are at the center of presidential debates every four years, Americans appear to be much more comfortable with state and local autonomy, perhaps a cultural remnant from the early days of the nation's history.

Another barrier to garnering support for strategies to reduce disparities is the focus of federal health policy on *cost containment*. With a growing deficit, policymakers are concerned by the nation's consistent increase in health care costs. Consequently, policies conveyed in terms of cost containment are favored over those addressing access and quality of health care, which creates a challenging political climate in which to address health disparities.

Given the nation's relative comfort with state and local intervention, could an expanded state role encourage strategies to improve health and reduce disparity? With regard to health insurance coverage, states have varying numbers of uninsured residents and varying state budget to address this issue. Often, the states with the most uninsured are the least able to afford expanding services to care for them, since lack of insurance is often tied to a lack of employment. Moreover, states cannot generally run budget deficits. When economic times are difficult, leading to higher uninsured rates and lower tax revenues, the states most affected by the economic downturns would find themselves the least able to help remedy the situation and would be forced to cut benefits when they were most needed. States can borrow money through loans and other mechanisms, but states in bad financial shape often do not have good credit and cannot bring in sufficient money. Furthermore, conspicuous differences in state health policies could lead to population redistribution as residents relocate to the states offering better health benefits.

Another challenge faced by the numerous programs reviewed is the difficult task of measuring outcomes. Particularly where social determinants are concerned, it is difficult to tease out the effects caused by the intervention and not by other economic, social, or health care influences. To reap the full benefit of an intervention's investment, it is essential to fully evaluate the programs and distribute the results to create a better understanding of the mechanisms linking vulnerable populations with poor outcomes.

Furthermore, communities feel they have been taken advantage of when they participate in research but never receive feedback or see benefits from their participation. Considering the value that community participation and partnership contribute to public health initiatives, it would be wise to strengthen the relationship through open communication.

Front-Line Experience: Building Healthy Communities

Anthony Iton, senior vice president of Healthy Communities at the California Endowment, explains how a large health care philanthropy in California has targeted root causes of health to develop a bold, multi-factorial approach to investing in the reduction of health disparities. Even though this project is early in its implementation, the concept of Building Healthy Communities exemplifies how an organization can rethink and reorganize its efforts to more effectively help vulnerable populations.

"Social justice is a matter of life and death. It affects the way people live, their consequent chance of illness, and their risk of premature death." So begins the recent report of the World Health Organization (WHO) Commission on the Social Determinants of Health. The Commission goes on to highlight that these avoidable inequities in health "arise because of the circumstances in which people grow, live, work, and age, and the systems put in place to deal with illness. The conditions in which people live and die are, in turn, shaped by political, social, and economic forces." Like this book, WHO and others are articulating the need to address local and system-level changes in tackling the root causes of poor health.

The California Endowment (TCE) has been at the leading edge of this public health thinking and practice for over a decade. After analyzing its history of grant-making and the steady evolution of public health understanding of the social determinants of health, TCE has designed the Building Healthy Communities Initiative (BHC). The BHC initiative is a ten-year initiative designed to help bring about transformational change in fourteen historically under-resourced California communities to make fundamental improvements in the health status of residents. The initiative will focus on big-picture, systems-change strategies that have the potential to sustainably alter the social, physical, and economic environments by investing in community advocacy, organizing, and youth engagement.

But systems are difficult to change. The bigger the system, the more resistant it is to change. Systems do respond to power, however, so a systems-change approach must address power inequities between the system and the people it is serving. TCE has embarked on this initiative with the recognition that success will require a fundamental systems-change in social norms. Changing norms through advocacy and organizing has proven itself to be a winning approach in public health and impressive victories have been achieved in tobacco control, drunk driving, seat belt and helmet use, and sexual harassment in the workplace. Similarly human rights campaigns on civil rights, women's rights, inter-racial marriage, and gay rights have been driven by social norms change strategies. Several of the core subject areas of our BHC initiative are very amenable to a purposeful social norms change strategy.

The initiative began with a nine- to twelve-month planning process during which a lead agency was selected in each community and key constituencies were invited to a central planning table to generate a community plan based on ten targeted health and social outcomes:

1. All children have health insurance coverage.
2. Families have improved access to a healthy home that supports healthy behaviors.
3. Health and family-focused human services shift resources toward prevention.
4. Residents live in communities with health-promoting land-use, transportation, and community development.
5. Children and their families are safe from violence in their homes and neighborhoods.
6. Communities support healthy youth development.
7. Neighborhood and school environments support improved health and healthy behaviors.
8. Community health improvements are linked to economic development.
9. Health gaps for boys and young men of color are narrowed.
10. California has a shared vision of community health.

Each community selected three to five priority outcomes for the first three years and designed a set of strategies to implement to drive progress towards the outcomes. More than 20,000 people participated in the planning phase through surveys, house meetings, block parties, community gatherings, e-mails, social networking, phone banking, and other modalities. Each of the fourteen sites generated a written community plan that was submitted to TCE.

We divided the ten years of the initiative into four phases to help focus the community strategies and develop meaningful milestones of progress. These phases can be summarized by what we call the *four Ps*: power, profile, policies, and products.

Phase 1: Building advocacy *power* among underrepresented low-income populations

Phase 2: Raising the *profile* of seminal health issues

Phase 3: Implementing new *policies*, practices, and assurance mechanisms

Phase 4: The end *product*, moving the needle on key outcomes

For instance, in the first twenty-four months, funding will be focused disproportionately on creating advocacy infrastructure. The goal is to build partnerships among systems players, community-based organizations, and residents. We will be looking for opportunities to break down silos, examine best practices from other communities and disciplines, and improve relationships between the key constituencies that are working in the various systems (schools, after-school, youth development, health programs, parks and recreation, land-use, and so forth). A major goal will be to build community resident power to examine, confront, and hold systems accountable for better performance and outcomes. This requires the creation and support of strong organizations that reflect resident interests and support the development of resident leaders. It will also require an investment in the development of communications tools and strategies that take advantage of local social networks.

As the BHC initiative enters the first phase, we are encountering some barriers that include an unprecedented poor fiscal environment, a policing ethos of crime suppression trumping prevention, evidence of entrenched social and political divisions, and few existing partnerships on which to build. However, our sites also have many new opportunities for youth engagement, an interest in developing new political and community leadership, and promising opportunities for local media engagement. We anticipate steady progress as we begin building capacity in each of our sites to do this necessary work, and we believe that our focus on root problems is essential to beginning to sustainably remedy entrenched health disparities. The "story" of BHC impact will lie in our communities' ability to harness, manage, and fuel this momentum going forward.

COURSE OF ACTION FOR RESOLVING DISPARITIES

The idea that underprivileged populations in the United States have poorer health status is not recent; however, Americans have not reacted strongly by advocating aggressively in a unified voice on behalf of these populations. It is not particularly difficult to explain the public's response. Americans have been known to tolerate high levels of inequality because they have a great faith in the nation's opportunities for individual upward mobility (Graham and Osawald, 2003). Many Americans may acknowledge these vast disparities, but they may also believe that social programs cannot be done without lapsing into socialism. Many Americans fear that having a government bureaucracy control the health care system would reduce personal freedoms in seeking health care or create large waiting lists for care (Navarro, 2003). Americans likely have a similarly resigned attitude toward the persistence of disparities in health as well as the likelihood that a truly integrated local and federal effort could eliminate them.

By examining social shifts in other developed countries that have successfully motivated an unresponsive public to take action, we can identify a course of action to move us toward our goal of changing the political and social climate to benefit vulnerable populations. In seeking to provide an agenda for placing public health issues higher on the public's agenda, we suggest the following course of action that consists of ten steps in four evolving stages.

In the preparation stage, efforts are made to enhance awareness, demonstrate severity, and establish the relevance of the issues. In the design stage, programs and initiatives are developed that focus on multiple major determinants of the problem, are integrated in nature, and are feasible. In the implementation stage, attention is given to applying effective implementation strategies, persevering, and making sure that incremental progress is guided by and built on efforts that have already proved successful and credible. In the post-implementation stage, programs and initiatives are evaluated.

Step 1: Enhance Awareness

Given the vast amount of research in the medical and social science literature on health care disparities in the United States and recent government reports addressing the problem of health disparities, one might be surprised to find that experts still consistently cite lack of problem recognition as a barrier to eliminating health disparities. Many individuals, including some policymakers, still think that Americans enjoy the best health care in the world and that our health status leads that of all other nations. The vast disparities presented in this book are not fully known or acknowledged. It is critical that the public and policymakers understand the true state of our health and the disparities among us.

Education can be used as a tool to raise awareness about health care disparities and to promote a climate of outrage and support for programmatic changes to eliminate such disparities. Education-based approaches generally fall into one of three categories: educating policymakers and the general public about health care disparities, educating vulnerable groups, and promoting better educational attainment in general as a strategy to eliminate health care barriers.

One way to draw attention to a public health issue such as disparity is to illustrate the issue's pervasiveness by using local, state, and national data.

There have been some efforts to bring the issue of health disparities to greater community and public attention. One noteworthy example is Healthy People 2020, which highlights the problem of health disparities and offers strategies for communities to build coalitions and alliances in order to address the issue. Even more such efforts are needed.

Statistics can often make the issue more compelling to a public that is unaware that such vulnerability is so widespread. Socioeconomic data are recorded at the local, state, and national levels, but they are not always analyzed. Examining untapped data resources for valuable metric contributions to the field of study will further promote a public health cause. The use of data can also be advanced by improving the way in which disparity is measured. It is challenging to establish clear and precise methods to measure complex and qualitative factors such as stress and discrimination; however, continued development of statistical methods to measure such factors could make a tremendous positive impact on disparity research. Improved metrics would also enable progress to be better tracked over time.

To go a step further, policy alternatives and quantitative goals need to be widely publicized. Technology has provided innumerable means for distributing information. A media campaign incorporating Internet, television, radio, and print ad channels with a simple, readable, and galvanizing message could reach and motivate a broad segment of the population. Policy alternatives, goals, and research, in particular, should also be well published in highly regarded academic publications in order to ensure consistent political pressure on policymakers.

Step 2: Demonstrate Severity

It is critical that the public and policymakers understand the severity of the problem. Policymakers are more likely to act when there is a clear public demand and a perceived crisis. One way to demonstrate severity is the publication of international rankings on key health and health care indicators. Taking advantage of national pride by highlighting a public health issue for which the United States performs poorly compared with other countries may motivate the public to take steps to improve their national ranking. This strategy has often been invoked to garner support for infant mortality interventions. The dismal ranking of the United States among OECD countries as the seventh highest in infant mortality continues to inspire outrage that a country with so many resources does not ensure adequate care for vulnerable citizens. Domestic ranking on health and disparities could also draw public attention. For example, the annual America's health rankings sponsored by the American Public Health Association, Partnership for Prevention and United Health Foundation have consistently drawn large press coverage and state responses (America's Health Rankings, 2010).

Step 3: Establish Relevance

Although most Americans are concerned about the plights of the vulnerable populations, relatively few have considered these to be their own problems. Fewer have the understanding that it is actually to their economic advantage to address the plights of vulnerable populations. A rational review of the costs and benefits associated with improving the health of vulnerable populations reveals the advantage of making such an investment. The consideration of costs to the nation resulting from poor health status among the vulnerable cannot evade the public's attention much longer.

Numerous studies have explored the costs of limited access to care and inadequate quality to the underserved populations and the cost to the general public as well. The American public does not seem to relate the suffering of vulnerable populations to the suffering of the nation or to associate wasted human potential with poor health status among vulnerable populations. Missed workdays, social and interpersonal violence, inefficient use of health care dollars, and compromised educational attainment are just a few of the factors putting America at a competitive disadvantage as a result of an insufficient health care system (Miller, 1995).

For example, depression, a condition that is much more common among vulnerable populations, costs employers $44 billion each year in lost labor time. Studies have also estimated that about 3 to 5 percent of hospital days used by the uninsured could have been prevented if the patients had been insured and received appropriate ambulatory or primary care (Stewart, Ricci, Chee, Hahn, and Morganstein, 2003; Stewart, Ricci, Chee, and Morganstein, 2003; Stewart, Ricci, Chee, Morganstein, and Lipton, 2003). Taking these and other factors into account, if vulnerable population groups had health status levels equivalent to nonvulnerable groups, our national earnings could improve by 10 to 30 percent (Hadley, 2002).

Every taxpayer is affected by the health status of vulnerable populations. The total cost of health care services used by the uninsured was estimated to be $98.9 billion for 2001. The Institute of Medicine's Committee on the Consequences of Uninsurance concluded that uninsured individuals create about $35 billion in uncompensated health care each year, the majority of it provided by federal, state, and local governments (Institute of Medicine Committee on the Consequences of Uninsurance, 2003). The committee also found that the aggregate cost of the poor health status and high mortality rate of uninsured Americans is between $65 and $130 billion for each year of health insurance forgone.

Communities are also affected by the health status of vulnerable populations, as they shoulder a disproportionate amount of the subsidized care that uninsured individuals receive. As a result, other health care services such as infectious disease control, immunization programs, and emergency preparedness that are dependent on the local tax revenue may be shortchanged to provide basic health needs to a community with many underprivileged residents. It is also important to consider the liability these communities face when service providers such as hospitals and clinics become financially insolvent as a result of providing uncompensated care. These service providers can no longer afford to offer services to anyone in the community.

Current data strongly suggest that the nation's health care system does not function cost-efficiently. While spending more money than any other OECD country, millions of residents in the United States have no dependable means to pay for their health care, and the nation's health system financing is deteriorating as a consequence. Does the nation have the resources to fix itself? And if so, how can the public and their policymakers be motivated to redistribute those resources? In the conclusion of lengthy analyses on the hidden costs of uninsurance in the United States, both a 2003 and 2009 Institute of Medicine report determined that the benefits of providing health insurance to residents currently uninsured would substantially outweigh the costs to be incurred (Institute of Medicine Committee on Health Insurance Status and Its Consequences, 2009; Institute of Medicine Committee on the Consequences of Uninsurance, 2003).

Step 4: Expand the Focus to Multiple Risk Factors

The United States needs to begin to develop a health policy agenda that reflects not just the impact of medical care services on health, but also, and more importantly, the impact of social and environmental factors. An examination of current health policy debates reveals that most debates center primarily on the financing of health care rather than health outcomes or social determinants of health. The United States should expand this focus on financing and issues of cost containment to include *health impact assessment*, which would estimate the influence of social, economic, and health care policies on population health, not just cost savings.

Based on our solutions-focused framework (Figure 6.4), interventions may not have a significant and long-lasting impact if they focus on only immediate determinants of health (such as quality of care) while neglecting more fundamental determinants of health such as personal and community levels of SES. Although it is much more difficult to change social and economic policies than to pass new regulations to monitor health care quality, it is necessary to examine and intervene, when possible, much earlier in the process of poor health development. Because many of these social factors are the root causes of poor health, tackling them will be paramount to resolving health disparities. As this book has repeated continually, most interventions used today are not comprehensive and instead focus on a single, narrowly defined problem or population segment. For example, programs have been developed specifically to serve individuals with HIV, natives of Hawaii or the Pacific Islands, those who are disabled, and those who are homeless, among others. These programs no doubt have had an important role in improving health for these groups, but they have a very limited focus and often have to compete among each other (even within government health departments) for the funding to sustain their efforts.

These programs often address only one aspect of what makes a group vulnerable. For example, homeless individuals have many vulnerable risk factors, including having low income, lacking a stable social support system and stable housing, and frequently are unemployed and so lack health insurance. They may be dealing with mental health and physical health issues that complicate and exacerbate these social problems. But programs serving homeless individuals are generally not sufficiently coordinated to affect substantial long-lasting and comprehensive changes.

Homeless shelters, for example, are generally funded through a network of local public and private partners and charities. The very best of these shelters offer referrals to health care and psychological counselors and have support programs for educating, training, and case management for these individuals for help in finding stable sources of social assistance, employment, and housing. More commonly, these shelters simply provide a roof for the night and have little influence on any of these other risk factors. Even the federal Health Care for the Homeless Program, which provides exceptional physical and mental health services on-site to many homeless individuals, has limitations in its mandate and cannot address the full range of risk factors that are present for homeless individuals.

What has evolved is an elaborate patchwork of local, state, and national programs and policies that have varying comprehensiveness and sustainability in serving vulnerable populations. If these programs could be synthesized or national efforts could be developed to provide more overarching guidance and direction to address these multiple risks simultaneously, these programs would have better chances of success in intervening in the creation of vulnerability. For example, addressing mental health issues among the homeless would bolster the successes of other areas, such as helping individuals to develop social support networks and to make use of education, training, and employment assistance. Combining these efforts would allow these more effective and comprehensive services to be touted to funding agencies as packages and could help to reduce levels of competition among programs serving these vulnerable populations.

Step 5: Stress the Multilevel Integration of Interventions

Invariably, for some vulnerable groups there are gaps in service provision, and for others there are major duplications. Building on the focus on multiple risk factors, efforts could be made toward unifying services across agencies and organizations with common goals. Domestic and foreign public health initiatives have shown greater promise when using the collective resources of public and private advocates. Recognizing common goals encourages multisector alliances and minimizes partisan or other political barriers.

Participation and empowerment at many political and community levels is another critical component of acceptance, success, and continuation of any set of interventions. For example, the National Commission to Prevent Infant Mortality is a successful joint public, private, and congressional effort to combat infant mortality in the United States. It is not a coincidence that this consortium, based on collaboration among organizations at many levels, has made substantially greater progress in reducing infant mortality than the United States has made in other areas.

Improving the health of vulnerable populations will require the participation of traditional health agencies and involvement from education, housing, environmental, criminal justice, and economic agencies. To achieve cross-agency collaboration, these agencies should create standing mechanisms for policy development among sectors, promote interdepartmental collaboration, and create networks among public and private agencies and particularly with advocates to study, evaluate, and disseminate policy options. These efforts should also include greater community involvement and leadership in priority setting and policy development.

Perhaps one of the best ways to include communities in decision making is to focus on community strengths and resources rather than community deficits or problems. Communities should be seen as action centers for development, progress, and change. Community members and community leaders should have a central role in planning and managing initiatives. Through community mobilization, skill building, and resource sharing, communities can be empowered to identify and meet their own needs, making them stronger advocates in supporting the vulnerable populations within and across their community boundaries.

Step 6: Ensure Feasibility

Making sure intervention is feasible is also critical to its success. Areas of feasibility to be considered include *technical feasibility* (whether the intervention can plausibly solve or reduce the problem as defined), *economic feasibility* (the costs and benefits of a given intervention from an economic standpoint), political feasibility (a proposed intervention must survive the test of political acceptability, which depends on support from key officials, other stakeholders inside and outside of government, and ultimately voters), and administrative feasibility (assessing how possible it would be to implement an intervention, given a variety of social, political, and administrative constraints).

Step 7: Apply Effective Implementation Strategies

In the implementation stage, proper use of strategies is critical to success. An approach that has been successful in Europe, restating the public health issue using different language, may attract new attention to an issue not previously compelling to the public or policymakers. In the past, advocates have used the *social justice* argument to persuade the public that inequality in the United States needs to be eliminated. Politicians in the Netherlands were more impressed by a discussion centering on "lost human potential" than inequality, and perhaps the same effect would be seen among Americans if the national conversation focused less on social justice. Furthermore, Moss recommends that the discussion not target special populations but include the whole spectrum of socioeconomic status, broadening the appeal of the policy issue (Moss, 2000).

Another strategy is to work on realistic intervention. This strategy is a call to action for academics, advocates, and associated organizations to investigate and construct policy options. Presenting the public with choices they can mobilize around reduces the frustration and resulting resignation brought about by a system of limited alternatives. Quantitative targets, like the ones established by Healthy People 2020, also help the public focus their efforts toward specific goals.

To ensure that public health issues remain on the policy agenda, it is essential for the public to be able to gauge an initiative's progress, or lack thereof. Promoting action steps using media channels will help keep the public engaged.

Foundations can be mobilized in shaping public opinion. Foundations provide a unique avenue for promoting scientific and policy discussion of a public health issue. In addition to providing the necessary financial resources to explore issues such as disparity, foundations can influence public opinion through publications and media and the discourse it inspires. The America's Health Rankings by United Health Foundation is a good example.

Behavior and lifestyle have been shown to have great contributions to health. Studies estimate that roughly one-quarter of socioeconomic differences in mortality are attributable to variations in lifestyle (Syme, 1989). One important strategy is to target health promotion campaigns to vulnerable populations. In doing so, there are important caveats to consider. Oldenburg cautions that "traditional health promotion and disease prevention efforts are not as effective in people from lower SES groups" (Oldenburg and others, 2000, p. 490). One way to address this is to have more community involvement in development of messages, more culturally appropriate materials, and media campaigns using local community groups and faith-based organizations.

However, there are other important factors to consider. Moss argues that "During the past 25 years, US government intervention to improve health has come almost entirely through initiatives aimed at changing individual behavior.… Individual behaviors are, to a large extent, shaped by social class position and the material environment" (Moss, 2000, p. 1631). In other words, it will take more than a focus on individual behavior modification campaigns in order to change individuals' behaviors. Interventions with a behavioral focus are more successful if the information and education are complemented by support and structural change. Through safe play and park areas, urban renewal projects to build safe and affordable housing, tax incentives to attract grocery stores to urban areas, and enforcement of existing legislation to promote cleaner air (to name just a few examples), urban planning, housing, and environmental policies can provide the structural support for healthy behaviors.

Step 8: Persevere

The vast disparities in health and health care that we experience today are the result of social, economic, and health policies, or the lack of, in the past several decades. It is naive to believe these disparities can be eliminated quickly, especially when some of our current policies and programs contribute toward widening the disparities. Although politicians like quick fixes and slogans (such as stating eliminating disparities in the Healthy People initiative), we have to be prepared for a long-term, sustained campaign.

Step 9: Use Guided Incrementalism

Given the nature of social and health policies in the United States, more success may be expected if we use guided *incrementalism* and build on initiatives that already have credibility. A new intervention is more likely to be taken seriously if its objective is integrated with an older initiative that has already achieved credibility. Although no longer in operation under this title, the Healthy Schools, Healthy Communities initiative provides an illustrative example. This national program, funded by the Bureau of Primary Health Care, began as a school-based initiative to provide primary care to vulnerable children. Over time, additional services were integrated into the program to address other public health needs of this population. The program expanded to include violence prevention, fitness, parenting groups, and self-esteem enhancement programs. It is likely that the integrity established early on by the Healthy Schools program encouraged participants to take advantage of new services of the program.

Step 10: Evaluate and Refine Programs and Initiatives

In the post-implementation stage, programs and initiatives should be thoroughly evaluated, modified, and continually improved. Evaluation, feedback, and refinement processes should be built into the funding of every intervention or policy, and the results of these analyses should guide future program and policy development. While a culture of continual process improvement should be developed, it will be important to judge the progress made by these interventions in a realistic way. Programs that are comprehensive in scope (addressing multiple risks) should be evaluated along multiple dimensions but should be appropriately evaluated against criteria that are feasible to obtain. In too many circumstances, health and social programs are judged on whether they have a direct impact on the health of their consumers, even though the program is funded for short-term cycles (just two or three years). If these results are possible over a longer period, programs must be held accountable to meeting their goals to improve health.

SUMMARY

Our hope is that considering these ten steps in any course of action will help promote the overcoming of health disparities to a more prominent position on the public agenda. It is essential to keep the public engaged and educated. Health disparities among vulnerable populations are not unavoidable. Interventions to eliminate socioeconomic and racial and ethnic disparities have been successful in the United States through health care delivery interventions (Fiscella, Franks, Gold, and Clancy, 2000). Integrated efforts in Canada and Australia have made progress outside the medical realm toward reducing health inequalities associated with the more socially based determinants of health (Dixon, Douglas, and Eckersley, 2000). Using these action steps and adapting them to the needs of the U.S. population are the requisite next steps to prevent the occurrence of and reduce the consequences of health vulnerability.

KEY TERMS

Community building

Community participatory decision making

Complementary or alternative medicine

Continuity of care

Cost containment

Economic feasibility

Health impact assessment

Health trajectories

Income redistribution

Incrementalism

Leading health indicators

Means tested

Medically underserved areas (MUAs)

Political feasibility

Single payer

Sliding fee scale

Social justice

Technical feasibility

REVIEW QUESTIONS

1. Healthy People 2010 and 2020 call for the elimination of disparities. What strategies can be used to achieve this goal?
2. Describe how one might resolve the nation's disparities using the framework presented in Figure 6.3.
3. What are the challenges and barriers in implementing strategies to resolve disparities?

ESSAY QUESTIONS

1. Healthy People 2010 and 2020 call for the elimination of health and health care disparities. What progress, if any, has been made toward reducing disparities in one of the following: infant mortality, cardiovascular disease, or adult mortality? To what can this progress, if any, be attributed to, and what strategies could be implemented to improve on the successes achieved so far?
2. Based on the book and your own research, what do you think are critical next steps to take to resolve health disparities in this country? Be specific, and provide the steps or strategies that should be taken for one well-known health disparity (for example, HIV infection rates across racial or ethnic groups). Consider preparation, design, implementation, and post-implementation steps.

REFERENCES

Abel, T. "Cultural Capital and Social Inequality in Health." *Journal of Epidemiology and Community Health*, 2008, *62*(7), e13.

Acevedo-Garcia, D., Lochner, K. A., Osypuk, T. L., and Subramanian, S. V. "Future Directions in Residential Segregation and Health Research: A Multilevel Approach." *American Journal of Public Health*, 2003, *93*(2), 215–221.

Adams, S. H., Husting, S., Zahnd, E., and Ozer, E. M. "Adolescent Preventive Services: Rates and Disparities in Preventive Health Topics Covered during Routine Medical Care in a California Sample." *Journal of Adolescent Health*, 2009, *44*(6), 536–545.

Aday, L., Fleming, G., and Andersen, R. *Access to Medical Care in the U.S.: Who Has It, Who Doesn't?* Chicago: Pluribus Press, 1984.

Aday, L. A. "Indicators and Predictors of Health Services Utilization." In S. J. Williams and P. R. Torrens (eds.), *Introduction to Health Services*. (4th ed.) Albany, New York: Delmar, 1993, pp. 46–70.

Aday, L. A. "Health Status of Vulnerable Populations." *Annual Review of Public Health*, *15*, 1994, 487–509.

Aday, L. A. *At Risk in America: The Health and Health Care Needs of Vulnerable Populations in the United States*. (2nd ed.) San Francisco: Jossey-Bass, 2001.

Aday, L. A., and Andersen, R. M. "Equity of Access to Medical Care: A Conceptual and Empirical Overview." *Medical Care*, 1981, *19*(12 Suppl), 4–27.

Adler, N., and others. "Social Status and Health: A Comparison of British Civil Servants in Whitehall-II with European- and African-Americans in CARDIA." *Social Science & Medicine*, 2008, *66*(5), 1034–1045.

Adler, N. E., and Ostrove, J. M. "Socioeconomic Status and Health: What We Know and What We Don't." *Annals of the New York Academy of Sciences*, 1999, *896*, 3–15.

Administration on Children and Families. *How the Performance Standards Support New Early Head Start Programs: Lessons Learned from Research*. Washington, D.C.: U.S. Department of Health and Human Services, 2009.

Agency for Healthcare Research and Quality. *National Healthcare Disparities Report*. Rockville, Md.: U.S. Department of Health and Human Services, Agency for Healthcare Quality Research, 2003.

Agency for Healthcare Research and Quality. *National Healthcare Disparities Report 2008*. Rockville, Md.: U.S. Department of Health and Human Services, Agency for Healthcare Research and Quality, 2009.

Ahmed, A. T., Mohammed, S. A., and Williams, D. R. "Racial Discrimination and Health: Pathways and Evidence." *Indian Journal of Medical Research*, 2007, *126*(4), 318–327.

Almeida, C., and others. "Methodological Concerns and Recommendations on Policy Consequences of the World Health Report 2000." *Lancet*, 2001, *357*(9269), 1692–1697.

America's Health Rankings. "About the Rankings," 2010. Retrieved January 25, 2010, from www.americashealthrankings.org.

American Medical Association. "Portraits of Major U.S. Racial/Ethnic Groups." In *Culturally Competent Health Care for Adolescents*. Chicago: American Medical Association, 1994, pp. 39–68.

Anda, R. F., and others. "Adverse Childhood Experiences and Smoking During Adolescence and Adulthood." *Journal of the American Medical Association*, 1999, *282*(17), 1652–1658.

Andersen, A. F., and others. "Life-Course Socio-Economic Position, Area Deprivation and Type 2 Diabetes: Findings from the British Women's Heart and Health Study." *Diabetic Medicine*, 2008, *25*(12), 1462–1468.

Andersen, R., and Aday, L. A. "Access to Medical Care in the U.S.: Realized and Potential." *Medical Care*, 1978, *16*(7), 533–546.

Anderson, G., Brook, R., and Williams, A. "A Comparison of Cost-Sharing versus Free Care in Children: Effects on the Demand for Office-Based Medical Care." *Medical Care*, 1991, *29*(9), 890–898.

Anderson, G. F., Reinhardt, U. E., Hussey, P. S., and Petrosyan, V. "It's the Prices, Stupid: Why the United States Is So Different from Other Countries." *Health Affairs (Millwood)*, 2003, *22*(3), 89–105.

Antonovsky, A. "Social Class, Life Expectancy and Overall Mortality." *Milbank Quarterly*, 1967, *45*(2), 31–73.

Armstrong, K., and others. "Differences in the Patterns of Health Care System Distrust Between Blacks and Whites." *Journal of General Internal Medicine*, 2008, *23*(6), 827–833.

Asch, S. M., and others. "Who Is at Greatest Risk for Receiving Poor-Quality Health Care?" *New England Journal of Medicine*, 2006, *354*(11), 1147–1156.

Ashman, S. B., and others. "Stress Hormone Levels of Children of Depressed Mothers." *Development and Psychopathology*, 2002, *14*(2), 333–349.

Association of Schools of Public Health. *Schools of Public Health Goals Towards Eliminating Racial and Ethnic Health Disparities*. Washington, D.C., 2006.

Avendano, M., Glymour, M. M., Banks, J., and Mackenbach, J. P. "Health Disadvantage in U.S. Adults Aged 50 to 74 Years: A Comparison of the Health of Rich and Poor Americans with That of Europeans." *American Journal of Public Health*, 2009, *99*(3), 540–548.

Ayanian, J. Z., Kohler, B. A., Abe, T., and Epstein, A. M. "The Relation Between Health Insurance Coverage and Clinical Outcomes Among Women with Breast Cancer." *New England Journal of Medicine*, 1993, *329*(5), 326–331.

Ayanian, J. Z., and others. "Unmet Health Needs of Uninsured Adults in the United States." *Journal of the American Medical Association*, 2000, *284*(16), 2061–2069.

Backlund, E., and others. "Income Inequality and Mortality: A Multilevel Prospective Study of 521, 248 Individuals in 50 U.S. States." *International Journal of Epidemiology*, 2007, *36*(3), 590–596.

Backlund, E., Sorlie, P. D., and Johnson, N. J. "A Comparison of the Relationships of Education and Income with Mortality: The National Longitudinal Mortality Study." *Social Science & Medicine*, 1999, *49*(10), 1373–1384.

Backus, L., and others. "Effect of Managed Care on Preventable Hospitalization Rates in California." *Medical Care*, 2002, *40*(4), 315–324.

Badura, M., Johnson, K., Hench, K., and Reyes, M. "Healthy Start Lessons Learned on Interconception Care." *Womens Health Issues*, 2008, *18*(6 Suppl), S61–66.

Barger, S. D., Donoho, C. J., and Wayment, H. A. "The Relative Contributions of Race/Ethnicity, Socioeconomic Status, Health, and Social Relationships to Life Satisfaction in the United States." *Quality of Life Research*, 2009, *18*(2), 179–189.

Barnett, E., Armstrong, D. L., and Casper, M. L. "Evidence of Increasing Coronary Heart Disease Mortality Among Black Men of Lower Social Class." *Annals of Epidemiology*, 1999, *9*(8), 464–471.

Barnett, W. S. "Long-Term Cognitive and Academic Effects of Early Childhood Education on Children in Poverty." *Preventive Medicine*, 1998, *27*(2), 204–207.

Barone, B. M., and others. "Commun-I-Care: Experience in the First Four Years." *Journal of the South Carolina Medical Association*, 1998, *94*(7), 318–322.

Basu, J., Friedman, B., and Burstin, H. "Managed Care and Preventable Hospitalization Among Medicaid Adults." *Health Services Research*, 2004, *39*(3), 489–510.

Basu, J., Friedman, B., and Burstin, H. "Preventable Hospitalization and Medicaid Managed Care: Does Race Matter?" *Journal of Health Care for the Poor and Underserved*, 2006, *17*(1), 101–115.

Baum, A., Garofalo, J. P., and Yali, A. M. "Socioeconomic Status and Chronic Stress: Does Stress Account for SES Effects on Health?" *Annals of New York Academy of Sciences*, 1999, *896*, 131–144.

Bell, J., and others. *Reducing Health Disparities Through a Focus on Communities*. Oakland, Calif.: PolicyLink, 2002.

Ben-Shlomo, Y., and Kuh, D. "A Life Course Approach to Chronic Disease Epidemiology: Conceptual Models, Empirical Challenges and Interdisciplinary Perspectives." *International Journal of Epidemiology*, 2002, *31*(2), 285–293.

Berkman, L. "The Role of Social Relations in Health Promotion." *Psychosomatic Medicine*, 1995, *57*, 245–254.

Berz, J. P., and others. "The Influence of Black Race on Treatment and Mortality for Early-Stage Breast Cancer." *Medical Care*, 2009, *47*(9), 986–992.

Betancourt, J. R., Green, A. R., Carrillo, J. E., and Ananeh-Firempong, O. "Defining Cultural Competence: A Practical Framework for Addressing Racial/Ethnic Disparities in Health and Health Care." *Public Health Reports*, 2003, *118*(4), 293–302.

Betancourt, J. R., Green, A. R., Carrillo, J. E., and Park, E. R. "Cultural Competence and Health Care Disparities: Key Perspectives and Trends." *Health Affairs (Millwood)*, 2005, *24*(2), 499–505.

Bierman, K. L., and others. "Promoting Academic and Social-Emotional School Readiness: The Head Start REDI Program." *Child Development*, 2008, *79*(6), 1802–1817.

Billings, J., Anderson, G. M., and Newman, L. S. "Recent Findings on Preventable Hospitalizations." *Health Affairs (Millwood)*, 1996, *15*(3), 239–249.

Bindman, A. B., and others. "Preventable Hospitalizations and Access to Health Care." *Journal of the American Medical Association*, 1995, *274*(4), 305–311.

Bird, C. E., and others. "Neighborhood Socioeconomic Status and Biological 'Wear & Tear' in a Nationally Representative Sample of U.S. Adults." *Journal of Epidemiology and Community Health*, 2009. http://www.ncbi.nlm.nih.gov/pubmed/19759056.

Black Women's Health Imperative REACH 2010. Retrieved December 30, 2009, from www.blackwomenshealth.org

Blackwell, D. L., and others. "Socioeconomic Status and Utilization of Health Care Services in Canada and the United States: Findings from a Binational Health Survey." *Medical Care*, 2009, *47*(11), 1136–1146.

Blanchard, J., and Lurie, N. "R-E-S-P-E-C-T: Patient Reports of Disrespect in the Health Care Setting and Its Impact on Care." *Journal of Family Practice*, 2004, *53*(9), 721–730.

Bodenheimer, T. "The Movement for Universal Health Insurance: Finding Common Ground." *American Journal of Public Health*, 2003, *93*(1), 112–115.

Brach, C., and Fraser, I. "Can Cultural Competency Reduce Racial and Ethnic Health Disparities? A Review and Conceptual Model." *Medical Care Research and Review*, 2000, *57 Suppl 1*, 181–217.

Bradford, P. T. "Skin Cancer in Skin of Color." *Dermatology Nursing*, 2009, *21*(4), 170–177, 206; quiz 178.

Braveman, P., Starfield, B., and Geiger, H. J. "World Health Report 2000: How It Removes Equity from the Agenda for Public Health Monitoring and Policy." *British Medical Journal*, 2001, *323*(7314), 678–681.

Brenneman, G., Rhoades, E., and Chilton, L. "Forty Years in Partnership: The American Academy of Pediatrics and the Indian Health Service." *Pediatrics*, 2006, *118*(4), e1257–1263.

Breslow, L. "Health Measurement in the Third Era of Health." *American Journal of Public Health*, 2006, *96*(1), 17–19.

Brown, L. D., and Sparer, M. S. "Poor Program's Progress: The Unanticipated Politics of Medicaid Policy." *Health Affairs (Millwood)*, 2003, *22*(1), 31–44.

Brown, T. N., Williams, D. R., and Jackson, J. S. "'Being Black and Feeling Blue': The Mental Health Consequences of Racial Discrimination." *Race and Society*, 2000, *2*, 117–131.

Bullard, R. (1994). "Urban Infrastructure: Social, Environmental and Health Risks to African-Americans." In I. Livingston (ed.), *Handbook of Black American Health: The Mosaic of Conditions, Issues, Policies, and Prospects*. Santa Barbara, Calif.: Greenwood Publishing Group, 1994.

Bureau of Labor Statistics. Data from the Current Population Survey, Table A1, 2009a. Retrieved November 19, 2009: http://www.bls.gov/cps/cpsatabs.htm

Bureau of Labor Statistics. Data from the Current Population Survey, Tables A2 and A3, 2009b. Retrieved November 19, 2009: www.bls.gov/cps/cpsatabs.htm

Bureau of Labor Statistics. International Unemployment Rates and Employment Indexes, Seasonally Adjusted, 2007–2009, Table 1, 2009c. Retrieved November 24, 2009: http://www.bls.gov/fls/intl_unemployment_rates_monthly.htm

Bureau of Labor Statistics. Labor Statistics from the Current Population Survey, Women in the Labor Force: A Databook, 2009d. Retrieved January 24, 2010: http://www.bls.gov/cps/wlf-databook2009.htm

Cable, G. "Income, Race, and Preventable Hospitalizations: A Small Area Analysis in New Jersey." *Journal of Health Care for the Poor and Underserved*, 2002, *13*(1), 66–80.

California Department of Public Health. *Strategic Plan 2008–2010*. Sacramento, Calif., 2008.

Calle, E. E., Flanders, W. D., Thun, M. J., and Martin, L. M. "Demographic Predictors of Mammography and Pap Smear Screening in U.S. Women." *American Journal of Public Health*, 1993, *83*(1), 53–60.

Campbell, J. A. *Health Insurance Coverage 1998* (No. P60–208): U.S. Census Bureau, 1999.

Caplan, R. L., Light, D. W., and Daniels, N. "Benchmarks of Fairness: A Moral Framework for Assessing Equity." *International Journal of Health Services*, 1999, *29*(4), 853–869.

Carpenter, W. R., and others. "Racial Differences in Trust and Regular Source of Patient Care and the Implications for Prostate Cancer Screening Use." *Cancer*, 2009, *115*(21), 5048–5059.

Carrillo, J. E., Green, A. R., and Betancourt, J. R. "Cross-Cultural Primary Care: A Patient-Based Approach." *Annals of Internal Medicine*, 1999, *130*(10), 829–834.

Casagrande, S. S., and others. "Perceived Discrimination and Adherence to Medical Care in a Racially Integrated Community." *Journal of General Internal Medicine*, 2007, *22*(3), 389–395.

Casper, M. L., and others. "Social Class and Race Disparities in Premature Stroke Mortality Among Men in North Carolina." *Annals of Epidemiology*, 1997, *7*(2), 146–153.

Centers for Disease Control and Prevention. *At a Glance: Racial and Ethnic Approaches to Community Health (REACH 2010). Addressing Disparities in Health.* Atlanta: Centers for Disease Control and Prevention, 2003.

Centers for Medicare & Medicaid Services. *FY 2008 CHIP Annual Enrollment Report.* Baltimore, Md., 2009.

Chernew, M. E., and Newhouse, J. P. "What Does the RAND Health Insurance Experiment Tell Us About the Impact of Patient Cost Sharing on Health Outcomes?" *American Journal of Managed Care*, 2008, *14*(7), 412–414.

Chichlowska, K. L., and others. "Individual and Neighborhood Socioeconomic Status Characteristics and Prevalence of Metabolic Syndrome: The Atherosclerosis Risk in Communities (ARIC) Study." *Psychosomatic Medicine*, 2008, *70*(9), 986–992.

Chin, M. H., Walters, A. E., Cook, S. C., and Huang, E. S. "Interventions to Reduce Racial and Ethnic Disparities in Health Care." *Medical Care Research and Review*, 2007, *64*(5 Suppl.), 7S-28S.

Cohen, S., Kessler, R. C., & Gordon, L. U. "Strategies for Measuring Stress in Studies of Psychiatric and Physical Disorders." In S. Cohen, R. C. Kessler, and L. U. Gordon (eds.), *Measuring Stress: A Guide for Health and Social Scientists.* New York: Oxford University Press, 1995, pp. 3–26.

Cole, R., and Deskins Jr., D. "Racial Factors in Site Location and Employment Patterns of Japanese Auto Firms in America." *California Management Review*, 1988, *31*, 9–22.

Colhoun, H., and others. "Ecological Analysis of Collectivity of Alcohol Consumption in England: Importance of Average Drinker." *British Medical Journal*, 1997, *314*(7088), 1164–1168.

Collins, K., and others. *Diverse Communities, Common Concerns: Assessing Health Care Quality For Minority Americans* (No. 523). New York: The Commonwealth Fund, 2002.

Common Ground. About Us. Retrieved January 11, 2010, from http://www.commonground. org/?page_id=24

Conry, C. M., and others. "Factors Influencing Mammogram Ordering at the Time of the Office Visit." *Journal of Family Practice*, 1993, *37*(4), 356–360.

Cooley, W. C. "Redefining Primary Pediatric Care for Children with Special Health Care Needs: The Primary Care Medical Home." *Current Opinion in Pediatrics*, 2004, *16*(6), 689–692.

Cooper, L., and Roter, D. "Patient-Provider Communication: The Effect of Race and Ethnicity on Process and Outcomes of Healthcare." In B. Smedley, A. Stith, and A. Nelson (eds.), *Unequal Treatment: Confronting Racial and Ethnic Disparities in Health Care.* Washington, D.C.: The National Academies Press, 2002.

Cooper, L. A., and Powe, N. *Disparities in Patient Experiences, Health Care Processes, and Outcomes: The Role of Patient-Provider Racial, Ethnic, and Language Concordance.* New York: The Commonwealth Fund, 2004.

Cooper-Patrick, L., and others. "Race, Gender, and Partnership in the Patient-Physician Relationship." *Journal of the American Medical Association*, 1999, *282*(6), 583–589.

Corbie-Smith, G., Flagg, E. W., Doyle, J. P., and O'Brien, M. A. "Influence of Usual Source of Care on Differences by Race/Ethnicity in Receipt of Preventive Services." *Journal of General Internal Medicine*, 2002, *17*(6), 458–464.

Council on Graduate Medical Education. *Seventeenth Report: Minorities in Medicine: An Ethnic and Cultural Challenge for Physician Training, an Update.* Rockville, Md.: U.S. Department of Health and Human Services, Bureau of Health Professions, 2005.

Cousineau, M. R., Stevens, G. D., and Pickering, T. A. "Preventable Hospitalizations Among Children in California Counties After Child Health Insurance Expansion Initiatives." *Medical Care*, 2008, *46*(2), 142–147.

Crenshaw, K. W. "Framing Affirmative Action." *Michigan Law Review*, 2007, *105*, 123.

Cross Cultural Health Care Program. About us. Retrieved January 25, 2010, from www.xculture.org/about.php.

Crump, R. L., Gaston, M. H., and Fergerson, G. "HRSA's Models That Work Program: Implications for Improving Access to Primary Health Care." *Public Health Reports*, 1999, *114*(3), 218–224.

Cunningham, P. J., Clancy, C. M., Cohen, J. W., and Wilets, M. "The Use of Hospital Emergency Departments for Nonurgent Health Problems: A National Perspective." *Medical Care Research and Review*, 1995, *52*(4), 453–474.

Cunningham, P. J., Reschovsky, J. D., and Hadley, J. "SCHIP, Medicaid Expansions Lead to Shifts in Children's Coverage." *Issue Brief: Center for Studying Health System Change*, 2002, (59), 1–6.

Cutler, D. M., and McClellan, M. "Is Technological Change in Medicine Worth It?" *Health Affairs (Millwood)*, 2001, *20*(5), 11–29.

Davidoff, A., Garrett, B., and Yemane, A. *Medicaid-Eligible Adults Who Are Not Enrolled: Who Are They and Do They Get the Care They Need?* (New Federalism: Issues and Options for States No. A-48). Washington, D.C.: Urban Institute, 2001.

Dawson, G., Ashman, S. B., and Carver, L. J. "The Role of Early Experience in Shaping Behavioral and Brain Development and Its implications for Social Policy." *Development and Psychopathology*, 2000, *12*(4), 695–712.

De Vogli, R., Mistry, R., Gnesotto, R., and Cornia, G. A. "Has the Relation Between Income Inequality and Life Expectancy Disappeared? Evidence from Italy and Top Industrialised Countries." *Journal of Epidemiology and Community Health*, 2005, *59*(2), 158–162.

DeLia, D. "Distributional Issues in the Analysis of Preventable Hospitalizations." *Health Services Research*, 2003, *38*(6 Pt. 2), 1761–1779.

DeNavas-Walt, C., Proctor, B., and Lee, C. *Income, Poverty, and Health Insurance Coverage in the United States: 2008* (Current Population Reports No. P60–231). Washington, D.C.: U.S. Census Bureau. (U.S.G.P. Office), 2009.

DeVoe, J. E., Fryer, G. E., Phillips, R., and Green, L. "Receipt of Preventive Care Among Adults: Insurance Status and Usual Source of Care. *Amican Journal of Public Health*, 2003, *93*(5), 786–791.

DeVoe, J. E., Saultz, J. W., Krois, L., and Tillotson, C. J. "A Medical Home versus Temporary Housing: The Importance of a Stable Usual Source of Care. *Pediatrics*, 2009, *124*(5), 1363–1371.

Dievler, A., and Giovannini, T. "Community Health Centers: Promise and Performance." *Medical Care Research and Review*, 1998, *55*(4), 405–431.

Diez Roux, A. V. "Residential Environments and Cardiovascular Risk." *Journal of Urban Health*, 2003, *80*(4), 569–589.

Diez Roux, A. V., Merkin, S. S., and others. "Neighborhood of Residence and Incidence of Coronary Heart Disease." *New England Journal of Medicine*, 2001, *345*(2), 99–106.

Diez-Roux, A. V., Nieto, F. J., Caulfield, L., and others. Neighbourhood Differences in Diet: The Atherosclerosis Risk in Communities (ARIC) Study." *Journal of Epidemiology and Community Health*, 1999, *53*(1), 55–63.

Diez-Roux, A. V., Nieto, F. J., Muntaner, C., and others. "Neighborhood Environments and Coronary Heart Disease: A Multilevel Analysis." *American Journal of Epidemiology*, 1997, *146*(1), 48–63.

Dixon, J. M., Douglas, R. M., and Eckersley, R. M. "Making a Difference to Socioeconomic Determinants of Health in Australia: A Research and Development Strategy." *Medical Journal of Australia*, 2000, *172*(11), 541–544.

Djojonegoro, B. M., Aday, L. A., Williams, A. F., and Ford, C. E. "Area Income as a Predictor of Preventable Hospitalizations in the Harris County Hospital District, Houston." *Texas Medicine*, 2000, *96*(1), 58–62.

Do, D. P. "The Dynamics of Income and Neighborhood Context for Population Health: Do Long-Term Measures of Socioeconomic Status Explain More of the Black/White Health Disparity Than Single-Point-in-Time Measures?" *Social Science & Medicine*, 2009, *68*(8), 1368–1375.

Do, D. P., and Finch, B. K. "The Link Between Neighborhood Poverty and Health: Context or Composition?" *American Journal of Epidemiology*, 2008, *168*(6), 611–619.

Doty, H. E., and Weech-Maldonado, R. "Racial/Ethnic Disparities in Adult Preventive Dental Care Use." *Journal of Health Care for the Poor and Underserved*, 2003, *14*(4), 516–534.

Draper, D. A., Hurley, R. E., Lesser, C. S., and Strunk, B. C. "The Changing Face of Managed Care." *Health Affairs (Millwood)*, 2002, *21*(1), 11–23.

Draper, D. A., Hurley, R. E., and Short, A. C. "Medicaid Managed Care: The Last Bastion of the HMO?" *Health Affairs (Millwood)*, 2004, *23*(2), 155–167.

Dressler, W. W. "Lifestyle, Stress, and Blood Pressure in a Southern Black Community." *Psychosomatic Medicine*, 1990, *52*(2), 182–198.

Druss, B. G., and others. "Trends in Care By Nonphysician Clinicians in the United States." *New England Journal of Medicine*, 2003, *348*(2), 130–137.

Du, X. L., Fang, S., and Meyer, T. E. "Impact of Treatment and Socioeconomic Status on Racial Disparities in Survival Among Older Women with Breast Cancer." *American Journal of Clinical Oncology*, 2008, *31*(2), 125–132.

Dubay, L., Guyer, J., Mann, C., and Odeh, M. "Medicaid at the Ten-Year Anniversary of SCHIP: Looking Back and Moving Forward." *Health Affairs (Millwood)*, 2007, *26*(2), 370–381.

Dubay, L., and Kenney, G. "The Impact of CHIP on Children's Insurance Coverage: An Analysis Using the National Survey of America's Families." *Health Services Research*, 2009, *44*(6).

Dusheiko, M., Gravelle, H., Yu, N., and Campbell, S. "The Impact of Budgets for Gatekeeping Physicians on Patient Satisfaction: Evidence from Fundholding." *Journal of Health Economics*, 2007, *26*(4), 742–762.

Dwyer, T., Blizzard, and others. "Cutaneous Melanin Density of Caucasians Measured by Spectrophotometry and Risk of Malignant Melanoma, Basal Cell Carcinoma, and Squamous Cell Carcinoma of the Skin." *American Journal of Epidemiology*, 2002, *155*(7), 614–621.

Dwyer, T., Prota, G., and others. "Melanin Density and Melanin Type Predict Melanocytic Naevi in 19–20 Year Olds of Northern European Ancestry." *Melanoma Research*, 2000, *10*(4), 387–394.

Earle, C. C., Burstein, H. J., Winer, E. P., and Weeks, J. C. "Quality of Non-Breast Cancer Health Maintenance Among Elderly Breast Cancer Survivors." *Journal of Clinical Oncology*, 2003, *21*(8), 1447–1451.

Erwin, P. C. "Poverty in America: How Public Health Practice Can Make a Difference." *American Journal of Public Health*, 2008, *98*(9), 1570–1572.

Escobar, G. J., Littenberg, B., and Petitti, D. B. "Outcome Among Surviving Very Low Birthweight Infants: A Meta-Analysis." *Archives of Disease in Childhood*, 1991, *66*(2), 204–211.

Evans, G. W., and Kantrowitz, E. "Socioeconomic Status and Health: The Potential Role of Environmental Risk Exposure." *Annual Review of Public Health*, 2002, *23*, 303–331.

Evans, R., Barer, M., and Marmor, T. *Why Are Some People Healthy and Others Not?* New York: Walter de Gruyter, Inc., 1994.

Federal Interagency Forum on Child and Family Statistics. *America's Children: Key National Indicators of Well-Being, 2009.* Washington, D.C.: Federal Interagency Forum on Child and Family Statistics (U.S.G.P. Office), 2009.

Felitti, V. J., and others. "Relationship of Childhood Abuse and Household Dysfunction to Many of the Leading Causes of Death in Adults: The Adverse Childhood Experiences (ACE) Study." *American Journal of Preventive Medicine*, 1998, *14*(4), 245–258.

Ferguson, W., and Candib, L. "Culture, Language, and the Doctor-Patient Relationship." *Family Medicine*, 2002, *34*(5), 353–361.

Ferris, T. G., and others. "Effects of Removing Gatekeeping on Specialist Utilization by Children in a Health Maintenance Organization." *Archives of Pediatrics and Adolescent Medicine*, 2002, *156*(6), 574–579.

Finch, B., Hummer, R., and Kolody, B. "The Role of Discrimination and Acculturative Stress in the Physical Health of Mexican-Origin Adults." *Hispanic Journal of Behavioral Sciences*, 23, 399–429.

Fiscella, K., Franks, P., Doescher, M. P., and Saver, B. G. "Disparities in Health Care By Race, Ethnicity, and Language Among the Insured: Findings from a National Sample." *Medical Care*, 2002, *40*(1), 52–59.

Fiscella, K., Franks, P., Gold, M., and Clancy, C. "Inequality in Quality: Addressing Socioeconomic, Racial, and Ethnic Disparities in Health Care." *Journal of the American Medical Association*, 2000, *283*(19), 2579–2584.

Fisher, T. L., and others. "Cultural Leverage: Interventions Using Culture to Narrow Racial Disparities in Health Care." *Medical Care Research and Review*, 2007, *64*(5 Suppl), 243S–282S.

Flaskerud, J. H., and Winslow, B. J. "Conceptualizing Vulnerable Populations Health-Related Research." *Nursing Research*, 1998, *47*(2), 69–78.

Flores, G., Abreau, M., Olivar, M., and Kastner, B. "Access Barriers to Health Care for Latino Children." *Archives of Pediatrics & Adolescent Medicine*, 1998, *152*(11), 1119–1125.

Flores, G., Olson, L., and Tomany-Korman, S. C. "Racial and Ethnic Disparities in Early Childhood Health and Health Care." *Pediatrics*, 2005, *115*(2), e183–193.

Flores, G., and Tomany-Korman, S. C. "Racial and Ethnic Disparities in Medical and Dental Health, Access to Care, and Use of Services in U.S. Children." *Pediatrics*, 2008, *121*(2), e286–298.

Flores, G., and Vega, L. R. "Barriers to Health Care Access for Latino Children: A Review." *Family Medicine*, 1998, *30*(3), 196–205.

Forrest, C. B., and others. "The Pediatric Primary-Specialty Care Interface: How Pediatricians Refer Children and Adolescents to Specialty Care." *Archives of Pediatrics & Adolescent Medicine*, 1999, *153*(7), 705–714.

Forrest, C. B., and Starfield, B. "Entry into Primary Care and Continuity: The Effects of Access." *American Journal of Public Health*, 1998, *88*(9), 1330–1336.

Franks, P., Campbell, T. L., and Shields, C. G. "Social Relationships and Health: The Relative Roles of Family Functioning and Social Support." *Social Science & Medicine*, 1992, *34*(7), 779–788.

Franks, P., Clancy, C., and Gold, M. "Health Insurance and Mortality: Evidence from a National Cohort." *Journal of the American Medical Association*, 1993, *270*(6), 737–741.

Friedman, B., and Basu, J. "Health Insurance, Primary Care, and Preventable Hospitalization of Children in a Large State." *American Journal of Managed Care*, 2001, 7(5), 473–481.

Fuller, K. E. "Low Birth-Weight Infants: The Continuing Ethnic Disparity and the Interaction of Biology and Environment." *Ethnicity & Disease*, 2000, *10*(3), 432–445.

Furstenberg, F. J., and others. *Urban Families and Adolescent Success.* Chicago: University of Chicago Press, 1999.

Gallo, L. C., and Matthews, K. A. "Do Negative Emotions Mediate the Association Between Socioeconomic Status and Health?" *Annals of the New York Academy of Sciences*, 1999, *896*, 226–245.

Gallo, L. C., and Matthews, K. A. "Understanding the Association Between Socioeconomic Status and Physical Health: Do Negative Emotions Play a Role?" *Psychological Bulletin*, 2003, *129*(1), 10–51.

Garg, A., Probst, J. C., Sease, T., and Samuels, M. E. "Potentially Preventable Care: Ambulatory Care-Sensitive Pediatric Hospitalizations in South Carolina in 1998." *Southern Medical Journal*, 2003, *96*(9), 850–858.

Gaskin, D. J., and Hoffman, C. "Racial and Ethnic Differences in Preventable Hospitalizations Across 10 States." *Medical Care Research and Review*, 2000, *57 Suppl 1*, 85–107.

Gecková, A., and others. "Influence of Social Support on Health Among Gender and Socio-Economic Groups of Adolescents." *European Journal of Public Health*, 2003, *13*(1), 44–50.

Gerald, D. E., and Hussar, W. J. *Projections of Education Statistics to 2013.* Washington, D.C.: National Center for Education Statistics, U.S. Department of Education, 2003.

Geronimus, A. T., and others. "Excess Mortality Among Blacks and Whites in the United States." *New England Journal of Medicine*, 1996, *335*(21), 1552–1558.

Giachello, A. L., and others. "Reducing Diabetes Health Disparities Through Community-Based Participatory Action Research: The Chicago Southeast Diabetes Community Action Coalition." *Public Health Reports*, 2003, *118*(4), 309–323.

Giles, W. *Addressing Racial and Ethnic Health Disparities: Racial and Ethnic Approaches to Community Health (REACH U.S.),* 2007. Paper presented at the Society for Public Health Education. Accessed 2007 from http://www.cdc.gov/reach/pdf/giles_sophe.pdf

Glascoe, F. P. "Parents' Evaluation of Developmental Status: How Well Do Parents' Concerns Identify Children with Behavioral and Emotional Problems?" *Clinical Pediatrics (Phila)*, 2003, *42*(2), 133–138.

Glazier, R. H., Agha, M. M., Moineddin, R., and Sibley, L. M. "Universal Health Insurance and Equity in Primary Care and Specialist Office Visits: A Population-Based Study." *Annals of Family Medicine*, 2009, *7*(5), 396–405.

Glick, S. M. "Equity in Health and Health Care Reforms." *Acta Oncologica*, 1999, *38*(4), 469–473.

Goel, M. S., and others. "Racial and Ethnic Disparities in Cancer Screening: The Importance of Foreign Birth as a Barrier to Care." *Journal of General Internal Medicine*, 2003, *18*(12), 1028–1035.

Gornick, M. E., and others. "Effects of Race and Income on Mortality and Use of Services Among Medicare Beneficiaries." *New England Journal of Medicine*, 1996, *335*(11), 791–799.

Grady, K. E., Lemkau, J. P., Lee, N. R., and Caddell, C. "Enhancing Mammography Referral in Primary Care." *Preventive Medicine*, 1997, *26*(6), 791–800.

Graham, C., and Osawald, A. *The View from Mars: The Missing Debate on Income Inequality in America.* Washington, D.C.: Brookings Institute, 2003.

Grann, V., and others. "Regional and Racial Disparities in Breast Cancer-Specific Mortality." *Social Science & Medicine*, 2006, *62*(2), 337–347.

Grant, E. N., Lyttle, C. S., and Weiss, K. B. "The Relation of Socioeconomic Factors and Racial/Ethnic Differences in U.S. Asthma Mortality." *American Journal of Public Health*, 2000, *90*(12), 1923–1925.

Gray, B. and Stoddard, J. J. "Patient-Physician Pairing: Does Racial and Ethnic Congruity Influence Selection of a Regular Physician?" *Journal of Community Health*, 1997, *22*(4), 247–259.

Gray, R., and Francis, E. "The Implications of U.S. Experiences with Early Childhood Interventions for the UK Sure Start Programme." *Child Care, Health and Development*, 2007, *33*(6), 655–663.

Grumbach, K., and others. "Primary Care Physicians' Experience of Financial Incentives in Managed-Care Systems." *Journal of American Medical Association*, 1998, *339*(21), 1516–1521.

Grutter v. Bollinger, 539 U.S. 306, 2003.

Guendelman, S., and Schwalbe, J. "Medical Care Utilization by Hispanic Children: How Does It Differ from Black and White Peers?" *Medical Care*, 1986, *24*(10), 1066–1071.

Guyll, M., Matthews, K. A., and Bromberger, J. T. "Discrimination and Unfair Treatment: Relationship to Cardiovascular Reactivity Among African American and European American Women." *Health Psychology*, 2001, *20*(5), 315–325.

Haan, M., Kaplan, G. A., and Camacho, T. "Poverty and Health: Prospective Evidence from the Alameda County Study." *American Journal of Epidemiology*, 1987, *125*(6), 989–998.

Hann, M. "Life Course Perspectives on Coronary Heart Disease, Stroke and Diabetes: Key Issues and Implications for Policy and Research." University of Michigan. Adapted from World Health Organization, *Summary Reports of a Meeting of Experts*, 2–4 May 2001. Accessed October 3, 2008, http://whqlibdoc.who.int/hq/2001/WHO_NMH_NPH_01.4.pdf.

Hadley, J. *Sicker and Poorer: The Consequences of Being Uninsured*. Washington, D.C.: The Kaiser Commission on Medicaid and the Uninsured, 2002.

Hadley, J., Steinberg, E. P., and Feder, J. "Comparison of Uninsured and Privately Insured Hospital Patients: Condition on Admission, Resource Use, and Outcome." *Journal of the American Medical Association*, 1991, *265*(3), 374–379.

Halfon, N., and Hochstein, M. "Life Course Health Development: An Integrated Framework for Developing Health, Policy, and Research. *Milbank Quarterly*, 2002, *80*(3), 433–479, iii.

Halfon, N., and Inkelas, M. "Optimizing the Health and Development of Children." *Journal of the American Medical Association*, 2003, *290*(23), 3136–3138.

Hall, A. G., Harman, J. S., and Zhang, J. "Lapses in Medicaid Coverage: Impact on Cost and Utilization Among Individuals with Diabetes Enrolled in Medicaid. *Medical Care*, 2008, *46*(12), 1219–1225.

Halm, E. A., Causino, N., and Blumenthal, D. "Is Gatekeeping Better Than Traditional Care? A Survey of Physicians' Attitudes." *Journal of the American Medical Association*, 1997, *278*(20), 1677–1681.

Hamburg, D. A., Elliott, G. R., Parron, D. L., and Institute of Medicine. *Health and Behavior: Frontiers of Research in the Biobehavioral Sciences*. Washington, D.C.: National Academy Press, 1982.

Han, Y., Williams, R. D., and Harrison, R. A. "Breast Cancer Screening Knowledge, Attitudes, and Practices Among Korean American Women." *Oncology Nursing Forum*, 2000, *27*(10), 1585–1591.

Hanks, C. A. "Social Capital in an Impoverished Minority Neighborhood: Emergence and Effects on Children's Mental Health." *Journal of Child and Adolescent Psychiatric Nursing*, 2008, *21*(3), 126–136.

Hannan, E. L., and others. "Access to Coronary Artery Bypass Surgery by Race/Ethnicity and Gender Among Patients Who Are Appropriate for Surgery." *Medical Care*, 1999, *37*(1), 68–77.

Hanson, K. L. "Patterns of Insurance Coverage Within Families with Children." *Health Affairs (Millwood)*, 2001, *20*(1), 240–246.

Hart, C. L., Smith, G. D., and Blane, D. "Inequalities in Mortality by Social Class Measured at 3 Stages of the Lifecourse." *American Journal of Public Health*, 1998, *88*(3), 471–474.

Hausmann, L. R., Jeong, K., Bost, J. E., and Ibrahim, S. A. "Perceived Discrimination in Health Care and Health Status in a Racially Diverse Sample." *Medical Care*, 2008, *46*(9), 905–914.

Hayward, M. D., and Heron, M. "Racial Inequality in Active Life Among Adult Americans." *Demography*, 1999, *36*(1), 77–91.

Hegarty, V., Burchett, B. M., Gold, D. T., and Cohen, H. J. "Racial Differences in Use of Cancer Prevention Services Among Older Americans." *Journal of the American Geriatrics Society*, 2000, *48*(7), 735–740.

Hertzman, C. "The Biological Embedding of Early Experience and Its Effects on Health in Adulthood." *Annals of the New York Acadamy of Sciences*, 1999, *896*, 85–95.

Hillis, S. D., and others. "Adverse Childhood Experiences and Sexually Transmitted Diseases in Men and Women: A Retrospective Study." *Pediatrics*, 2000, *106*(1), E11.

Hochstein, M., Halfon, N., and Inkelas, M. "Creating Systems of Developmental Health Care for Children." *Journal of Urban Health*, 1998, *75*(4), 751–771.

Hodgkin, D., and others. "Does Type of Gatekeeping Model Affect Access to Outpatient Specialty Mental Health Services?" *Health Services Research*, 2007, *42*(1 Pt. 1), 104–123.

Hoilette, L. K., Clark, S. J., Gebremariam, A., and Davis, M. M. "Usual Source of Care and Unmet Need Among Vulnerable Children: 1998–2006. *Pediatrics*, 2009, *123*(2), e214–219.

Holohan, J., Dubay, L., and Kenney, M. "Which Children Are Still Uninsured and Why." *The Future of Children*, 2003, *13*(1), 55–79.

Holt, P. G., and Sly, P. D. "Allergic Respiratory Disease: Strategic Targets for Primary Prevention During Childhood." *Thorax*, 1997, *52*(1), 1–4.

Holt, P. G., and Sly, P. D. "Prevention of Adult Asthma By Early Intervention During Childhood: Potential Value of New Generation Immunomodulatory Drugs. *Thorax*, 2000, *55*(8), 700–703.

Horbar, J. D., and others. "Trends in Mortality and Morbidity for Very Low Birth Weight Infants, 1991–1999." *Pediatrics*, 2002, *110*(1 Pt. 1), 143–151.

Horn, L. *Placing College Graduation Rates in Context: How Four-Year College Graduation Rates Vary with Selectivity and the Size of Low-Income Enrollment.* U.S. Department of Education. Washington, D.C.: National Center for Education Statistics, 2006.

Horner, D., Lazarus, W., and Morrow, B. "Express Lane Eligibility." *The Future of Children*, 2003, *13*(1), 224–229.

House, J. S., Landis, K. R., and Umberson, D. "Social Relationships and Health." *Science*, 1988, *241*(4865), 540–545.

House, J. S., Robbins, C., and Metzner, H. L. "The Association of Social Relationships and Activities with Mortality: Prospective Evidence from the Tecumseh Community Health Study. *American Journal of Epidemiology*, 1982, *116*(1), 123–140.

Howell, E., Almeida, R., Dubay, L., and Kenney, G. *Early Experience with Covering Uninsured Parents Under SCHIP* (Series A, No. A-51). Washington, D.C.: The Urban Institute, 2002.

Howell, E. M., and Trenholm, C. "The Effect of New Insurance Coverage on the Health Status of Low-Income Children in Santa Clara County." *Health Services Research*, 2007, *42*(2), 867–889.

Hseih, C., and Pugh, M. "Poverty, Income Inequality, and Violent Crime: A Meta-Analysis of Recent Aggregate Data Studies." *Criminal Justice Review*, 1993, *18*, 182–202.

Huisman, M., and Oldehinkel, A. J. "Income Inequality, Social Capital and Self-Inflicted Injury and Violence-Related Mortality." *Journal of Epidemiology and Community Health*, 2009, *63*(1), 31–37.

Hurley, R. E., and Draper, D. A. "Health Plan Responses to Managed Care Regulation." *Managed Care Quarterly*, 2002, *10*(4), 30–42.

Institute of Medicine Committee for the Study of the Future of Public Health. *The Future of Public Health.* Washington, D.C.: National Academy Press, 1988.

Institute of Medicine Committee on Health and Behavior: Research Practice and Policy. *Health and Behavior: The Interplay of Biological, Behavioral, and Societal Influences.* Washington, D.C.: National Academy Press, 2001.

Institute of Medicine Committee on Health Insurance Status and Its Consequences. *America's Uninsured Crisis: Consequences for Health and Health Care.* Washington, D.C.: National Academies Press, 2009.

Institute of Medicine Committee on Quality of Health Care in America. *Crossing the Quality Chasm: A New Health System for the 21st Century.* Washington, D.C.: National Academy Press, 2001.

Institute of Medicine Committee on the Consequences of Uninsurance. *Care Without Coverage: Too Little, Too Late.* Washington, D.C.: National Academy Press, 2002.

Institute of Medicine Committee on the Consequences of Uninsurance. *Hidden Costs, Value Lost: Uninsurance in America.* Washington, D.C.: National Academies Press, 2003.

Institute of Medicine Committee on the Consequences of Uninsurance. *Insuring America's Health Principles and Recommendations.* Washington, D.C.: National Academies Press, 2004.

Isaacs, S. L., and Schroeder, S. A. "Class—The Ignored Determinant of the Nation's Health." *New England Journal of Medicine*, 2004, *351*(11), 1137–1142.

Jackson, J. S., and others. "Racism and the Physical and Mental Health Status of African Americans: A Thirteen-Year National Panel Study. *Ethnicity & Disease*, 1996, *6*(1–2), 132–147.

James, S. A., LaCroix, A. Z., Kleinbaum, D. G., and Strogatz, D. S. "John Henryism and Blood Pressure Differences Among Black Men. II. The Role of Occupational Stressors." *Journal of Behavioral Medicine*, 1984, *7*(3), 259–275.

Johnson, J., and Hall, E. "Class, Work and Health." In B. Amick III, S. Levine, and A. Tarlov (eds.), *Society and Health*. New York: Oxford University Press, 1995.

Jones, A. R., Caplan, L. S., and Davis, M. K. "Racial/Ethnic Differences in the Self-Reported Use of Screening Mammography." *Journal of Community Health*, 2003, *28*(5), 303–316.

Jones, C. P. "Levels of Racism: A Theoretic Framework and a Gardener's Tale." *American Journal of Public Health*, 2000, *90*(8), 1212–1215.

Jones-Webb, R., and others. "Race, Socioeconomic Status, and Premature Mortality." *Minnesota Medicine*, 2009, *92*(2), 40–43.

Kaiser Commission on Medicaid and the Uninsured. *Health Coverage of Children: The Role of Medicaid and CHIP*. Washington, D.C., 2009a.

Kaiser Commission on Medicaid and the Uninsured. *Health Insurance Coverage in America, 2008 Online Chartbook*. Washington, D.C., 2009b.

Kaiser Commission on Medicaid and the Uninsured. *Medicaid: A Primer. Key Information on the Nation's Health Program for Low-Income People*. Washington, D.C., 2009c.

Kaiser Commission on Medicaid and the Uninsured. *State Fiscal Conditions and Medicaid* (No. 7580–05). Washington, D.C., 2009d.

Kaiser Commission on Medicaid and the Uninsured. (2010). *Medicare at a Glance*. Washington, D.C., 2010.

Kaler, S. G., and Rennert, O. M. "Reducing the Impact of Poverty on Health and Human Development: Scientific Approaches." *Annals of the New York Academy of Sciences*, 2008, *1136*, xi–xii.

Kaplan, D., and others. "A Comparison Study of an Elementary School–Based Health Center: Effects on Health Care Access and Use." *Archives of Pediatrics & Adolescent Medicine*, 1999, *153*(3), 235–243.

Kaplan, G. A., and others. "Inequality in Income and Mortality in the United States: Analysis of Mortality and Potential Pathways." *British Medical Journal*, 1996, *312*(7037), 999–1003.

Kaplan, J. R., and Manuck, S. B. "Status, Stress, and Atherosclerosis: The Role of Environment and Individual Behavior." *Annals of the New York Academy of Sciences*, 1999, *896*, 145–161.

Karasek, R. *Healthy Work: Stress, Productivity, and the Reconstruction of Working Life*. New York: Basic Books, 1990.

Karlsen, S., and Nazroo, J. Y. "Agency and Structure: The Impact of Ethnic Identity and Racism on the Health of Ethnic Minority People." *Sociology of Health & Illness*, 2002a, *2002*(24), 1–20.

Karlsen, S., and Nazroo, J. Y. "Relation Between Racial Discrimination, Social Class, and Health Among Ethnic Minority Groups." *American Journal of Public Health*, 2002b, *92*(4), 624–631.

Kasarda, J. D. "Urban Industrial Transition and the Underclass." *Annals of the American Academy of Political and Social Science*, 1989, *501*, 26–47.

Kawachi, I. "Social Capital and Community Effects on Population and Individual Health." *Annals of the New York Academy of Sciences*, 1999, *896*, 120–130.

Kawachi, I., and Kennedy, B. P. "Health and Social Cohesion: Why Care About Income Inequality?" *British Medical Journal*, 1997, *314*(7086), 1037–1040.

Kawachi, I., and Kennedy, B. P. "Income Inequality and Health: Pathways and Mechanisms." *Health Services Research*, 1999, *34*(1 Pt. 2), 215–227.

Kawachi, I., Kennedy, B. P., and Glass, R. "Social Capital and Self-Rated Health: A Contextual Analysis." *American Journal of Public Health*, 1999, *89*(8), 1187–1193.

Kawachi, I., Kennedy, B. P., Lochner, K., and Prothrow-Stith, D. "Social Capital, Income Inequality, and Mortality." *American Journal of Public Health*, 1997, *87*(9), 1491–1498.

Kessler, R. C., Mickelson, K. D., and Williams, D. R. "The Prevalence, Distribution, and Mental Health Correlates of Perceived Discrimination in the United States." *Journal of Health and Social Behavior*, 1999, *40*(3), 208–230.

Kilbourne, A. M., Switzer, G. E., Hyman, K., Crowley-Matoka, M., and Fine, M. "Advancing Health Disparities Research Within the Health Care System: A Conceptual Framework." *American Journal of Public Health*, 2006, *96*(12), 2113–2121.

King, G., and Williams, D. "Race and Health: A Multidimensional Approach to African-American Health." In B. Amick III, S. Levine, A. Tarlov, and D. Chapman Walsh (eds.), *Society and Health* (pp. 93–130). New York: Oxford University Press, 1995.

Kingsdale, J. "Implementing Health Care Reform in Massachusetts: Strategic Lessons Learned." *Health Affairs (Millwood)*, 2009, *28*(4), w588–594.

Kirschenman, J., and Neckerman, K. "'We'd Love to Hire Them, But…': The Meaning of Race for Employers." In C. Jencks and P. Peterson (eds.), *The Urban Underclass* (pp. 203–232). Washington, D.C.: Brookings Institution, 1991.

Klag, M. J., and others. "The Association of Skin Color with Blood Pressure in U.S. Blacks with Low Socioeconomic Status." *Journal of the American Medical Association*, 1991, *265*(5), 599–602.

Klein, J. D., and others. "Access to Medical Care for Adolescents: Results from the 1997 Commonwealth Fund Survey of the Health of Adolescent Girls." *Journal of Adolescent Health*, 1999, *25*(2), 120–130.

Klein, R. "Presumptive Eligibility." *The Future of Children*, 2003, *13*(1), 230–237.

Krieger, N. "Racial and Gender Discrimination: Risk Factors for High Blood Pressure? *Social Science & Medicine*, 1990, *30*(12), 1273–1281.

Krieger, N., and Sidney, S. "Racial Discrimination and Blood Pressure: The CARDIA Study of Young Black and White Adults." *American Journal of Public Health*, 1996, *86*(10), 1370–1378.

Kruger, M. Affordable Health Care for America Act. 2009. Retrieved January 25, 2010, from http://edlabor.house.gov/blog/2009/10/affordable-health-care.shtml

Laditka, J. N., and Laditka, S. B. "Insurance Status and Access to Primary Health Care: Disparate Outcomes for Potentially Preventable Hospitalization." *Journal of Health & Social Policy*, 2004, *19*(2), 81–100.

Lalonde, M. *A New Perspective on the Health of Canadians*. Ottawa: Ministry of National Health and Welfare, 1974.

Landon, B. E., Schneider, E. C., Normand, S. L., Scholle, S. H., Pawlson, L. G., and Epstein, A. M. "Quality of Care in Medicaid Managed Care and Commercial Health Plans." *Journal of the American Medical Association*, 2007, *298*(14), 1674–1681.

Landrine, H., and Klonoff, E. A. "Racial Discrimination and Cigarette Smoking Among Blacks: Findings from Two Studies." *Ethnicity & Disease*, 2000, *10*(2), 195–202.

Lang, I. A., and others. "Neighborhood Deprivation, Individual Socioeconomic Status, and Frailty in Older Adults." *Journal of the American Geriatrics Society*, 2009, *57*(10), 1776–1780.

Lansky, D. "Creating the New Health Care Consumer: An Interview with David Lansky. Interview by Ed Rabinowitz." *Healthplan*, 2003, *44*(4), 29–30.

Lantz, P. M., and others. "Socioeconomic Factors, Health Behaviors, and Mortality: Results from a Nationally Representative Prospective Study of U.S. Adults." *Journal of the American Medical Association*, 1998, *279*(21), 1703–1708.

Larson, K., Russ, S. A., Crall, J. J., and Halfon, N. "Influence of Multiple Social Risks on Children's Health." *Pediatrics*, 2008, *121*(2), 337–344.

Lasser, K. E., Himmelstein, D. U., and Woolhandler, S. "Access to Care, Health Status, and Health Disparities in the United States and Canada: Results of a Cross-National Population-Based Survey." *American Journal of Public Health*, 2006, *96*(7), 1300–1307.

LaVeist, T., and others. "Exploring Health Disparities in Integrated Communities: Overview of the EHDIC Study." *Journal of Urban Health*, 2008, *85*(1), 11–21.

LaVeist, T. A. "Beyond Dummy Variables and Sample Selection: What Health Services Researchers Ought to Know About Race as a Variable." *Health Services Research*, 1994, *29*(1), 1–16.

LaVeist, T. A. *Minority Populations and Health: An Introduction to Health Disparities in the U.S.* San Francisco: Jossey-Bass, 2005.

LaVeist, T. A., and Carroll, T. "Race of Physician and Satisfaction with Care Among African-American Patients." *Journal of the National Medical Association*, 2002, *94*(11), 937–943.

Laveist, T. A., Isaac, L. A., and Williams, K. P. "Mistrust of Health Care Organizations Is Associated with Underutilization of Health Services." *Health Services Research*, 2009, *44*(6), 2093-2105.

LaVeist, T. A., Sellers, R., and Neighbors, H. W. "Perceived Racism and Self and System Blame Attribution: Consequences for Longevity." *Ethnicity Disease*, 2001, *11*(4), 711–721.

LaVeist, T. A., Thorpe, R. J., Jr., and others. "Environmental and Socio-Economic Factors as Contributors to Racial Disparities in Diabetes Prevalence." *Journal of General Internal Medicine*, 2009, *24*(10), 1144–1148.

Lear, J. G. "Health at School: A Hidden Health Care System Emerges from the Shadows." *Health Affairs (Millwood)*, 2007, *26*(2), 409–419.

Lear, J. G., Barnwell, E. A., and Behrens, D. "Health-Care Reform and School-Based Health Care." *Public Health Reports*, 2008, *123*(6), 704–708.

LeClere, F. B., Rogers, R. G., and Peters, K. "Neighborhood Social Context and Racial Differences in Women's Heart Disease Mortality." *Journal of Health and Social Behavior*, 1998, *39*(2), 91–107.

Lee, R., and others. "Impact of Race on Morbidity and Mortality in Patients with Congestive Heart Failure: A Study of the Multiracial Population in Singapore." *International Journal of Cardiology*, 2009, *134*(3), 422–425.

Lee, R. E., and Cubbin, C. "Neighborhood Context and Youth Cardiovascular Health Behaviors." *American Journal of Public Health*, 2002, *92*(3), 428–436.

Leibowitz, A., and others. "Effect of Cost-Sharing on the Use of Medical Services by Children: Interim Results from a Randomized Controlled Trial." *Pediatrics*, 1985, *75*(5), 942–951.

Lemelin, E. T., and others. "Life-Course Socioeconomic Positions and Subclinical Atherosclerosis in the Multi-Ethnic Study of Atherosclerosis." *Social Science & Medicine*, 2009, *68*(3), 444–451.

Lewit, E., Bennett, T., and Behrman, R. "Health Insurance for Children: Analysis and Recommendations." *The Future of Children*, *2003*, *13*(1), 5–29.

Lillie-Blanton, M., and others. *Racial/Ethnic Disparities in Access to Care Among Children: How Does Medicaid Do in Closing the Gaps?* Washington, D.C.: The Henry J. Kaiser Family Foundation, 2009.

Lillie-Blanton, M., Rushing, O., and Ruiz, S. *Key Facts: Race, Ethnicity & Medical Care.* Menlo Park, California: Kaiser Family Foundation, 2003.

Lindstrom, M. "Marital Status, Social Capital, Material Conditions and Self-Rated Health: A Population-Based Study. *Health Policy*, 2009, *93*(2–3), 172–179.

Link, C. L., and McKinlay, J. B. "Disparities in the Prevalence of Diabetes: Is It Race/Ethnicity or Socioeconomic Status? Results from the Boston Area Community Health (BACH) Survey." *Ethnicity and Disease*, 2009, *19*(3), 288–292.

Lischko, A. M., Bachman, S. S., and Vangeli, A. "The Massachusetts Commonwealth Health Insurance Connector: Structure and Functions." *Issue Brief (Commonwealth Fund)*, 2009, *55*, 1–14.

Lobe, J. "U.S. Admits to UN That Racism Persists." *IPS Daily Journal of the UN*, 2000, *25*(8), p. 175.

Lopez, S. Smart-spending skid row program saves lives. February 11, 2009, *Los Angeles Times*, from http://articles.latimes.com/2009/feb/11/local/me-lopez11

Lowe, R. A., McConnell, K. J., Vogt, M. E., and Smith, J. A. "Impact of Medicaid Cutbacks on Emergency Department Use: The Oregon Experience." *Annals of Emergency Medicine*, 2008, *52*(6), 626–634.

Lu, M. C., and Halfon, N. "Racial and Ethnic Disparities in Birth Outcomes: A Life-Course Perspective." *Maternal and Child Health Journal*, 2003, *7*(1), 13–30.

Ludwig, J., and Phillips, D. A. "Long-Term Effects of Head Start on Low-Income Children." *Annals of the New York Academy Sciences*, 2008, *1136*, 257–268.

Lundberg, U. "Stress Responses in Low-Status Jobs and Their Relationship to Health Risks: Musculoskeletal Disorders." *Annals of the New York Academy of Sciences*, 1999, *896*, 162–172.

Lurie, N., Ward, N. B., Shapiro, M. F., and Brook, R. H. "Termination from Medi-Cal—Does It Affect Health?" *New England Journal of Medicine*, 1984, *311*(7), 480–484.

Lurie, N., and others. "Termination of Medi-Cal Benefits: A Follow-Up Study One Year Later." *New England Journal of Medicine*, 1986, *314*(19), 1266–1268.

Macinko, J., and Starfield, B. "The Utility of Social Capital in Research on Health Determinants." *Milbank Quarterly*, 2001, *79*(3), 387–427, IV.

Macinko, J., Starfield, B., and Shi, L. "The Contribution of Primary Care Systems to Health Outcomes Within Organization for Economic Cooperation and Development (OECD) Countries, 1970–1998." *Health Services Research*, 2003, *38*(3), 831–865.

Mackenbach, J. P., and others. "Socioeconomic Inequalities in Health in 22 European Countries." *New England Journal of Medicine*, 2008, *358*(23), 2468–2481.

Mangione-Smith, R., and others. "Racial/Ethnic Variation in Parent Expectations for Antibiotics: Implications for Public Health Campaigns." *Pediatrics*, 2004, *113*(5), e385–394.

Mansyur, C., Amick, B. C., Harrist, R. B., and Franzini, L. "Social Capital, Income Inequality, and Self-Rated Health in 45 Countries." *Social Science & Medicine*, 2008, *66*(1), 43–56.

Marmot, M. "Epidemiological Approach to the Explanation of Social Differentiation in Mortality: The Whitehall Studies." *Sozial- und Präventivmedizin*, 1993, *38*(5), 271–279.

Marmot, M. "The Influence of Income on Health: Views of an Epidemiologist: Does Money Really Matter? Or Is It a Marker for Something Else? *Health Affairs (Millwood)*, 2002, *21*(2), 31–46.

Marmot, M., and Theorell, T. "Social Class and Cardiovascular Disease: The Contribution of Work." *International Journal of Health Services*, 1988, *18*(4), 659–674.

Marmot, M. G. "Improvement of Social Environment to Improve Health." *Lancet*, 1998, *351*(9095), 57–60.

Marmot, M. G., and others. "Contribution of Job Control and Other Risk Factors to Social Variations in Coronary Heart Disease Incidence." *Lancet*, 1997, *350*(9073), 235–239.

Marmot, M. G., Shipley, M. J., Hemingway, H., Head, J., and Brunner, E. J. "Biological and Behavioural Explanations of Social Inequalities in Coronary Heart Disease: The Whitehall II Study." *Diabetologia*, 2008, *51*(11), 1980–1988.

Marmot, M. G., Smith, G. D., and others. "Health Inequalities Among British Civil Servants: The Whitehall II Study." *Lancet*, 1991, *337*(8754), 1387–1393.

Marshall, K. J., Urrutia-Rojas, X., Mas, F. S., and Coggin, C. "Health Status and Access to Health Care of Documented and Undocumented Immigrant Latino Women." *Health Care for Women International*, 2005, *26*(10), 916–936.

Martin, L. M., Calle, E. E., Wingo, P. A., and Heath, C. W., Jr. "Comparison of Mammography and Pap Test Use from the 1987 and 1992 National Health Interview Surveys: Are We Closing the Gaps?" *American Journal of Preventive Medicine*, 1996, *12*(2), 82–90.

McBean, A. M., and Gornick, M. "Differences by Race in the Rates of Procedures Performed in Hospitals for Medicare Beneficiaries." *Health Care Financing Review*, 1994, *15*(4), 77–90.

McCord, C., and Freeman, H. P. "Excess Mortality in Harlem." *New England Journal of Medicine*, 1990, *322*(3), 173–177.

McDonough, J. E., Hager, C. L., and Rosman, B. "Health Care Reform Stages a Comeback in Massachusetts." *New England Journal of Medicine*, 1997, *336*(2), 148–151.

McGee, D. L., Liao, Y., Cao, G., and Cooper, R. S. "Self-Reported Health Status and Mortality in a Multiethnic U.S. Cohort." *American Journal of Epidemiology*, 1999, *149*(1), 41–46.

McKeown, T. *The Role of Medicine: Dream, Mirage or Nemesis.* London: Nuffield Provincial Hospitals Trust, 1976.

Mechanic, D. "The Rise and Fall of Managed Care." *Journal of Health and Social Behavior*, 2004, *45 Suppl*, 76–86.

Mechanic, D., and Schlesinger, M. "The Impact of Managed Care on Patients' Trust in Medical Care and Their Physicians." *Journal of the American Medical Association*, 1996, *275*(21), 1693–1697.

Mechanic, D., and Tanner, J. "Vulnerable People, Groups, and Populations: Societal View." *Health Affairs (Millwood)*, 2007, *26*(5), 1220–1230.

Meghani, S. H., and others. "Patient-Provider Race-Concordance: Does It Matter in Improving Minority Patients' Health Outcomes?" *Ethnicity & Health*, 2009, *14*(1), 107–130.

Meissner, H. I., and others. "Which Women Aren't Getting Mammograms and Why? (United States)." *Cancer Causes & Control*, 2007, *18*(1), 61–70.

Merkin, S. S., Stevenson, L., and Powe, N. "Geographic Socioeconomic Status, Race, and Advanced-Stage Breast Cancer in New York City." *American Journal of Public Health*, 2002, *92*(1), 64–70.

Merrick, E. L., and others. "Changing Mental Health Gatekeeping: Effects on Performance Indicators." *Journal of Behavioral Health Services & Research*, 2008, *35*(1), 3–19.

Miller, J. E. "The Effects of Race/Ethnicity and Income on Early Childhood Asthma Prevalence and Health Care Use." *American Journal of Public Health*, 2000, *90*(3), 428–430.

Miller, R., and Luft, H. "Managed Care Plan Performance Since 1980: A Literature Analysis." *Journal of American Medical Association*, 1994, *271*(19), 1512–1519.

Miller, R. H., and Luft, H. S. "Does Managed Care Lead to Better or Worse Quality of Care?": *Health Affairs (Millwood)*, 1997, *16*(5), 7–25.

Miller, R. H., and Luft, H. S. "HMO Plan Performance Update: An Analysis of the Literature, 1997–2001." *Health Affairs (Millwood)*, 2002, *21*(4), 63–86.

Miller, S. M. "Thinking Strategically About Society and Health." In B. C. Amick, S. Levine, A. R. Tarlov, and D. C. Walsh (eds.), *Society and Health* (pp. 342–358). New York: Oxford University Press, 1995.

Mills, R., and Bhandari, S. *Health Insurance Coverage in the United States, 2002* (No. P60–223). Rockville, Md.: U.S. Census Bureau, 2003.

Minkler, M., Fuller-Thomson, E., and Guralnik, J. M. "Gradient of Disability Across the Socioeconomic Spectrum in the United States." *New England Journal of Medicine*, 2006, *355*(7), 695–703.

Mistry, R., and others. "Parenting-Related Stressors and Self-Reported Mental Health of Mothers with Young Children." *American Journal of Public Health*, 2007, *97*(7), 1261–1268.

Mitchell, E. A., Hutchison, L., and Stewart, A. W. "The Continuing Decline in SIDS Mortality." *Archives of Disease in Childhood*, 2007, *92*(7), 625–626.

Mohanty, S. A., and others. "Health Care Expenditures of Immigrants in the United States: A Nationally Representative Analysis." *American Journal of Public Health*, 2005, *95*(8), 1431–1438.

Morone, J. A. *Hellfire Nation: The Politics of Sin in American History.* New Haven, Connecticut: Yale University Press, 2003.

Morone, J. A. "Morality, Politics, and Health Policy." In D. Mechanic, L. B. Rogut, D. C. Colby, and J. R. Knickman (eds). *Policy Challenges in Modern Health Care.* New Brunswick, New Jersey: Rutgers University Press, 2005, 13–25.

Moss, N. "Socioeconomic Disparities in Health in the U.S.: An Agenda for Action. *Social Science & Medicine*, 2000, *51*(11), 1627–1638.

Mossakowski, K. N. "The Influence of Past Unemployment Duration on Symptoms of Depression Among Young Women and Men in the United States." *American Journal of Public Health*, 2009, *99*(10), 1826–1832.

Muntaner, C., and Lynch, J. "Income Inequality, Social Cohesion, and Class Relations: A Critique of Wilkinson's Neo-Durkheimian Research Program." *International Journal of Health Services*, 1999, *29*(1), 59–81.

Nandi, A., and others. "Access to and Use of Health Services Among Undocumented Mexican Immigrants in a U.S. Urban Area." *American Journal of Public Health*, 2008, *98*(11), 2011–2020.

National Center for Chronic Disease Prevention and Health Promotion. Behavioral Risk Factor Surveillance System, Environmental Quality and Metropolitan Area Data, 2006. Retrieved November 26, 2009, from Centers for Disease Control and Prevention: http://www.cdc.gov/brfss/cde/index.htm.

National Center for Complementary and Alternative Medicine. *The Use of Complementary and Alternative Medicine in the United States.* Bethesda, Md.: National Center for Complementary and Alternative Medicine, U.S. Department of Health and Human Services, 2008.

National Center for Health Statistics. *Health, United States 1998, with Socioeconomic Status and Health Chartbook.* Hyattsville, Md.: Centers for Disease Control, 1998.

National Center for Health Statistics. *Health, United States 2003.* Hyattsville, Md.: Centers for Disease Control, 2003.

National Center for Health Statistics. *Health, United States 2008* (No. 2009–1232). Hyattsville, Md.: Centers for Disease Control, National Center for Health Statistics, 2009.

National Conference of State Legislators. Health Disparities 2009 Overview. Retrieved December 28, 2009, from http://www.ncsl.org/?tabid=14494#statewide

National Governors Association. *MCH Update 2002: State Health Coverage for Low-Income Pregnant Women, Children and Parents.* Washington, DC: National Governors Association, 2003.

Navarro, V. "Assessment of the World Health Report 2000." *Lancet*, 2000, *356*(9241), 1598–1601.

Navarro, V. "Policy Without Politics: The Limits of Social Engineering." *American Journal of Public Health*, 2003, *93*(1), 64–67.

Navarro, V., and Shi, L. "The Political Context of Social Inequalities and Health." *Social Science & Medicine*, 2001, *52*(3), 481–491.

Neckerman, K., & Kirschenman, J. "Hiring Strategies, Racial Bias, and Inner-City Workers." *Social Problems*, 1991, *38*, 433–447.

Neumark, D., and Wascher, W. *Using the EITC to Help Poor Families: New Evidence and a Comparision with the Minimum Wage*. Washington, D.C.: Center on Budget and Policy Priorities, 2000.

Newacheck, P., Jameson, W. J., and Halfon, N. "Health Status and Income: The Impact of Poverty on Child Health." *Journal of School Health*, 1994, *64*(6), 229–233.

Newacheck, P. W. "Poverty and Childhood Chronic Illness." *Archives of Pediatrics & Adolescent Medicine*, 1994, *148*(11), 1143–1149.

Newacheck, P. W., and others. "The Unmet Health Needs of America's Children." *Pediatrics*, 2000, *105*(4 Pt. 2), 989–997.

Newacheck, P. W., Hughes, D.C., and Stoddard, J. J. "Children's Access to Primary Care: Differences by Race, Income, and Insurance Status." *Pediatrics*, 1996, *97*(1), 26–32.

Newacheck, P. W., Hung, Y. Y., Hochstein, M., and Halfon, N. "Access to Health Care for Disadvantaged Young Children." *Journal of Early Intervention*, 2002, *25*(1), 1–11.

O'Malley, M. S., and others. "The Association of Race/Ethnicity, Socioeconomic Status, and Physician Recommendation for Mammography: Who Gets the Message About Breast Cancer Screening?" *American Journal of Public Health*, 2001, *91*(1), 49–54.

Oksanen, T., and others. "Social Capital at Work as a Predictor of Employee Health: Multilevel Evidence from Work Units in Finland. *Social Science & Medicine*, 2008, *66*(3), 637–649.

Oldenburg, B. F., McGuffog, I. D., and Turrell, G. "Making a Difference to the Socioeconomic Determinants of Health: Policy Responses and Intervention Options." *Asia-Pacific Journal of Public Health*, 2000, *12 Suppl*, S51–54.

Olson, L. M., Tang, S. F., and Newacheck, P. W. "Children in the United States with Discontinuous Health Insurance Coverage." *New England Journal of Medicine*, 2005, *353*(4), 382–391.

Orfield, G., and Eaton, S. *Dismantling Desegregation: The Quiet Reversal of Brown v. Board of Education*. New York: New Press, 1996.

Organisation for Economic Co-operation and Development. OECD Health Data 2009. Retrieved November 21, 2009: http://www.ecosante.org/index2.php?base=OCDE&langs=ENG&langh=ENG

Patel, D., and others. "Feasibility of Using Risk Factors to Screen for Psychological Disorder During Routine Breast Care Nurse Consultations." *Cancer Nursing*, 2010, *33*(1), 19–27.

Patton, G. A. "The Two-Edged Sword: How Technology Shapes Medical Practice." *Physician Executive*, 2001, *27*(2), 42–49.

Perry, M., Williams, R. L., Wallerstein, N., and Waitzkin, H. "Social Capital and Health Care Experiences Among Low-Income Individuals." *American Journal of Public Health*, 2008, *98*(2), 330–336.

Peterson, E. D., Shah, B. R., and others. "Trends in Quality of Care for Patients with Acute Myocardial Infarction in the National Registry of Myocardial Infarction from 1990 to 2006." *American Heart Journal*, 2008, *156*(6), 1045–1055.

Peterson, E. D., Shaw, L. K., and others. "Racial Variation in the Use of Coronary-Revascularization Procedures: Are the Differences Real? Do They Matter?" *New England Journal Medicine*, 1997, *336*(7), 480–486.

Pincus, T., Esther, R., DeWalt, D. A., and Callahan, L. F. "Social Conditions and Self-Management Are More Powerful Determinants of Health Than Access to Care." *Annals of Internal Medicine*, 1998, *129*(5), 406–411.

Poehlmann, J., Schwichtenberg, A. J., Bolt, D., and Dilworth-Bart, J. "Predictors of Depressive Symptom Trajectories in Mothers of Preterm or Low Birth Weight Infants." *Journal of Family Psychology*, 2009, *23*(5), 690–704.

Popp, T. K., Spinrad, T. L., and Smith, C. L. "The Relation of Cumulative Demographic Risk to Mothers' Responsivity and Control: Examining the Role of Toddler Temperament." *Infancy*, 2008, *13*(5), 496–518.

Power, C., and Matthews, S. "Origins of Health Inequalities in a National Population Sample." *Lancet*, 1997, *350*(9091), 1584–1589.

Power, C., Matthews, S., and Manor, O. "Inequalities in Self-Rated Health: Explanations from Different Stages of Life." *Lancet*, 1998, *351*(9108), 1009–1014.

Prentice, J. C., and Pizer, S. D. "Delayed Access to Health Care and Mortality." *Health Services Research*, 2007, *42*(2), 644–662.

Rahman, S. M., Dignan, M. B., and Shelton, B. J. "Factors Influencing Adherence to Guidelines for Screening Mammography Among Women Aged 40 Years and Older." *Ethnicity & Diseases*, 2003, *13*(4), 477–484.

Ramsay, S. E., and others. "Is Socioeconomic Position Related to the Prevalence of Metabolic Syndrome?: Influence of Social Class Across the Life Course in a Population-Based Study of Older Men." *Diabetes Care*, 2008, *31*(12), 2380–2382.

Rand Health. *Taking the Pulse of Health Care in America: Research Highlights*. Santa Monica, Calif.: RAND, 1999.

Raphael, S., and Stoll, M. *Modest Progress: The Narrowing Spatial Mismatch Between Blacks and Jobs in the 1990s*. Washington, D.C.: The Brookings Institute Center on Urban and Metropolitan Policy, 2002.

Rebok, G., and others. "Elementary School-Aged Children's Reports of Their Health: A Cognitive Interviewing Study." *Quality Life Research*, 2001, *10*(1), 59–70.

Reede, J. Y. "A Recurring Theme: The Need for Minority Physicians." *Health Affairs (Millwood)*, 2003, *22*(4), 91–93.

Remote Area Medical Volunteer Corps. Remote Area Medical News, 2009. Retrieved January 22, 2010, from http://www.ramusa.org/

Rhoades, E. R., D'Angelo, A. J., and Hurlburt, W. B. "The Indian Health Service Record of Achievement." *Public Health Reports*, 1987, *102*(4), 356–360.

Roberts, R. E., Roberts, C. R., and Chan, W. "One-Year Incidence of Psychiatric Disorders and Associated Risk Factors Among Adolescents in the Community." *The Journal of Child Psychology and Psychiatry*, 2009, *50*(4), 405–415.

Rodriguez, H. P., and others. "Physician Effects on Racial and Ethnic Disparities in Patients' Experiences of Primary Care." *Journal of General Internal Medicine*, 2008, *23*(10), 1666–1672.

Rodriguez, M. A., Bustamante, A. V., and Ang, A. "Perceived Quality of Care, Receipt of Preventive Care, and Usual Source of Health Care Among Undocumented and Other Latinos. *Journal of General Internal Medicine*, 2009, *24 Suppl 3*, 508–513.

Rogers, A. C. "Vulnerability, Health and Health Care." *Journal of Advanced Nursing*, 1997, *26*(1), 65–72.

Ronsaville, D. S., and Hakim, R. B. "Well Child Care in the United States: Racial Differences in Compliance with Guidelines." *American Journal of Public Health*, 2000, *90*(9), 1436–1443.

Rosen, H., and others. "Lack of Insurance Negatively Affects Trauma Mortality in U.S. Children." *Journal of Pediatric Surgery*, 2009, *44*(10), 1952–1957.

Rosenbach, M., and others. "Characteristics, Access, Utilization, Satisfaction, and Outcomes of Healthy Start Participants in Eight Sites." *Maternal and Child Health Journal, 2009.*

Rosenbaum, S., and others. "The Children's Hour: The State Children's Health Insurance Program." *Health Affairs (Millwood)*, 1998, *17*(1), 75–89.

Ross, C. E., and Mirowsky, J. "Family Relationships, Social Support and Subjective Life Expectancy." *Journal of Health and Social Behavior*, 2002, *43*(4), 469–489.

Ross, D., and Cox, L. *Enrolling Children and Families in Health Coverage: The Promise of Doing More.* Washington, D.C.: The Kaiser Commission on Medicaid and the Uninsured, 2002.

Ross, N. A., and others. "Relation Between Income Inequality and Mortality in Canada and in the United States: Cross Sectional Assessment Using Census Data and Vital Statistics." *British Medical Journal*, 2000, *320*(7239), 898–902.

Saha, S., Arbelaez, J. J., and Cooper, L. A. "Patient-Physician Relationships and Racial Disparities in the Quality of Health Care." *American Journal of Public Health*, 2003, *93*(10), 1713–1719.

Saha, S., Komaromy, M., Koepsell, T., and Bindman, A. "Patient-Physician Racial Concordance and the Perceived Quality and Use of Health Care." *Archives of Internal Medicine*, 1999, *159*(9), 997–1004.

Salihu, H. M., and others. "Healthy Start Program and Feto-Infant Morbidity Outcomes: Evaluation of Program Effectiveness." *Maternal and Child Health Journal*, 2009, *13*(1), 56–65.

Sambamoorthi, U., and McAlpine, D. D. "Racial, Ethnic, Socioeconomic, and Access Disparities in the Use of Preventive Services Among Women." *Preventive Medicine*, 2003, *37*(5), 475–484.

Sameroff, A. J., and others. "Intelligence Quotient Scores of 4-Year-Old Children: Social-Environmental Risk Factors." *Pediatrics*, 1987, *79*(3), 343–350.

Sanders, J. State health care bind: Fixing inequities can be expensive. *Sacramento Bee*, December 22, 2002.

Satcher, D. "Eliminating Racial and Ethnic Disparities in Health: The Role of the Ten Leading Health Indicators." *Journal of the National Medical Association*, 2000, *92*(7), 315–318.

Sato, T., and others. "Effects of Social Relationships on Mortality of the Elderly: How Do the Influences Change with the Passage of Time?" *Archives of Gerontology and Geriatrics*, 2008, *47*(3), 327–339.

Schnittker, J., and Bhatt, M. "The Role of Income and Race/Ethnicity in Experiences with Medical Care in the United States and United Kingdom." *International Journal of Health Services*, 2008, *38*(4), 671–695.

Schoen, C., and others. "In Chronic Condition: Experiences of Patients with Complex Health Care Needs, in Eight Countries, 2008." *Health Affairs (Millwood)*, 2009, *28*(1), w1–16.

Schulman, K. A., Rubenstein, L. E., Chesley, F. D., and Eisenberg, J. M. "The Roles of Race and Socioeconomic Factors in Health Services Research. *Health Services Research*, 1995, *30*(1 Pt. 2), 179–195.

Schultz, J., Corman, H., Noonan, K., and Reichman, N. E. "Effects of Child Health on Parents' Social Capital." *Social Science & Medicine*, 2009, *69*(1), 76–84.

Schulz, A., and others. "Social Inequalities, Stressors and Self-Reported Health Status Among African American and White Women in the Detroit Metropolitan Area." *Social Science & Medicine*, 2000, *51*(11), 1639–1653.

Schulz, A. J., and others. "Discrimination, Symptoms of Depression, and Self-Rated Health Among African American Women in Detroit: Results from a Longitudinal Analysis." *American Journal of Public Health*, 2006, *96*(7), 1265–1270.

Schulz, A. J., Williams, D. R., Israel, B. A., and Lempert, L. B. "Racial and Spatial Relations as Fundamental Determinants of Health in Detroit." *Milbank Quarterly*, 2002, *80*(4), 677–707, iv.

Secretary's Advisory Committee on National Health Promotion and Disease Prevention Objectives for 2020. *Phase I Report: Recommendations for the Framework and Format of Healthy People 2020*. Washington, D.C.: U.S. Department of Health and Human Services, 2008.

Seeman, M., and Lewis, S. "Powerlessness, Health and Mortality: A Longitudinal Study of Older Men and Mature Women." *Social Science & Medicine*, 1995, *41*(4), 517–525.

Seeman, T. E., and Crimmins, E. "Social Environment Effects on Health and Aging: Integrating Epidemiologic and Demographic Approaches and Perspectives." *Annals of the New York Academy of Sciences*, 2001, *954*, 88–117.

Seid, M., Varni, J. W., Cummings, L., and Schonlau, M. "The Impact of Realized Access to Care on Health-Related Quality of Life: A Two-Year Prospective Cohort Study of Children in the California State Children's Health Insurance Program." *Journal of Pediatrics*, 2006, *149*(3), 354–361.

Selden, T. M., Banthin, J. S., and Cohen, J. W. "Waiting in the Wings: Eligibility and Enrollment in the State Children's Health Insurance Program." *Health Affairs (Millwood)*, 1999, *18*(2), 126–133.

Shea, S., and others. "Predisposing Factors for Severe, Uncontrolled Hypertension in an Inner-City Minority Population." *New England Journal of Medicine*, 1992, *327*(11), 776–781.

Shi, L. "The Relationship Between Primary Care and Life Chances." *Journal of Health Care for the Poor and Underserved*, 1992, *3*(2), 321–335.

Shi, L. "Primary Care, Specialty Care, and Life Chances." *International Journal of Health Services*, 1994, *24*(3), 431–458.

Shi, L. "Balancing Primary versus Specialty Care." *Journal of the Royal Society of Medicine*, 1995, *88*(8), 428–432.

Shi, L. "Experience of Primary Care By Racial and Ethnic Groups in the United States." *Medical Care*, 1999, *37*(10), 1068–1077.

Shi, L. "Type of Health Insurance and the Quality of Primary Care Experience." *American Journal of Public Health*, 2000, *90*(12), 1848–1855.

Shi, L., Forrest, C. B., Von Schrader, S., and Ng, J. "Vulnerability and the Patient-Practitioner Relationship: The Roles of Gatekeeping and Primary Care Performance." *American Journal of Public Health*, 2003, *93*(1), 138–144.

Shi, L., and Macinko, J. "Changes in Medical Care Experiences of Racial and Ethnic Groups in the United States, 1996–2002.: *International Journal of Health Services*, 2008, *38*(4), 653–670.

Shi, L., Macinko, J., and others. "Primary Care, Income Inequality, and Stroke Mortality in the United States: A Longitudinal Analysis, 1985–1995." *Stroke*, 2003, *34*(8), 1958–1964.

Shi, L., Macinko, J., and others. "Primary Care, Infant Mortality, and Low Birth Weight in the States of the USA." *Journal of Epidemiology and Community Health*, 2004, *58*(5), 374–380.

Shi, L., Regan, J., Politzer, R. M., and Luo, J. "Community Health Centers and Racial/Ethnic Disparities in Healthy Life." *International Journal of Health Services*, 2001, *31*(3), 567–582.

Shi, L., and Starfield, B. "Primary Care, Income Inequality, and Self-Rated Health in the United States: A Mixed-Level Analysis." *International Journal of Health Services*, 2000, *30*(3), 541–555.

Shi, L., Starfield, B., Kennedy, B., and Kawachi, I. "Income Inequality, Primary Care, and Health Indicators." *Journal of Family Practice*, 1999, *48*(4), 275–284.

Shi, L., Stevens, G. D., and Politzer, R. M. "Access to Care for U.S. Health Center Patients and Patients Nationally: How Do the Most Vulnerable Populations Fare?" *Medical Care*, 2007, *45*(3), 206–213.

Shi, L., Stevens, G. D., Wulu, J. T., and others. "America's Health Centers: Reducing Racial and Ethnic Disparities in Perinatal Care and Birth Outcomes." *Health Services Research*, 2004, *39*(6 Pt 1), 1881–1901.

Shihadeh, E., and Flynn, N. "Segregation and Crime: The Effect of Black Social Isolation on the Rates of Black Urban Violence." *Social Forces*, 1996, *74*, 1325–1352.

Shishehbor, M. H., Gordon-Larsen, P., Kiefe, C. I., and Litaker, D. "Association of Neighborhood Socioeconomic Status with Physical Fitness in Healthy Young Adults: The Coronary Artery Risk Development in Young Adults (CARDIA) Study." *American Heart Journal*, 2008, *155*(4), 699–705.

Short, L. J., and others. "Disparities in Medical Care Among Commercially Insured Patients with Newly Diagnosed Breast Cancer: Opportunities for Intervention." *Cancer*, 2009, *116*(1), 193–202.

Siddiqi, A., Zuberi, D., and Nguyen, Q. C. "The Role of Health Insurance in Explaining Immigrant versus Non-Immigrant Disparities in Access to Health Care: Comparing the United States to Canada." *Social Science & Medicine*, 2009, *69*(10), 1452–1459.

Siegel, B., and Nolan, L. "Leveling the Field—Ensuring Equity Through National Health Care Reform." *New England Journal of Medicine*, 2009, *25*(361), 2401–2403.

Sims, M., and others. "Development and Psychometric Testing of a Multidimensional Instrument of Perceived Discrimination Among African Americans in the Jackson Heart Study." *Ethnicity & Disease*, 2009, *19*(1), 56–64.

Smedley, B., Stith, A., and Nelson, A. (eds.). *Unequal Treatment: Confronting Racial and Ethnic Disparities in Health Care*. Washington, D.C.: National Academy Press, 2002.

Smeeding, T. M., Phillips, K. R., and O'Connor, M. "The EITC: Expectation, Knowledge, Use, and Economic and Social Mobility." *National Tax Journal*, 1999, *53*, 1187–1219.

Smith-Bindman, R., and others. "Does Utilization of Screening Mammography Explain Racial and Ethnic Differences in Breast Cancer?" *Annals of Internal Medicine*, 2006, *144*(8), 541–553.

Snelgrove, J. W., Pikhart, H., and Stafford, M. "A Multilevel Analysis of Social Capital and Self-Rated Health: Evidence from the British Household Panel Survey." *Social Science & Medicine*, 2009, *68*(11), 1993–2001.

Sorlie, P., and others. "Mortality in the Uninsured Compared with That in Persons with Public and Private Health Insurance." *Archives of Internal Medicine*, 1994, *154*, 2409–2416.

Stafford, M., De Silva, M., Stansfeld, S., and Marmot, M. "Neighbourhood Social Capital and Common Mental Disorder: Testing the Link in a General Population Sample." *Health & Place*, 2008, *14*(3), 394–405.

Starfield, B. "Health Services Research: A Working Model." *New England Journal of Medicine*, 1973, *289*(3), 132–136.

Starfield, B. "The Promise of HMOs: Primary Care, Prevention, Research and Education." *HMO Practice*, 1993, *7*(3), 103–109.

Starfield, B. "Primary Care: Is It Essential?" *Lancet*, 1994, *344*(8930), 1129–1133.

Starfield, B. "The Future of Primary Care in a Managed Care Era." *International Journal of Health Services*, 1997, *27*(4), 687–696.

Starfield, B. *Primary Care: Balancing Health Needs, Services, and Technology.* New York: Oxford University Press, 1998.

Starfield, B. "Equity in Health." *Journal of Epidemiology and Community Health*, 2002, *56*(7), 483–484.

Starfield, B. "Equity, Social Determinants, and Children's Rights: Coming to Grips with the Challenges." *Ambulatory Pediatrics*, 2005, *5*(3), 134–137.

Starfield, B., Riley, A. W., Witt, W. P., and Robertson, J. "Social Class Gradients in Health During Adolescence." *Journal of Epidemiology and Community Health*, 2002, *56*(5), 354–361.

Starfield, B., Robertson, J., and Riley, A. W. "Social Class Gradients and Health in Childhood." *Ambulatory Pediatrics*, 2002, *2*(4), 238–246.

Starfield, B., and Shi, L. "Determinants of Health: Testing of a Conceptual Model." *Annals of the New York Academy of Sciences*, 1999, *896*, 344–346.

Steenland, K., and others. "Research Findings Linking Workplace Factors to CVD Outcomes." *Occupational Medicine*, 2000, *15*(1), 7–68.

Steinhauer, J. California plan for health care would cover all. *New York Times,* January 9. 2007.

Steptoe, A., and Appels, A. *Stress, Personal Control, and Health.* New York: John Wiley & Sons. 1989.

Stevens, G. D. "Gradients in the Health Status and Developmental Risks of Young Children: The Combined Influences of Multiple Social Risk Factors." *Maternal and Child Health Journal*, 2006, *10*(2), 187–199.

Stevens, G. D., Pickering, T. A., Seid, M., and Tsai, K. Y. "Disparities in the National Prevalence of a Quality Medical Home for Children with Asthma. *Academic of Pediatrics*, 2009, *9*(4), 234–241.

Stevens, G. D., Rice, K., and Cousineau, M. R. *Challenges Facing the Children's Health Initiatives in a Down Economy.* Alhambra, Calif.: USC Center for Community Health Studies, 2009.

Stevens, G. D., Seid, M., and Halfon, N. "Enrolling Vulnerable, Uninsured But Eligible Children in Public Health Insurance: Association with Health Status and Primary Care Access." *Pediatrics*, 2006, *117*(4), e751–759.

Stevens, G. D., Seid, M., Mistry, R., and Halfon, N. "Disparities in Primary Care for Vulnerable Children: The Influence of Multiple Risk Factors." *Health Services Research*, 2006, *41*(2), 507–531.

Stevens, G. D., Seid, M., Pickering, T. A., and Tsai, K. Y. "National Disparities in the Quality of a Medical Home for Children." *Maternal and Child Health Journal*, 2010, *14*(4), 580–589.

Stevens, G. D., and Shi, L. "Effect of Managed Care on Children's Relationships with Their Primary Care Physicians: Differences by Race." *Archives of Pediatrics & Adolescent Medicine*, 2002a, *156*(4), 369–377.

Stevens, G. D., and Shi, L. "Racial and Ethnic Disparities in the Quality of Primary Care for Children." *Journal of Family Practice*, 2002b, *51*(6), 573.

Stevens, G. D., and Shi, L. "Racial and Ethnic Disparities in the Primary Care Experiences of Children: A Review of the Literature." *Medical Care Research and Review*, 2003, *60*(1), 3–30.

Stevens, G. D., Shi, L., and Cooper, L. A. "Patient-Provider Racial and Ethnic Concordance and Parent Reports of the Primary Care Experiences of Children." *Annals of Family Medicine*, 2003, *1*(2), 105–112.

Stevens, G. D., West-Wright, C. N., and Tsai, K. Y. "Health Insurance and Access to Care for Families with Young Children in California, 2001–2005: Differences by Immigration Status." *Journal of Immigrant and Minority Health*, 2008, *12*(3), 273–81.

Stewart, S. H., and Silverstein, M. D. "Racial and Ethnic Disparity in Blood Pressure and Cholesterol Measurement." *Journal of General Internal Medicine*, 2002, *17*(6), 405–411.

Stewart, W. F., Ricci, J. A., Chee, E., Hahn, S. R., and Morganstein, D. "Cost of Lost Productive Work Time Among U.S. Workers with Depression." *Journal of the American Medical Association*, 2003, *289*(23), 3135–3144.

Stewart, W. F., Ricci, J. A., Chee, E., and Morganstein, D. "Lost Productive Work Time Costs from Health Conditions in the United States: Results from the American Productivity Audit." *Journal of Occupational and Environmental Medicine*, 2003, *45*(12), 1234–1246.

Stewart, W. F., Ricci, J. A., Chee, E., Morganstein, D., and Lipton, R. "Lost Productive Time and Cost Due to Common Pain Conditions in the U.S. Workforce." *Journal of the American Medical Association*, 2003, *290*(18), 2443–2454.

Stoddard, J. J., St Peter, R. F., and Newacheck, P. W. "Health Insurance Status and Ambulatory Care for Children." *New England Journal of Medicine*, 1994, *330*(20), 1421–1425.

Subramanian, S. V., Lochner, K. A., and Kawachi, I. "Neighborhood Differences in Social Capital: A Compositional Artifact or a Contextual Construct?" *Health & Place*, 2003, *9*(1), 33–44.

Syme, S. "Control and Health: A Personal Perspective." In A. Steptoe and A. Appels (eds.), *Stress, Personal Control and Health*. New York: John Wiley & Sons, 1989.

Syme, S. L., and Berkman, L. F. "Social Class, Susceptibility and Sickness." *American Journal of Epidemiology*, 1976, *104*(1), 1–8.

Szilagyi, P. G. "Managed Care for Children: Effect on Access to Care and Utilization of Health Services." *The Future of Children*, 1998a, *8*(2), 39–59.

Szilagyi, P. G. "Medicaid Managed Care and Childhood Immunization Delivery." *Journal of Public Health Management and Practice*, 1998b, *4*(1), 67–72.

Szilagyi, P. G., and others. "Improved Asthma Care After Enrollment in the State Children's Health Insurance Program in New York." *Pediatrics*, 2006, *117*(2), 486–496.

Szilagyi, P. G., and others. "Improved Access and Quality of Care After Enrollment in the New York State Children's Health Insurance Program (SCHIP)." *Pediatrics*, 2004, *113*(5), e395–404.

Szilagyi, P. G., Rodewald, L. E., and Roghmann, K. J. "Managed Health Care for Children." *Journal of Ambulatory Care Management*, 1993, *16*(1), 57–70.

Tang, T. S., Solomon, L. J., and McCracken, L. M. "Cultural Barriers to Mammography, Clinical Breast Exam, and Breast Self-Exam Among Chinese-American Women 60 and Older." *Preventive Medicine*, 2000, *31*(5), 575–583.

Task Force on Black and Minority Health. *Report of the Secretary's Task Force on Black and Minority Health*. Washington, D.C.: Department of Health and Human Services, 1985.

Taylor, G. B., Katz, V. L., and Moos, M. K. "Racial Disparity in Pregnancy Outcomes: Analysis of Black and White Teenage Pregnancies." *Journal of Perinatology*, 1995, *15*(6), 480–483.

Taylor, S. "Wealth, Health and Equity: Convergence to Divergence in Late 20th Century Globalization." *British Medical Bulletin*, 2009, *91*, 29–48.

Taylor, S. E., Repetti, R. L., and Seeman, T. "Health Psychology: What Is an Unhealthy Environment and How Does It Get Under the Skin?" *Annual Review of Psychology*, 1997, *48*, 411–447.

Taylor, S. E., and Seeman, T. E. "Psychosocial Resources and the SES-Health Relationship." *Annals of the New York Academy of Sciences*, 1999, *896*, 210–225.

Terwilliger, S. "Early Access to Health Care Services Through a Rural School-Based Health Center." *Journal of School Health*, 1994, *64*(7), 284–289.

Thompson, J. R., and others. "A Population-Based Study of the Effects of Birth Weight on Early Developmental Delay or Disability in Children." *American Journal of Perinatology*, 2003, *20*(6), 321–332.

Thorpe, R. J., Jr., Brandon, D. T., and LaVeist, T. A. "Social Context as an Explanation for Race Disparities in Hypertension: Findings from the Exploring Health Disparities in Integrated Communities (EHDIC) Study." *Social Science & Medicine*, 2008, *67*(10), 1604–1611.

Tooker, J. "Affordable Health Insurance for All Is Possible by Means of a Pragmatic Approach." *American Journal of Public Health*, 2003, *93*(1), 106–109.

Tsoukalas, T. H., and Glantz, S. A. "Development and Destruction of the First State-Funded Anti-Smoking Campaign in the USA." *Tobacco Control*, 2003, *12*(2), 214–220.

Tu, S. P., Taplin, S. H., Barlow, W. E., and Boyko, E. J. "Breast Cancer Screening by Asian-American Women in a Managed Care Environment." *American Journal of Preventive Medicine*, 1999, *17*(1), 55–61.

University of California Regents v. Bakke. 438 U.S. 265. (1978).

U.S. Census Bureau. Current Population Survey, annual social and economic supplement. Historical poverty table #2, 2009a. Retrieved November 19, 2009: www.census.gov/hhes/www/poverty/histpov/perindex.html

U.S. Census Bureau. Current Population Survey, annual social and economic supplement. Educational attainment in the United States, 2008, 2009b. Table A2. Retrieved November 19, 2009: http://www.census.gov/population/www/socdemo/educ-attn.html

U.S. Census Bureau News. *More Than 300 Counties Now "Majority-Minority." 2007.*

U.S. Census Bureau Population Division. Projections of the population by Sex, Race, and Hispanic Origin for the United States: 2010 to 2050, 2008. Retrieved November 19, 2009: www.census.gov/population/www/projections/summarytables.html

U.S. Department of Health and Human Services. *Healthy People.* Washington, D.C.: U.S. Government Printing Office, 1979.

U.S. Department of Health and Human Services. *Healthy People in Healthy Communities.* Washington, DC: U.S. Government Printing Office, 2001.

U.S. Department of Health and Human Services. *Healthy People 2010: Understanding and Improving Health.* Washington, D.C.: U.S. Government Printing Office, 2000.

U.S. Department of Health and Human Services. *Annual Update of the HHS Poverty Guidelines.* U.S. Government Printing Office 73:3971–3972, 2008.

U.S. Department of Health and Human Services. *Annual Update of the HHS Poverty Guidelines.* U.S. Government Printing Office 74:4199–4201, 2009.

U.S. Office of Management and Budget. *Statistical Directive No. 15: Race and Ethnic Standards for Federal Agencies and Administrative Reporting.* Federal Register 43:19269–19270, 1978.

United Nations Development Programme. *Human Development Report 2009: Overcoming Barriers: Human Development and Mobility*. New York: Palgrave Macmillan, 2009.

Urban, N., Anderson, G. L., and Peacock, S. "Mammography Screening: How Important Is Cost as a Barrier to Use?" *American Journal of Public Health*, 1994, *84*(1), 50–55.

Valdez, R., and others. "Consequences of Cost-Sharing for Children's Health." *Pediatrics*, 1985, *75*(5), 952–961.

van Ryn, M. "Research on the Provider Contribution to Race/Ethnicity Disparities in Medical Care." *Medical Care*, 2002, *40*(1 Suppl), 140–151.

van Ryn, M., and Burke, J. "The Effect of Patient Race and Socio-Economic Status on Physicians' Perceptions of Patients." *Social Science & Medicine*, 2000, *50*(6), 813–828.

van Ryn, M., and Fu, S. S. "Paved with Good Intentions: Do Public Health and Human Service Providers Contribute to Racial/Ethnic Disparities in Health?" *American Journal of Public Health*, 2003, *93*(2), 248–255.

Viera, A. J., Pathman, D. E., and Garrett, J. M. "Adults' Lack of a Usual Source of Care: A Matter of Preference?" *Annals of Family Medicine*, 2006, *4*(4), 359–365.

Wagner, E. H. "The Role of Patient Care Teams in Chronic Disease Management." *British Medical Journal*, 2000, *320*(7234), 569–572.

Wallace, R. "Urban Desertification, Public Health and Public Order: 'Planned Shrinkage,' Violent Death, Substance Abuse and AIDS in the Bronx." *Social Science & Medicine*, 1990, *31*(7), 801–813.

Wallace, R. "Expanding Coupled Shock Fronts of Urban Decay and Criminal Behavior." *Journal of Quantitative Criminology*, 1991, *7*, 333–356.

Warshaw, C., Gugenheim, A. M., Moroney, G., and Barnes, H. "Fragmented Services, Unmet Needs: Building Collaboration Between the Mental Health and Domestic Violence Communities." *Health Affairs (Millwood)*, 2003, *22*(5), 230–234.

Wei, H. G., and Camargo, C. A., Jr. "Patient Education in the Emergency Department." *Academic Emergency Medicine*, 2000, *7*(6), 710–717.

Weinick, R., and Krauss, N. "Racial and Ethnic Differences in Children's Access to Care." *American Journal of Public Health*, 2000, *90*(11), 1771–1774.

Weinick, R. M., and Drilea, S. K. "Usual Sources of Health Care and Barriers to Care, 1996." *Statistical Bulletin, Metropolitan Insurance Co.*, 1998, *79*(1), 11–17.

Weissman, J. S., Gatsonis, C., and Epstein, A. M. "Rates of Avoidable Hospitalization by Insurance Status in Massachusetts and Maryland." *Journal of the American Medical Association*, 1992, *268*(17), 2388–2394.

Whitaker, R. C., Gooze, R. A., Hughes, C. C., and Finkelstein, D. M. "A National Survey of Obesity Prevention Practices in Head Start." *Archives of Pediatrics & Adolescent Medicine*, 2009, *163*(12), 1144–1150.

Wilkinson, R. *Unhealthy Societies: The Afflictions of Inequality*. London: Routledge, 1996.

Wilkinson, R. G. "Comment: Income, Inequality, and Social Cohesion." *American Journal of Public Health*, 1997, *87*(9), 1504–1506.

Wilkinson, R. G., and Pickett, K. E. "Income Inequality and Socioeconomic Gradients in Mortality." *American Journal of Public Health*, 2008, *98*(4), 699–704.

Williams, D. R. "Race, Socioeconomic Status, and Health: The Added Effects of Racism and Discrimination." *Annals of the New York Academy of Sciences*, 1999, *896*, 173–188.

Williams, D. R., and Collins, C. "Racial Residential Segregation: A Fundamental Cause of Racial Disparities in Health." *Public Health Reports*, 2001, *116*(5), 404–416.

Williams, D. R., and Mohammed, S. A. "Discrimination and Racial Disparities in Health: Evidence and Needed Research." *Journal of Behavioral Medicine*, 2009, *32*(1), 20–47.

Williams, D. R., Neighbors, H. W., and Jackson, J. S. "Racial/Ethnic Discrimination and Health: Findings from Community Studies." *American Journal of Public Health*, 2003, *93*(2), 200–208.

Williams, D. R., Neighbors, H. W., and Jackson, J. S. "Racial/Ethnic Discrimination and Health: Findings from Community Studies." *American Journal of Public Health*, 2008, *98*(9 Suppl), S29–37.

Williams, R. L., Flocke, S. A., and Stange, K. C. "Race and Preventive Services Delivery Among Black Patients and White Patients Seen in Primary Care." *Medical Care*, 2001, *39*(11), 1260–1267.

Williams, T. V., Zaslavsky, A. M., and Cleary, P. D. "Physician Experiences with, and Ratings of, Managed Care Organizations in Massachusetts." *Medical Care*, 1999, *37*(6), 589–600.

Willms, D. *Inequalities in Literacy Skills Among Youth in Canada and the United States*. (No. 89–552-MIE99006). Canada: National Literacy Secretariat/Human Resources Development, 1999.

Wilper, A. P., and others. "Health Insurance and Mortality in U.S. Adults." *American Journal of Public Health*, 2009, *99*(12), 2289–2295.

Wilson, W. *The Truly Disadvantaged*. Chicago: University of Chicago Press, 1987.

Wilson, W. *When Work Disappears: The World of the New Urban Poor*. New York: Alfred A. Knopf, 1996.

Winkleby, M. A., Cubbin, C., Ahn, D. K., and Kraemer, H. C. "Pathways By Which SES and Ethnicity Influence Cardiovascular Disease Risk Factors." *Annals of the New York Academy of Sciences*, 1999, *896*, 191–209.

Wise, P. H., Wampler, N. S., Chavkin, W., and Romero, D. "Chronic Illness Among Poor Children Enrolled in the Temporary Assistance for Needy Families Program." *American Journal of Public Health*, 2002, *92*(9), 1458–1461.

Wood, P. R., and others. "Relationships Between Welfare Status, Health Insurance Status, and Health and Medical Care Among Children with Asthma." *American Journal of Public Health*, 2002, *92*(9), 1446–1452.

World Health Organization. "Constitution of the World Health Organization." In *Basic Documents*. Geneva: World Health Organization, 1948.

World Health Organization. *World Health Report 2000: Health System Performance*. Geneva, Switzerland: World Health Organization, 2000.

World Health Organization. *World Conference Against Racism, Racial Discrimination, Xenophobia and Related Intolerance: Health and Freedom from Discrimination*. Geneva, Switzerland: World Health Organization, 2001.

Wright, R. A., Andres, T. L., and Davidson, A. J. "Finding the Medically Underserved: A Need to Revise the Federal Definition." *Journal of Health Care for the Poor and Underserved*, 1996, *7*(4), 296–307.

Xu, K. T. "Usual Source of Care in Preventive Service Use: A Regular Doctor versus a Regular Site." *Health Services Research*, 2002, *37*(6), 1509–1529.

Yarcheski, A., Mahon, N. E., and Yarcheski, T. J. "Social Support and Well-Being in Early Adolescents: The Role of Mediating Variables." *Clinical Nursing Research*, 2001, *10*(2), 163–181.

Yarcheski, T. J., Mahon, N. E., and Yarcheski, A. "Social Support, Self-Esteem, and Positive Health Practices of Early Adolescents." *Psychological Reports*, 2003, *92*(1), 99–103.

Yen, I. H., and Kaplan, G. A. "Poverty Area Residence and Changes in Physical Activity Level: Evidence from the Alameda County Study." *American Journal of Public Health*, 1998, *88*(11), 1709–1712.

Yen, I. H., Ragland, D. R., Greiner, B. A., and Fisher, J. M. "Racial Discrimination and Alcohol-Related Behavior in Urban Transit Operators: Findings from the San Francisco Muni Health and Safety Study." *Public Health Reports*, 1999a, *114*(5), 448–458.

Yen, I. H., Ragland, D. R., Greiner, B. A., and Fisher, J. M. "Workplace Discrimination and Alcohol Consumption: Findings from the San Francisco Muni Health and Safety Study." *Ethnicity Disease*, 1999b, *9*(1), 70–80.

Young, T., D'angelo, S., and Davis, J. "Impact of a School-Based Health Center on Emergency Department Use By Elementary School Students." *Journal of School Health*, 2001, *71*(196–8).

Yu, M. Y., Hong, O. S., and Seetoo, A. D. "Uncovering Factors Contributing to Under-Utilization of Breast Cancer Screening by Chinese and Korean Women Living in the United States." *Ethnicity & Disease*, 2003, *13*(2), 213–219.

Zuckerman, S., Haley, J., Roubideaux, Y., and Lillie-Blanton, M. "Health Service Access, Use, and Insurance Coverage Among American Indians/Alaska Natives and Whites: What Role Does the Indian Health Service Play?" *American Journal of Public Health*, 2004, *94*(1), 53–59.

Zuvekas, A. *Measuring Farmworker and Homeless Patients Experiences in Community Health Centers*. Bethesda, Md.: National Association of Community Health Centers, 2002.

INDEX

Page references followed by *fig* indicate an illustrated figure; followed by *t* indicate a table; followed by *e* indicate an exhibit.

A

Academy of General Dentistry, 228

Aday's framework for studying vulnerable populations, 15–16*fig*, 17

Advocates for Youth programs, 244

Affirmative action policies, 235–236

Affordable Care Act, 251

African Americans: children living in poverty among, 58; college completion rates among, 60, 61*fig*; fair or poor health status of, 164*fig*; health care access by, 95*fig*–98; health care quality and, 98–103; health data kept on, 32; health status of, 103–110; high school completion rates among, 60, 61*fig*; infant mortality by maternal education and, 168*fig*; infant mortality rates among, 105*fig*–106; Medicaid program participation by, 79; multiple factors impacting health care access of, 142*fig*–151*fig*; national risk factor prevalence of, 154*t*; national trends in poverty/income distribution and, 53–58; poverty rates among, 4; regular source of care (RSC) of, 95*fig*; risk factors and preventive services in past year, 155*t*; risk profiles and preventive services in past year, 157*t*; smoking rates among, 109, 243; social class and health disparities of Whites and, 168–169*t*; unemployment rates among, 63*fig*–64. *See also* Race/ethnicity differences

Afterschool.gov, 238

Agency for Healthcare Research and Quality (AHRQ), 143, 153, 160, 185, 236, 265

Aligning Forces for Quality, 196

Ambulatory care sensitive conditions (ACS), 114, 126–127

American Academy of Pediatrics (AAP), 250

American College of Cardiology, 101

American Heart Association, 101

American Indians/Alaskan Natives (AIANs): alcohol use rates of, 243; children living in poverty among, 58; fair or poor health status of, 164*fig*; health care access by, 95*fig*–98; health data kept on, 32; health status of, 103–110; Indian Health Service (IHS) agency working with, 183, 188–189, 196–198; infant mortality by maternal education and, 168*fig*; infant mortality rates among, 105*fig*–106; multiple factors impacting health care access of, 143–144; regular source of care (RSC) of, 95*fig*; smoking rates among, 109. *See also* Race/ethnicity differences

American Legacy Foundation's Quit Plan, 243

American Medical Association (AMA), 228

American Public Health Association, 274

America's Health Rankings, 274, 279

Antismoking media campaign (Minnesota), 268

Appropriate access to care, 27*e*

Appropriate care, 28*e*

Area Health Education Center (AHEC), 262

Asians: college completion rates among, 60, 61*fig*; cultural factors and vulnerability of, 43; fair or poor health status of, 164*fig*; health care access by, 95*fig*–98; health care quality and, 98–103; health data kept on, 32; high school completion rates among, 60, 61*fig*; infant mortality by maternal education and, 168*fig*; infant mortality rates among, 105*fig*–106; low birth weight rates among, 106*fig*; Medicaid program participation by, 79; multiple factors impacting health care access of, 149*t*–151*fig*; national risk factor prevalence of, 154*t*; national trends in poverty/

Asians: (*continued*)
income distribution and, 53–58; poverty rates among, 4; regular source of care (RSC) of, 95*fig*; risk factors and preventive services in past year, 155*t*; risk profiles and preventive services in past year, 158*t*; smoking rates among, 109; unemployment rates among, 63*fig*–64. *See also* Race/ethnicity

Association of Schools of Public Health/Kellogg Taskforce, 181, 193

Association of SIDS and Infant Mortality Program, 250

B

BadgerCare program, 253–254

Bakke, University of California Regents v., 37

Balanced Budget Act (1997), 80

Beneficiaries: gatekeeping practice and, 83; health plan influences on, 84–85

Black Women's Health Imperative (BWHI), 242

Blacks. *See* African Americans

Blue Shield of California, 255

Bollinger, Grutter v., 235

Breast cancer: race/ethnicity differences in treatment of, 101; race/ethnicity mortality rates from, 107*fig*

Building Healthy Communities Initiative (BHC), 270–272

Bureau of Indian Affairs, 189

Bureau of Labor Statistics, 63

Bureau of Primary Health Care (BPHC), 189, 202, 204, 280

C

California: Children's Health Initiatives (CHIs), 140–141, 181, 212, 215; Department of Public Health, 192; Department of Public Health Strategic Plan, 181, 191–192; efforts to reform health care, in, 255; Medicaid cutbacks in, 133; risk factors and health literacy in, 162*t*; TCE (The California Endowment), 270–272

California Endowment's Building Healthy Communities Initiative, 181, 193–194, 196

California Health Interview Survey (CHIS), 139, 161

California State University, Fresno, 248

CAM (complementary or alternative medicine), 240–242

Canadian universal health insurance, 260

Cancer screening, 100–101

Capitation, 84

CEEDs (Centers of Excellence in the Elimination of Disparities), 187

Center on Budget and Policy Priorities study (1998), 245

Center for Health Care Rights, 267

Center for Health and Health Care in Schools (CHHCS), 181, 205–206

Centers for Disease Control and Prevention (CDC), 118, 187, 243, 265

Centers of Excellence Programs, 188

Centers for Medicare & Medicaid Services, 81

Central/South American infant mortality rates, 105*fig*

Children: development risk of, 106, 172*t*–173*t*, 174*fig*; Head Start program for, 55, 182, 201–202, 209, 245–246, 264; health insurance coverage and health needs of, 125–126; health insurance coverage and mortality risk of, 131–132; Healthy Start program for, 183, 190, 196, 264; incrementally expanding public insurance coverage for, 253–254; multiple risk factors and health status of, 166*t*–167*t*; no healthcare visits by race/ethnicity/insurance coverage, 145*fig*–146; overlap of three risk factors for, 138*fig*; risk factor combinations and development risk for under 3 years, 174*fig*; risk factors/profiles with health status/development risk for under 3 years, 172*t*–173*t*; sociodemographic risks with preventive care for, 159–160

Children's Alliance (Washington), 255

Children's Health Initiatives (CHIs), 140–141, 181, 212, 215

Children's Health Insurance Program (CHIP): coverage provided through, 209–210, 263–264; eligibility for, 78; encouraging enrollment for eligible individuals, 251–252; expansion of eligible population by, 249; health care reform initiated by, 6; incrementally expanding public insurance coverage through, 252–254; poverty thresholds used by, 55; SES of participants in, 41; social stigma of, 84–85; strengths and weaknesses of, 213–215. *See also* Federal initiatives; Health insurance coverage; Safety net programs; State Children's Health Insurance Program

Children's Health Insurance Program Reauthorization Act (2009), 249

Citizenship status, children eleven years and under health status and, 166*t*–167*t*

Civil Rights Act (1964), 6, 37

Clinical practice focus on vulnerability: cultural competence to improve care, 196, 238–240, 250; individual risk factors and, 133–135; intervention programs to reduce health disparities, 30–31; multiple risk factors and, 175–176; Project 50, 216–217. *See also* Vulnerability

Coalition for Natural Health, 242

Commission on the Social Determinants of Health (WHO), 270

Commonwealth Fund 2001 International Health Policy Survey, 115

Commonwealth Fund Health Care Quality Survey, 97

Communicable diseases/SES disparities, 120

Community building strategies, 246–247

Community environmental exposures model, 14

Community health center (CHC) program, 75, 189, 199, 208

Community Implementation Program, 228

Community medically underserved model, 14–15

Community and Migrant Health Centers, 182

Community partnerships, 258–259

Community social resources model, 12–13

Community Tracking Study Household Survey, 94, 160

Community vulnerability determinants/mechanisms: health insurance as, 72–85; individual SES and relative deprivation as, 68–69; interconnections between cycling of vulnerability and, 85–87; race and ethnicity as, 36–49; SES (socioeconomic status) as, 49–71

Community-based interventions: to resolve health insurance disparities, 255–256; to resolve race/ethnic disparities, 236–238; to resolve SES disparities, 246–248

Complementary Alternative Medicine Association, 242

Complementary or alternative medicine (CAM), 240–242

Consumer Coalition for Quality Health Care, 267

Consumer Price Index, 55

Contextual Community Health Profile, 242

Continuity of care, 163

Cost containment issue, 269

Cost sharing, 83

Council on Graduate Medical Education, 240

Crime environmental circumstance, 13

Cross-Cultural Health Care Program (CCHCP), 240

Cuban infant mortality rates, 105*fig*

Cultural competence: description and importance of, 196; health care interventions with, 238–240; patient response to, 250

Cultural factors: providing linguistically appropriate services, 196; race/ethnicity vulnerability and, 43; *respeto* (Hispanic culture), 43

D

Dartmouth Atlas of Health Care, 134

Dental care: multiple risk factors and delayed, 151*fig*; risk factors and receipt of, 155*t*–156*t*

Developed countries: Gini Index of income inequality for, 59*fig*; health care spending percentage of GDP among, 50*fig*; illiterate rates among, 62; universal

health coverage offered by, 72. *See also* OECD countries

Development risk: children under 3 years risk factors/ profiles with health status and, 172*t*–173*t*; low-birth-weight rates associated with, 106; risk factor combinations for children under 3 years, 174*fig*

DHHS. *See* U.S. Department of Health and Human Services (DHHS)

Diabetes: community based interventions for, 236–237; race/ethnicity mortality rates from, 107*fig*

Discrimination: based on negative racial stereotypes, 52; Civil Rights Act (1964) on, 6, 37; negative behavior patterns and self-reported, 44–45; race/ ethnicity linked to health care, 43–45. *See also* Race/ ethnicity

Diversity national trends, 39–40*fig*

Domestic Violence and Mental Health Policy Initiative (DVMHPI), 248–249

Don't Let Another Year Go Up in Smoke (CDC), 243

E

Earned Income Tax Credit (EITC), 244–245

East Side House Settlement project (NYC), 259

Ecological risk factors: enabling, 24*e*, 25–26; need factors, 25*e*, 26; overview of, 24–26; predisposing, 24*e*–25

Economic feasibility, 278

Economic Opportunity Act (1964), 199

Education: contribution to health through, 256–257; resolving health disparities by enhancing, 256–258

Educational levels: children eleven years and under health status and, 166*t*–167*t*; college completion rates by race/ethnicity, 61*fig*; health risk behaviors by, 119*fig*; high school completion rates by race/ ethnicity, 61*fig*; infant mortality by race/ethnicity and maternal, 168*fig*; national trends in race/ethnicity, 60–62; regular source of care (RSC) and, 111–112; reported mental distress by, 118*fig*–119; risk factors and preventive services in past year by, 155*t*

Effectiveness of programs, 36

Efficient and safe care, 28*e*

Elderly patients: Program for All Inclusive Care of the Elderly (PACE), 195–196; vulnerability of, 194–195

Emergency department (ED) visits, 125

Emotional health. *See* Mental health

Employment: reported mental distress by, 118*fig*–119; trends in the U.S. occupations and, 62–64. *See also* Unemployment rates

Enabling factors: ecological level, 24*e*, 25–26; individual level, 22*e*

Entitlement programs, 75

Environmental circumstances: racial and ethnic segregation as, 51–53; violence and crime as, 13

Equity: definition of, 5; vulnerability inconsistency with, 5–6

Experiences in care, 28*e*

F

Families USA, 267

Family-centered care, 163

Feasible intervention, 278

Federal initiatives: CEEDs (Centers of Excellence in the Elimination of Disparities), 187; CHC (community health center) program, 75, 189, 199, 208; to eliminate racial and ethic disparities, 186–190; to eliminate socioeconomic disparities in health, 198–202; Head Start, 55, 182, 201–202, 209, 245–246, 264; Health Care for the Homeless (HCH) Program, 182, 201; Healthy Start, 183, 190, 196, 264; Indian Health Service (IHS), 183, 188–189, 196–198; migrant health centers (MHCs), 189–190, 196–197; National Health Service Corps (HPSA), 184, 199–200; National Institutes of Health (NIH), 188; Public Housing Primary Care (PHPC) Program, 184, 200–201, 209; REACH 2010, 187, 191, 197, 198, 236–238; U.S. Office of Minority Health (OMH), 186–187. *See also* Children's Health Insurance Program (CHIP); Medicaid; Medicare

Federal poverty level (FPL): CHIP eligibility and, 55; Head Start eligibility tied to, 202; health care access and, 141–147*t*; Health Howard Health Plan eligibility tied to, 203; risk factors for poor child health and, 170; uninsured individuals at the, 253–254. *See also* Poverty rates

Fee-for-service (FFS) coverage, 81

Flu shots: combinations of risk factors and receipt of, 159*fig*; risk factors and receipt of, 155*t*–156*t*

Food Stamp Program, 55

Framework: action model to achieve Healthy People 2020 goals, 227*fig*; definition of, 3; Healthy People 2020 conceptual, 225*fig*; introduction to vulnerability model, 18–32; linking health insurance coverage with health care, 82*fig*; linking race/ethnicity and health care, 42*fig*; linking SES with health, 65*fig*

Front-line experience: Building Healthy Communities Initiative (BHC), 270–272; Children's Health Initiative (CHI), 140–141; L.A. Care Health Plan, 6–8; South Carolina Primary Health Care Association, 122–124; TCE (The California Endowment), 270–272; Weingart Foundation's

Center for Community Health, 47–49; working with vulnerable seniors, 194–195

"The Future of Public Health" (IOM), 6

G

Gatekeeping practice, 83

Gender differences: mortality rates among Black/White populations and, 169*t*; SES disparities and disease/morality, 120; smoking rates among, 109

George Washington University School of Public Health and Health Services, 192

Gini Index: description of, 58; of income inequality for developed countries, 59*fig*

Gradient for vulnerability: description of, 14; documentation on SES as, 67–68

Grutter v. Bollinger, 235

Guided incrementalism, 280

H

Harlem Children's Zone, 247

Head Start, 55, 182, 201–202, 209, 245–246, 264

Health: conceptual model linking SES with, 65*fig*; leading health indicators (LHIs) in the U.S., 229*t*; life course development of, 262–265; WHO definition of, 27–29. *See also* Mental health

Health care: conceptual model linking health insurance coverage with, 82*fig*; conceptual model linking race/ethnicity and, 42*fig*; cost containment issue of, 269; RSC (regular source of care), 95*fig*–97, 111–112, 125. *See also* Health inequalities

Health care access: across racial and ethic lines, 36; appropriate, 27*e*; community resources available for, 14–15; multiple risk factors and, 141–151*fig*; national risk factor prevalence by race/ethnicity (2007), 148*t*; national risk factors (2006) and, 147*t*; potential, 27*e*; racial and ethnic disparities of, 95*fig*–98; realized, 27*e*; SES (socioeconomic status) disparities and, 110–117; socioeconomic status (SES) and, 70–71. *See also* Medical services

Health Care for the Homeless (HCH) Program, 182, 201, 277

Health care interventions: challenges/barriers in implementing strategies for, 267–270; cultural competence in, 238–242; integrative approaches to resolving disparities, 256–267; to resolve disparities by health insurance, 250–256; to resolve race/ethnic disparities, 234–244; to resolve SES disparities, 248–250; TCE (The California Endowment) example of, 270–272

Health care quality: appropriate, 28*e*; efficient and safe, 28*e*; experiences in, 28*e*; health insurance coverage and, 127*fig*–130*fig*; health insurance disparities and, 127*fig*–130*fig*; L.A. Care Health Plan efforts to improve, 7; multiple risk factors and, 152–163; national risk factor prevalence by race/ethnicity, 154*t*; racial and ethnic disparities of, 98–103; satisfaction with, 28*e*; SES and percentage reporting satisfaction with, 116*fig*

Health care system: developed countries GDP percentage spent on, 50*fig*; primary care in the, 70–71, 122–124, 128–129, 260–262; race/ethnicity differences in experience with, 46–47, 102*fig*–103; SES differentials and, 70–71; SES and percentage reporting satisfaction with, 116*fig*

Health Careers Opportunity Program, 236

Health Foundation of Greater Cincinnati, 206

Health Howard Health Plan, 203

Health impact assessment, 276

Health inequalities: community determinants and mechanism of, 36–91; contact information for major programs focused on, 181*e*–185*e*; ecological level of risk for, 24–26; improving national monitoring of disparities and, 265–267; individual risk factors for, 21–24, 94–135; multiple risk factors for, 138–176, 276–277; social cohesion role in, 69–70; War on Poverty to eliminate, 6, 199. *See also* Health care; Resolving health disparities

Health insurance coverage: children eleven years and under health status and, 166*t*–167*t*; as community vulnerability determinant/mechanism, 72–85; conceptual model linking health care with, 82*fig*; historical development of importance of, 72, 75; individual risk factors and disparities in, 124–135; national trends in public and private, 75–81; no healthcare visits by children by race/ethnicity and, 145*fig*–146; percentage of individuals without (2007), 77*fig*; regular source of care (RSC) and, 95*fig*; theoretical pathways of, 81–85; uninsured rates among nonelderly by state (2007-2008), 78*fig*; uninsured rates among working adults, 76*fig*; universal, 6, 72, 73*e*–74*e*, 254–255, 260; as vulnerable populations factor, 31–32. *See also* Children's Health Insurance Program (CHIP); Health plan policies; Medicaid; Medicare

Health insurance disparities: federal initiatives to eliminate, 209–210; private initiatives to eliminate, 211–212; state and local initiatives to eliminate, 210–211; strategies to resolve, 250–256; strengths/weaknesses of programs addressing, 212–215

Health literacy, 162*t*

Health maintenance organizations (HMOs): description of, 81; Healthcare Group (HCG) of Arizona

administration through, 182, 211; patient satisfaction with, 129*fig*–130*fig*

Health needs: ecological level, 25*e*, 26; health insurance coverage and children's, 125–126; individual level, 22*e*; race/ethnicity and, 45; risk factors predicting unmet, 149*t*–150*t*; unmet health care needs, 97; vulnerable populations, 3–4

Health plan policies: influences on beneficiaries, 84–85; influences on providers, 84; overview and types of, 81, 83; patient satisfaction and, 130*fig*. *See also* Health insurance coverage

Health Resources and Services Administration (HRSA), 189, 236

Health risk behaviors: ecological level of, 24–26; by educational status, 119*fig*; multiple, 138*fig*–176, 276–277; SES gradient in, 67–68; vulnerable populations and, 10–11. *See also* Individual risk factors; Socioeconomic status (SES)

Health status: children under 3 years and risk for development and, 172*t*–173*t*; fair or poor health status by race/ethnicity/income, 164*fig*; health insurance disparities and, 130–133; multiple risk factors and, 164*fig*–174*fig*; multiple risk factors and childrens,' 166*t*–167*t*; national risk factors, income levels, and self-reported, 165*t*; patient-provider relationships ratings by, 161*fig*; racial and ethnic disparities of, 103–110; self-reported by race/ethnicity, 104*fig*; SES (socioeconomic status) disparities and, 117–122; vulnerable populations health outcomes and, 3–4

Health trajectories, 263

Healthcare Effectiveness Data and Information Set (HEDIS), 266

Healthcare Group (HCG) of Arizona, 182, 211, 214

Healthy California program, 255

Healthy Howard Health Plan, 182

Healthy Kids program, 212

Healthy People: The Surgeon General's Report on Health Promotion and Disease Prevention (1979), 222

Healthy People 1990, 222

Healthy People 2000, 2, 32, 222–223

Healthy People 2010, 2, 6, 32, 222

Healthy People 2020: action model to achieve overarching goals of the, 227*fig*; conceptual framework for the, 225*fig*; federal program funding to meet goals of, 197; framework to resolve disparities supporting, 230*fig*–234; health goals established by, 6, 32, 223–224*fig*, 279; Healthy People Consortium partnership with, 227; origins and history of, 222–223; overview of the, 224–226; strategies and partnerships to achieve objectives, 226–229; tracking

Healthy People 2020 (*continued*)
    progress in achieving objectives of, 229. *See also*
    Resolving health disparities
Healthy People Consortium, 223, 227
Healthy People in Healthy Communities, 228
Healthy People Information Access Project, 228
Healthy People initiatives, 103
Healthy Start, 183, 190, 196, 264
Healthy Workforce (publication), 228
Heart disease mortality, 108
Hispanic Federation (New York), 255–256
Hispanics: college completion rates among, 60, 61*fig*;
    cultural factors and vulnerability of, 43; fair or
    poor health status of, 164*fig*; health care access by,
    95*fig*–98; health care quality and, 98–103; health
    center programs for migrant/seasonal farm workers
    among, 189–190, 196–197; health status of, 103–110;
    high school completion rates among, 60, 61*fig*;
    infant mortality by maternal education and, 168*fig*;
    infant mortality rates among, 105*fig*–106; Medicaid
    program participation by, 79; multiple factors
    impacting health care access of, 141–151*fig*; national
    risk factor prevalence of, 154*t*; national trends in
    poverty/income distribution and, 53–58; poverty
    rates among, 4; risk factors and preventive services in
    past year, 155*t*; risk profiles and preventive services
    in past year, 157*t*–158*t*; smoking rates among, 109;
    unemployment rates among, 63*fig*–64. *See also* Puerto
    Ricans; Race/ethnicity differences
HIV/AIDS: disproportionate racial/ethnic minorities
    with, 243; race/ethnicity differences in mortality
    rates, 106–107*fig*; SES disparities and, 120. *See also*
    Sexually transmitted diseases (STDs)
Homeless: Health Care for the Homeless (HCH)
    Program, 182, 201, 277; health care services for the,
    47–49; Project 50 program for the, 216–217
Homicide mortality, 107*fig*
Howard County General Hospital, 203
Human capital: definition of, 10; vulnerability
    determined by, 9–10

I

Incidence-vulnerability relationship, 9
Income levels: fair or poor health status by, 164*fig*;
    Gini Index for developed countries distribution
    of, 58, 59*fig*; mortality rates among Black/White
    populations and different, 169*t*; national risk factors
    and self-reported health status, 165*fig*; national
    trends in racial/ethnicity, 53–58; patient-provider
    relationships ratings by, 161*fig*; reported mental
    distress by, 118*fig*–119; risk factors, health literacy,

and, 162*t*; risk factors and preventive services in past
    year by, 155*t*; trends in inequality of, 58, 60. *See also*
    Poverty rates
Incrementalism (guided), 280
Indian Health Service (IHS), 183, 188–189, 196–198
Indian Self-Determination and Education Assistance
    Act, 189
Individual and community interaction model, 15–17
Individual determinants model, 8–9
Individual risk factors: enabling, 22*e*, 23–24; health
    insurance disparities and, 124–135; health needs,
    22*e*, 23–24; overview of, 21–24; predisposing, 22*e*,
    23–24; racial and ethnic disparities in, 94–110;
    socioeconomic status disparities and, 110–124. *See*
    also Health risk behaviors
Individual social resources model, 9–10
Individual-level interventions: to resolve race/ethnic
    disparities, 242–244; to resolve SES disparities, 250
Infant mortality rates: as MUA factor, 15; by race/
    ethnicity and maternal education, 105*fig*–106, 168*fig*;
    SES disparities and, 120; of the United States, 274.
    See also Mortality rates
Initiative to Expand Access to Health Care (2004), 208
Institute of Medicine (IOM): Committee on the
    Consequences of Uninsurance, 32, 131, 275, 276;
    Committee on Health Insurance Status and Its
    Consequences, 32, 125, 131, 276; Committee on
    Quality of Health Care in America, 27; Committee
    for the Study of the Future of Public Health, 6; "The
    Future of Public Health" report of, 6; on health
    risk behaviors and illness, 11; on racial/ethnicity
    vulnerability, 44
Integration of care, 206

J

Johns Hopkins Bloomberg School of Public Health, 194
Johns Hopkins Geriatrics Education Center, 194
Johnson & Johnson Community Health Care Program,
    183, 206–207

K

Kaiser Commission on Medicaid and the Uninsured,
    79, 80, 214
Kansas City TeleKidcare, 183, 204
King's Fund report [1995], 256

L

L.A. Care Health Plan, 6–8
L.A. Care's Healthy Kids, 7
Latino Center for Medical Education and
    Research, 248

Latino Health Research Center (University of Illinois), 236

Latinos in Leadership Action and Change, 259

Latinos. *See* Hispanics

Leading health indicators (LHIs), 229*t*

Legal citations: *Grutter v. Bollinger,* 235; *University of California Regents v. Bakke,* 37

Legislation: Affordable Care Act, 251; Balanced Budget Act (1997), 80; Children's Health Insurance Program Reauthorization Act (2009), 249; Civil Rights Act (1964), 6, 37; Economic Opportunity Act (1964), 199; Indian Self-Determination and Education Assistance Act, 189; Migrant Health Act (1962), 189; Minnesota's Alternative Health Care Freedom of Access Act, 241; No Child Left Behind Act (2001), 245. *See also* United States

Life course health development, 262–265

Life expectancy, 223

Linguistically appropriate services, 196

Local initiatives. *See* State and local initiatives

Los Angeles mobile clinics, 90*e*

Low birth weight rates, maternal race/ethnicity and, 106*fig*

Low-Income Home Energy Assistance Program, 55

M

MacArthur Network on SES and Health, 64

Maine Dirigo Health program, 254–255

Managed care organizations (MCOs): balancing primary and specialty care in, 261; description of, 83; health plan influences on, 84; investing in vulnerable populations by, 6–8; poorer patient-provider relationships in, 83

Massachusetts Commonwealth Health Insurance Connector Authority, 183, 210–211, 214, 215

MassHealth Family Assistance Program, 210

Material deprivation, 64, 66

Maternal and Child Health Bureau, 190

Means tested, 251–252

Medicaid: coverage provided through, 209–210; cutbacks in California's, 133; eligibility for, 76, 78; encouraging enrollment for eligible individuals, 251–252; health care reform initiated by, 6; health status of participants of, 131; incrementally expanding public insurance coverage through, 252–254; overview of, 79; participants likely to visit ED, 125; poverty thresholds used by, 55; Program for All Inclusive Care of the Elderly (PACE) and eligibility for, 195–196; racial/ethnicity differences in participants of, 41; risk factors and preventive services in past year of participants in, 155*t*; social stigma of,

84–85; strengths and weaknesses of, 213–215. *See also* Federal initiatives; Health insurance coverage; Safety net programs

Medical Expenditure Panel Survey (MEPS), 94, 96, 103, 126, 131, 139, 146, 153

Medical services: community resources available for, 14–15; no healthcare visits by children by race/ethnicity/insurance coverage, 145*fig*–146; RSC (regular source of care) for, 95*fig*–97. *See also* Health care access; Preventive care

Medically underserved areas (MUAs): current federal definition of, 15; health care interventions serving, 248

Medicare: coverage provided through, 209–210; health care reform initiated by, 6; overview of, 79–80; risk factors and preventive services in past year of participants in, 155*t*; strengths and weaknesses of, 212–215. *See also* Federal initiatives; Health insurance coverage

Medicare Part A, 79–80

Medicare Part B, 79–80

Medicare Part C, 80

Medicare Part D, 80

MEDLINE, 94

Mental distress, 118

Mental health: maternal, 171–172; measurements for, 29; multiple risk factor studies on, 171–172; types of psychiatric disorders and, 171. *See also* Health

Mexican infant mortality rates, 105*fig*

Migrant Health Act (1962), 189

Migrant health centers (MHCs), 189–190, 196–197

Minnesota antismoking media campaign (1990s), 268

Minnesota Department of Health (MDH), 191

Minnesota's Alternative Health Care Freedom of Access Act, 241

Minnesota's Eliminating Health Disparities Initiative, 183, 191, 197

Minority race/ethnicity: definition of, 9; historical development of SES and, 51–53. *See also* Race/ethnicity

Mobile clinics (Los Angeles Forum), 90*e*

Models That Work Campaign, 202, 204

Morality rates: by race and ethnicity, 106–107*fig*; SMR (standardized mortality ratio) of, 108; uninsured children and higher risk of, 131–132

Morbidity rates predictors, 13

Mortality rates: among Black/White populations in selected geographical areas, 169*t*; Geronimus study on standardized, 168; poverty rates as predictors of, 13; SES disparities and, 120–122. *See also* Infant mortality rates

Multiple risk factors: description of, 138–139; health care access and, 141–151*fig*; health care quality and, 152–163; health status and, 164*fig*–174*fig*; mental health and, 171–172; overlap of three risk factors, 138*fig*; predicting unmet needs, 149*t*–150*t*; resolving health disparities by expanding focus on, 276–277; risk profiles and delayed dental care (2007), 151*fig*; vulnerability in clinical practice and, 175–176

Multivariate analysis, 168

N

National Advisory Council on Complementary and Alternative Medicine (NCCAM), 240

National Association of Community Health Centers, 197

National Center for Complementary and Alternative Medicine, 240

National Center for Health Statistics (NCHS), 32, 45, 79, 94, 107, 120, 125, 173, 229, 243

National Center for Homeopathy, 242

National Center on Minority Health and Health Disparities, 184, 188, 196

National Commission to Prevent Infant Mortality, 278

National Committee for Quality Assurance (NCQA), 266

National Conference of State Legislators, 191

National Health Care Disparities Report, 160

National Health Interview Survey (NHIS), 94, 125, 139, 143, 146

National Health Service Corps (HPSA), 184, 199–200

National Healthcare Disparities Report, 143

National Institutes of Health (NIH), 188, 236, 265

National Library of Medicine, 228

National Lunch Program, 55

National Recreation and Parks Association, 228

National resources: community social resources model on, 12–13; socioeconomic status (SES) and availability to, 49, 51; vulnerability linked to, 4–5

National Rural Health Association (NRHA), 242

National School Lunch Program, 252

National Science Foundation, 236

National Survey of America's Families, 144

National Survey of Children's Health, 163, 170

National Survey of Early Childhood Health, 173

National Trauma Data Bank, 132

Native Americans. *See* American Indian/Alaskan Native

Native Hawaiian poverty rates, 58

New Jersey Cancer Registry, 132

New York's Hispanic Federation, 255–256

No Child Left Behind Act (2001), 245

Non-Hispanic whites: children living in poverty among, 58; college completion rates among, 60, 61*fig*; health status of, 103–110; high school completion rates among, 60, 61*fig*; infant mortality rates among, 105*fig*–106; low birth weight rates among, 106*fig*; multiple factors impacting health care access of, 142*fig*–151*fig*; poverty rates among, 4; regular source of care (RSC) of, 95*fig*; unemployment rates among, 63*fig*–64. *See also* Whites

NULITES (National Urban League Incentives to Excel and Succeed), 238

O

Obesity life course, 264*fig*

Occupation: social class defined by, 168; trends in the U.S., 62–64; unemployment rates associated with types of, 64; unemployment rates by race and ethnicity, 63*fig*–64

Occupational Safety and Health Administration (OSHA), 246

OECD countries: illiterate rates of, 62; U.S. infant mortality rating among, 274; U.S. membership as, 269. *See also* Developed countries

Office of Disease Prevention and Health Promotion (DHHS), 228

Office of Minority Health (OMH), 184, 196, 197

Older patients: Program for All Inclusive Care of the Elderly (PACE), 195–196; vulnerability of, 194–196

P

Pacific Islanders: children living in poverty among, 58; college completion rates among, 60, 61*fig*; health data kept on, 32; high school completion rates among, 60, 61*fig*; infant mortality by maternal education and, 168*fig*; infant mortality rates among, 105*fig*–106; low birth weight rates among, 106*fig*; national trends in poverty/income distribution and, 54; unemployment rates among, 63*fig*–64. *See also* Race/ethnicity differences

Participatory action research, 237*t*

Partners in Information Access for the Public Health Workforce, 228

Partnership for Prevention, 274

Pathways to Freedom: Winning the Fight Against Tobacco (CDC), 243

Patient satisfaction: health insurance plan type and, 130*fig*; health insurance status and, 129*fig*

Patient-provider relationships: MCO plans and poorer, 83; physician-reported perceptions of patients according to SES, 115*fig*, 117; qualitative experiences of, 98; ratings by race/ethnicity, income/ and health status, 161*fig*

Physician-to-population ratio, 15

Point of service (POS) plans, 81

Policy interventions: cost containment issue of, 269; to resolve health insurance disparities, 251–255; to resolve race/ethnic disparities, 235–236; to resolve SES disparities, 244–246

Political feasibility programs, 254

Potential access to care, 27*e*

Poverty rates: children eleven years and under health status and, 166*t*–167*t*; as morbidity/mortality predictors, 13; as MUA factor, 15; national trends in racial/ethnicity, 53–58; racial/ethnic differences in, 4; regular source of care (RSC) and poverty status, 95*fig*, 111; risk factors, health literacy, and, 162*t*. *See also* Federal poverty level (FPL); Income levels

Predictors: of morbidity/mortality, 13; risk factors for unmet needs, 149*t*–150*t*

Predisposing factors: ecological level, 24*e*, 25; individual level, 22*e*

Preferred provider organizations (PPOs), 81

Preventive care: effectiveness of programs for, 36; flu shots, 155*t*–156*t*, 159*fig*; health insurance coverage and, 127*fig*–128; L.A. Care Health Plan efforts to improve, 7; multiple risk factors for lack of, 152–163; racial/ethnicity differences in, 99*fig*–100; risk factors by race/ethnicity, 155*t*–156*t*; risk factors of uninsured for, 155*t*–156*t*; risk profiles for, 157*t*–158*t*; vaccination, 100, 249. *See also* Medical services

Preventive counseling, 160

Primary care: balancing specialty care and, 260–262; definition of, 70–71; insurance coverage and experiences with, 128–129; partnership building to improve, 122–124

Private initiatives: Association of Schools of Public Health/Kellogg Taskforce, 181, 193; California Children's Health Initiatives (CHIs), 140–141, 181, 212; California Endowment's Building Healthy Communities Initiative, 181, 193–194; Center for Health and Health Care in Schools (CHHCS), 181, 205–206; to eliminate disparities in health insurance, 211–212; to eliminate racial and ethic disparities, 190–192; to eliminate socioeconomic disparities in health, 204–207; Health Foundation of Greater Cincinnati, 206; Healthy Kids, 212; Johnson & Johnson Community Health Care Program, 183, 206–207; Project HEALTH, 184, 204–205; Robert Wood Johnson Foundation Aligning Forces for Quality Project, 185, 192

Program for All Inclusive Care of the Elderly (PACE), 195–196

Programs. *See* Vulnerable population programs

Project 50, 216–217

Project HEALTH, 184, 204–205

Prostate cancer mortality rates, 107*fig*

Providers: health plan policies influences on, 84; race/ethnicity and, 45–46

Proxy measure, 91

Public Health Foundation, 228

Public Housing primary Care (PHPC) Program, 184, 200–201, 209

PubMed database, 229

Puerto Ricans: infant mortality rates among, 105*fig*; low birth weight rates among, 106*fig*. *See also* Hispanics

Puget Sound Health Alliance (Seattle), 192

Q

Qualitative experiences, 98

Quality of care. *See* Health care quality

R

Race/ethnicity: access to care across, 36; as community determinants/mechanisms of vulnerability, 36–49; cultural factors of, 43; defining, 37–39; fair or poor health status by, 164*fig*; health needs and, 45; historical development of importance of, 36–37; as key risk factor, 31; provider factors and, 45–46; as proxy measure, 91; U.S. Census coding for, 38–39. *See also* Discrimination; Minority race/ethnicity

Race/ethnicity differences: cancer screening and, 100–101; children eleven years and under health status and, 166*t*–167*t*; health care system experiences and, 46–47, 102*fig*–103; health care system factors and, 46–47; historical development of SES and, 51–53; household monetary income (1967-2008) by, 54*fig*; income distribution trends and, 53–58; individual risk factors and, 94–110; infant mortality rates by, 105*fig*–106, 168*fig*; low birth weight rates by maternal, 106*fig*; Medicaid program participation, 79; multiple factors impacting health care access and, 141–151*fig*; national education trends among, 60–62; national risk factor prevalence (2007) by, 148*t*; national risk factor prevalence for health care quality by, 154*t*; national trends in diversity and, 39–40*fig*; no healthcare visits by children by insurance coverage and, 145*fig*–146; patient-provider relationships ratings by, 161*fig*; poverty rates and, 4; receipt of preventive care by, 99*fig*–100; regular source of care (RSC) by, 95*fig*; risk factors and preventive services by, 155*t*–156*t*; risk profiles for preventive services

Race/ethnicity differences (*continued*)
by, 157*t*–158*t*; SES (socioeconomic status) and, 41; strategies to resolve disparities in, 234–244; unemployment rates and, 63*fig*–64; unemployment rates by, 63*fig*. *See also* African Americans; American Indians/Alaskan Natives (AIANs); Asians; Hispanics; Pacific Islanders

Race/ethnicity vulnerability: community determinants/mechanisms of, 36–49; conceptual model linking health care and, 42*fig*; homeless health care services and, 47–49; theoretical pathways of, 40–41

Racial and Ethnic Approaches to Community Health Across the United States, 185

Racial stereotype discrimination, 52

Racial/ethnic disparities in health: federal initiatives to eliminate, 186–190; HIV/AIDS and, 106–107*fig*, 243; private initiatives to eliminate, 192–194; programs for vulnerable seniors, 194–195; scope and reach of programs for eliminating, 196–197; state and local initiatives to eliminate, 190–192; strategies to resolve, 234–244; strengths and weaknesses of programs addressing, 196–198

Racism-health association, 44–45

RAND Corporation, 265

REACH 2010, 187, 191, 197, 198, 236–238

REACH-sponsored South Carolina coalition, 198

Realized access to care, 27*e*

Regular source of care (RSC): by educational level (2005), 111–112; poverty and association with, 111; by race/ethnicity, poverty status, and insurance coverage, 95*fig*; racial/ethnicity differences in, 95–97; uninsured status and, 125

Remote Area Medical (RAM), 88–89*e*

Research: community-based interventions and, 236–238; traditional compared to participatory action, 237*t*

Resolving disparities actions: step 1: enhance awareness, 273–274; step 2: demonstrate severity, 274; step 3: establish relevance, 275–276; step 4: expand the focus to multiple risk factors, 276–277; step 5: stress the multilevel integration of interventions, 277–278; step 6: ensure feasibility, 278; step 7: apply effective implementation strategies, 279–280; step 8: persevere, 280; step 9: use guided incrementalism, 280; step 10: evaluate and refine programs and initiatives, 280–281

Resolving disparities integrative strategies: balancing primary care and specialty care, 260–262; Benzeval UK framework for addressing disparities, 256; community social cohesion, 258–259; enhancing education, 256–258; improving national monitoring of disparities, 265–267; life course health development, 262–265

Resolving health disparities: Building Healthy Communities Initiative (BHC) for, 270–272; course of action for, 272–281; framework used for, 230*fig*–234; programs eliminating health insurance disparities, 209–215; programs eliminating racial/ethnic disparities, 185–198; programs eliminating socioeconomic disparities, 198–209; strategies for, 234–270. *See also* Health inequalities; Healthy People 2020

Resolving health disparities strategies: challenges and barriers to implementing, 267–270; integrative approaches to, 256–267; to resolve disparities by health insurance, 250–256; to resolve racial/ethnic disparities, 234–244; to resolve SES disparities, 244–250

Resolving health insurance disparities: community-based interventions for, 255–256; encouraging enrollment for eligible individuals for, 251–252; health care reform legislation for, 251; incrementally expanding public insurance coverage, 252–254; policy interventions for, 251; unique state approaches to providing universal coverage for, 254–255

Resolving racial/ethnic disparities: community-based interventions for, 236–238; health care interventions for, 238–242; individual-level interventions for, 242–244; policy interventions for, 235–236

Respeto (Hispanic culture), 43

Risk behaviors. *See* Health risk behaviors

Risk profiles, 163

Robert Wood Johnson Foundation Aligning Forces for Quality Project, 185, 192

Robert Wood Johnson Foundation (RWJF), 205, 206, 247

S

Safety net programs: Community health center (CHC) program, 199, 208; definition of, 31; eligibility for, 78; encouraging enrollment for eligible individuals, 251–252; "express lane eligibility" for, 252; health care interventions through, 248–250; incrementally expanding public insurance coverage through, 252–254. *See also* Children's Health Insurance Program (CHIP); Medicaid

Satisfaction in care, 28*e*

Secretary's Advisory Committee on National Health Promotion and Disease Prevention Objectives for 2020, 2008, 32, 103, 224

Self-efficacy, 110

Sexually transmitted diseases (STDs), 243. *See also* HIV/AIDS

SIDS Alliance, 250

Single payer insurance programs, 255

Sinners and victims social policy model, 17–18

Slavery abolition (1865), 5

Sliding fee scale, 255

Smokefree.gov, 243

Smoking: African American males' rate of, 243; Antismoking media campaign (Minnesota), 268; race/ethnicity differences and, 109

Social capital: definition of, 10; vulnerability determined by, 9–10

Social class: African American/White health disparities and, 168–169*t*; defined by occupation, 168; vulnerability tied to, 9

Social cohesion: definition of, 69; health inequality role of, 69–70

Social health measurements, 29

Social justice argument, 279

Social participation: social/emotional health measured through, 29; socioeconomic status (SES) and, 64, 67–68

Social Security Administration, 54

Social status-vulnerability relationship, 9, 10

Social support-health risk behavior relationship, 11

Sociedad Latina, 259

Socioeconomic disparities in health: federal initiatives to eliminate, 198–202; private initiatives to eliminate, 204–207; state and local initiatives to eliminate, 202–204; strategies to resolve, 244–250; strengths and weaknesses of programs addressing, 207–209

Socioeconomic status (SES): community and relative deprivation and, 68–69; conceptual model linking health with, 65*fig*; definition of, 11; health care system access and, 70–71; historical development of the importance of, 51–53; individual risk factors and disparities in, 110–124; individual socioeconomic status model (SES) focus on, 11–12; material deprivation and, 64, 66; national trends in income/poverty distribution and, 53–58; physician-reported perceptions of patients according to, 115*fig*, 117; programs to eliminate disparities in health, 198–209; resources availability and, 49, 51; social cohesion and, 69–70; social participation and, 64, 67–68; theoretical pathways of vulnerability and, 64–66; trends in education and, 60–62; trends in income equality, 58–60; trends in occupation and, 62–64; as vulnerable populations factor, 3, 31, 49–71. *See also* Health risk behaviors

South Carolina Primary Health Care Association, 122–124

South Carolina Welvista Program, 185, 202–203

Special Supplemental Nutrition Program for Women, Infants, and Children, 252

Standardized mortality rates, 168

Standardized mortality ratio (SMR), 108

State Children's Health Insurance Program, 6, 80. *See also* Children's Health Insurance Program (CHIP)

State and local initiatives: California Children's Health Initiatives (CHIs), 140–141, 181, 212, 215; California Department of Public Health Strategic Plan, 191–192; Center for Health and Health Care in Schools (CHHCS), 205–206; to eliminate disparities in health insurance, 210–211; to eliminate racial and ethic disparities, 190–192; to eliminate socioeconomic disparities in health, 202–204; Health Howard Health Plan, 203; Healthcare Group (HCG) of Arizona, 182, 211, 214; Kansas City TeleKidcare, 183, 204; Massachusetts Commonwealth Health Insurance Connector Authority, 183, 210–211, 214, 215; Minnesota's Eliminating Health Disparities Initiative, 183, 191; South Carolina Welvista Program, 202–203

Steps to a Healthier US program, 228

Strengthening Primary Care Providers for the Poor, 185

Sudden infant death syndrome (SIDS), 250

Supplemental Nutrition Assistance Program, 55

T

TCE (The California Endowment), 270–272

Technical feasibility, 278

Technology: medical treatment options broadened through, 260–262; telemedicine, 204

Teen pregnancy, 17–18

Telemedicine, 204

Temporary Assistance to Needy Families (TANF), 244

Third National Health and Nutrition Examination Survey, 131

Turning Point program, 247–248

U

Unemployment rates: fluctuations in the U.S., 62–64; occupations with the lowest, 64; by race and ethnicity, 63*fig*–64. *See also* Employment

Uninsured: among the nonelderly by state (2007-2008), 78*fig*; population percentage (2007) of, 77*fig*; rates among working adults, 76*fig*; regular source of care (RSC) of, 125; risk factors for preventive services of, 156*t*; risk factors and preventive services in past year of participants in, 156*t*

United Health Foundation, 274, 279

United Kingdom King's Fund report (1995), 256

United Nations, 37

United Nations Development Programme, 60

United States: challenges and barriers to resolving health disparities in the, 267–270; increasing prevalence of vulnerability in the, 4; infant mortality rates of, 274; leading health indicators (LHIs) in the, 229*t*; life expectancy in the, 223; projected population size by race/ethnicity, 40*fig*; projected race/ethnicity distribution in, 41*fig*; public and private insurance trends in the, 75–81; trends in education in the, 60–62; trends in income inequality in the, 58–60; trends in income and poverty distribution in the, 53–58; trends in occupation in the, 62–64; unemployment rates by race/ethnicity in the, 63*fig*. *See also* Legislation

Universal health insurance: Canadian's, 260; health care reform (2010) moving toward, 6; unique state approaches for providing, 254–255; U.S. lack of, 72; WHO ranking of countries with, 73*e*–74*e*

University of California Regents v. Bakke, 37

University of Illinois at Chicago, 236

Unmet health care needs, 97

Urban League, 238

U.S. Census Bureau, 38–39, 110

U.S. Census Bureau Population Division, 4

U.S. Declaration of Independence, 5

U.S. Department of Health and Human Services (DHHS): Agency for Healthcare Research and Quality (AHRQ), 143, 153, 160, 185, 236, 265; annual reports of U.S. health by, 32; community support grant programs established by, 228; Health Resources and Services Administration (HRSA) of the, 189; healthy people initiative of, 2, 6, 32, 197, 222–229, 279; Indian Health Service (IHS) transferred to, 189; Office of Disease Prevention and Health Promotion of, 228; poverty threshold reported by, 55; reducing health disparities goal of, 222; vulnerable populations identified by, 2

U.S. Environmental Protection Agency (EPA), 110

U.S. Food and Drug Administration, 265

U.S. Office of Management and Budget, 32

U.S. Public Health Service, 250

U.S. State Department, 37

V

Vaccination: CDC Vaccines for Children program for, 249; race/ethnicity differences in, 100

Violence environmental circumstance, 13

Viva La Cultura Club, 259

Vocational Foundation, Inc. (VFI), 247

Vulnerability: traditional models: Aday's individual and community interaction model, 15–16*fig*, 17; community environmental exposures model, 14; community medically underserved model, 14–15; community social resources model, 12–13; individual determinants model, 8–9; individual health behaviors model, 10–11; individual social resources model, 9–10; individual socioeconomic status model, 11–12; sinners and victims social policy model, 17–18

Vulnerability: clinical practice focus on, 30–31; gradient for, 14, 67–68; Healthy People 2020 definition of, 2; increasing prevalence in the U.S., 4; interconnections between risk factors and cycling of, 85–87; research measurement of, 29–30; traditional definition of, 2. *See also* Clinical practice focus on vulnerability

Vulnerability community risk factors: children eleven years and under health status and, 166*t*–167*t*; health insurance as, 72–85; individual SES and relative deprivation as, 68–69; interconnections between cycling of vulnerability and, 85–87; SES (socioeconomic status) as, 49–71

Vulnerability model: components of, 21–32; distinctive characteristics of, 20–21; illustrated diagram of, 19*fig*; overview of new conceptual framework of, 18–20

Vulnerability model components: consequences of vulnerability, 26–29; ecological risk factors, 24*e*–26; individual risk factors, 21–24; measuring vulnerability in research, 29–31; race and ethnicity as, 36–49; three key risk factors, 31–32

Vulnerable population programs: clinical practice focus on, 216–217; contact information for current major, 181*e*–185; to eliminate disparities in health insurance, 209–215; to eliminate racial and ethnic disparities, 185–198; to eliminate socioeconomic disparities in health, 198–209

Vulnerable populations: elderly patients as, 194–196; establishing trust among, 140–141; five reasons for study of, 3–6; homeless, 47–49, 182, 201, 216–217; lack for consensus on what constitutes, 2; managed care investment in study of, 6–8; seniors or older patients, 194–195; traditional research focus on subpopulations of, 2. *See also specific populations*

W

War on Poverty (1960s), 6, 199

Washington's Children's Alliance, 255

Weingart Foundation's Center for Community Health, 47–49

Well-child care, 99

Whites: fair or poor health status of, 164*fig*; health care quality and, 98–103; health data kept on, 32; infant mortality by maternal education and, 168*fig*; Medicaid program participation by, 79; multiple factors impacting health care access of, 142*fig*–151*fig*; national risk factor prevalence of, 154*t*; national trends in poverty/income distribution and, 53–58; risk profiles and preventive services in past year, 157*t*; social class and health disparities of African Americans and, 168–169*t*. *See also* Non-Hispanic whites

W.K. Kellogg Foundation, 193, 247
Women's suffrage (1920), 5–6
World Health Organization (WHO): Commission on the Social Determinants of Health of, 270; health as defined by, 27–29; on medical care across racial and ethnic lines, 36; rankings of international health systems by, 72, 73*e*

Y
You Can Quit Smoking Consumer Guide (CDC), 243